G. Hasenfuss E. Marbán (Eds.)

Molecular Approaches to Heart Failure Therapy

G. Hasenfuss
E. Marbán
(Eds.)

Molecular Approaches to Heart Failure Therapy

With 114 Figures
in 174 Separate Illustrations
and 16 Tables

SPRINGER-VERLAG
BERLIN HEIDELBERG GMBH

Prof. Dr. med. GERD HASENFUSS
Georg-August-Universität Göttingen
Zentrum Innere Medizin, Abt. Kardiologie und Pneumologie
Robert-Koch-Straße 40
D-37075 Göttingen

EDUARDO MARBÁN, M.D., Ph.D.
Professor of Medicine and Physiology
Section of Molecular and Cellular Cardiology
844 Ross Building
The Johns Hopkins University
Baltimore MD 21205, USA

ISBN 978-3-642-63332-4 ISBN 978-3-642-57710-9 (eBook)
DOI 10.1007/978-3-642-57710-9

Die Deutsche Bibliothek – CIP-Einheitsaufnahme
A catelogue record for this publication is available from Die Deutsche Bibliothek

Originally published by Steinkopff-Verlag Darmstadt in 2000
Softcover reprint of the hardcover 1st edition 2000

Medical Editor: Sabine Ibkendanz – English Editor: Mary Gossen
Production: Klemens Schwind
Cover Design: Erich Kirchner, Heidelberg
Typesetting: K + V Fotosatz GmbH, Beerfelden

SPIN 10759504 85/7231-5 4 3 2 1 0 – Printed on acid-free paper

Table of Contents

List of Contributors

Prof. Dr. med. D. J. BEUCKELMANN
Klinik III für Innere Medizin
der Universität zu Köln
Josef-Stelzmann-Str. 9
D-50294 Köln

W. S. COLUCCI, MD
Dept. of Cardiology
Boston Medical Center
88 East Newton Street
Boston, MA 02118, USA

Prof. W. H. DILLMANN, MD
Division of Endocrinology/
Metabolism
University of California, San Diego
9500 Gilman Drive, BSB/5063
La Jolla, CA 92093-0618, USA

K. J. DONAHUE, MD
University of Cardiology
Johns Hopkins University
School of Medicine
720 N. Rutland Ave. (844 Ross Bldg).
Baltimore, MD 21205-2179, USA

Prof. Dr. T. ESCHENHAGEN
Institut für Experimentelle
und Klinische Pharmakologie
Universität Erlangen/Nürnberg
Fahrstr. 17
D-91054 Erlangen

L. J. FIELD, MD
Wells Center for Pediatric Research
James Withcomb Riley Hospital
for Children
702 Barnhill Drive, Room 2666
Indianapolis, IN 46202-5225, USA

Dr. med. W.-M. FRANZ
Medizinische Universität Lübeck
Medizinische Klinik II
Ratzeburger Allee 160
D-23538 Lübeck

R. J. HAJJAR, MD
Assistant Professor of Medicine
Massachusetts General Hospital
Cardiovascular Research Center
149 13th Street, Room 4215
Charlestown, MA 02129-2060, USA

A. HAUNSTETTER, MD
Beth Israel Diaconess
Medical Center
330 Brookline Ave. SL-201
Boston, MA 02215, USA

Prof. Dr. med. J. HOLTZ
Martin-Luther-Universität
Halle-Wittenberg
Medizinische Fakultät
Institut für Pathophysiologie
Magdeburger Str. 18
D-06097 Halle (Saale)

U. C. HOPPE, MD
Section of Molecular
and Cellular Cardiology
844 Ross Building
The Johns Hopkins University
School of Medicine
720 N. Rutland Ave.
Baltimore, MD 2105, USA

G. Inesi, MD
Dept. of Biochemistry Molecular Biology
University of Maryland
School of Medicine
108 N Green St.
Baltimore, MD 21201-1503, USA

S. Izumo, MD
Beth Israel Deaconess Medical Center - Cardiovascular Division
330 Brookline Avenue SL-201
Boston MA 02215, USA

Dr. med. P.M.L. Janssen
Georg-August-Universität
Zentrum Innere Medizin
Abt. Kardiologie
und Pneumonologie
Robert-Koch-Str. 40
D-37075 Göttingen

D.A. Kass, MD
Profressor of Medicine and Biomedical Engineering
Cardiology Division
Johns-Hopkins Hospital
Halsted 500
600 N. Wolfe Street
Baltimore, MD 21287, USA

Prof. Dr. med. M.J. Lohse
Universität Würzburg
Abteilung Pharmakologie
Versbacher Str. 9
D-97078 Würzburg

E. Marbán, MD, PhD
Professor of Medicine
and Physiology
Section of Molecular
and Cellular Cardiology
844 Ross Building
The Johns-Hopkins University
Baltimore, MD 21205, USA

F. del Monte, MD
Massachusetts General Hospital
Cardiovascular Research Center
149 13th Street
Boston, MA 02129-2060, USA

Prof. Dr. med. I. Morano
Molekulare Medizin
Max-Dellbrück-Zentrum
Robert-Roessle-Str. 10
D-13122 Berlin

C.E. Murry, MD, PhD
Dept. of Pathology
Box 357470, Room E-520 HSB
University of Washington
Seattle, WA 98195-7335, USA

K.B.S. Pasumarthi, MD
Wells Center for Pediatric Research
James Withcomb Riley Hospital
for Children
702 Barnhill Drive, Room 2600
Indianapolis, JN 46202-5225, USA

Priv.-Doz. Dr. med. B. Pieske
Georg-August-Universität
Zentrum Innere Medizin
Abt. Kardiologie
und Pneumonologie
Robert-Koch-Str. 40
D-37075 Göttingen

Dr. med. J. Prestle
Georg-August-Universität
Zentrum Innere Medizin
Abt. Kardiologie
und Pneumologie
Robert-Koch-Str. 40
D-37075 Göttingen

H. Reinecke, PhD
Dept. of Pathology
Box 357470, E-520 HSB
University of Washington
Seattle, WA 98195-7335, USA

D.B. Sawyer, MD, PhD
Dept. of Cardiology
Boston Medical Center
88 East Newton Street
Boston, MA 02118, USA

A.G. Schmidt, MD
Department of Pharmacology
and Cell Biophysis
University of Cincinnati
College of Medicine
Cincinnati, OH 45267-0575, USA

Introduction

G. Hasenfuss, E. Marbán

Heart failure embodies the central irony of modern medicine. As we have become increasingly adept at treating the major proximate causes of death in Western society, we have effectively converted acute illness into chronic malady. The last twenty years have witnessed a revolution in the treatment of acute coronary syndromes, myocardial infarction in particular. Patients who reach the hospital now have every expectation of leaving alive, but not necessarily well. Our ability to blunt the edge of ischemic insults has engendered new problems: a new cohort of patients whose hearts function well enough to enable short-term survival, but at the cost of decreased exercise tolerance, dyspnea and increased long-term mortality. The irony is compounded by our increasingly sophisticated pharmacopeia for the treatment of heart failure, which, by slowing the progression of ventricular dysfunction, has created a chronic illness. The fact of its chronicity makes heart failure no less deadly. In symptomatic patients, mortality exceeds 5–10% per year even with the best contemporary therapy. Not all heart failure is ischemic, of course, but the final common phenotype is eerily concordant regardless of the proximate cause. No wonder, then, that heart failure is the leading cause of hospitalization in America and in Western Europe and that the prevalence of the disease continues to rise.

Drugs have indeed revolutionized heart failure therapy, ACE inhibitors and beta-adrenergic blockers having the most outstanding records to date. The utility of these and other blockers of humoral stress pathways illuminates a central truism – that the disease may be dominated by the body's own limited repertoire of innate responses to circulatory insufficiency. What is good in the short run becomes maladaptive in the long run. No one would argue that catecholamines are bad in acute cardiogenic shock, for example; however, if the body's response to stress continues unchecked, beta receptors become downregulated and desensitized, perpetuating a downward spiral. Hence the paradoxical benefit of beta blockers in heart failure: the vicious cycle is broken. However, antagonists of various autocoids have their own limitations. Most notably, such drugs will not suffice to negate the initial insult and its impact on circulatory function. We now know that the heart failure syndrome cannot be completely attributed to the body's maladaptive efforts to defend central circulation. Our clinical experience with patients who have been supported by left ventricular assist devices (LVADs) is particularly instructive. While on such external support, autocoid reactions subside, and the programs of gene expression that underlie the heart failure phenotype revert to those characteristic of normal healthy hearts. One might then have reason to hope that, having "rested" the heart with an LVAD and broken the vicious cycle, heart failure might not recur once the machine is removed. Not so. These patients generally re-develop heart failure once removed from the LVAD. This experience means that we will have to pay attention not only to blocking the reactions to heart failure but also to reversing the initial injury.

To reverse the injury will require new approaches, in which we are currently limited by a conceptual gap. While palliative therapy is ever-improving, we simply do not know enough to be able to reverse the disease. The way we now approach end-stage heart failure serves to illustrate the current sad state of affairs. Until patients become bedridden, we push autocoid-blocking therapy to the limits of tolerance. At that point, in desperation, we begin subjecting patients to infusions of catecholamines and phosphodiesterase inhibitors. We know these therapies actually decrease survival in heart failure patients. Nevertheless, the obvious short-term hemodynamic benefits provide bridges to the most extreme of heart failure treatments, cardiac transplantation. While transplantation may become practical after we overcome immunological and infectious obstacles to xenotransplants, the enormous expense and limited success of the procedure as it now stands relegates it to a therapy of last recourse.

The present book grew out of a conference which was held in order to confront the conceptual gap and to explore ways of potentially overcoming the impass we now face. The various chapters address molecular approaches to the therapy of heart failure based on careful analysis of the pathophysiological alterations occurring in failing heart. This includes alterations of the myocyte phenotype as well as of the extracellular matrix. Furthermore, the current status of myocardial gene transfer techniques is addressed.

Based on the finding that altered excitation-contraction coupling is of significant relevance for the pathophysiology of human heart failure, inotropic stimulation by targeting various components of the calcium cycling system seems promising. This includes overexpression of the β-adrenoceptor system, stimulation of sarcoplasmic reticulum calcium accumulation by overexpressing the calcium pump or targeting its inhibitory protein, phospholamban, or by manipulating the sarcoplamic reticulum calcium release channel. One caution in inotropic therapy is the possibility that it may paradoxicall decrease survival, as seen with milrinone and with beta-adrenergic agonists.

The harmful effects of oxidative stress in myocardial ischemia have been extensively investigated. Only recently, however, has oxidative stress been considered to be a major player contributing to the transition from compensated to decompensated heart failure. Likewise, although its relevance in heart failure is not completely understood, apoptosis may be relevant for the manifestation and progression of heart failure, and different possibilities are suggested to interrupt the pro-apoptotic or support the anti-apoptotic pathways.

Besides pump failure, almost half of the patients with congestive heart failure die of bradycardic and tachycardic arrhythmias. Malignant ventricular arrhythmias are at least partially based on altered expression of potassium channels which may therefore represent another important target for gene therapy strategies.

As an alternative to correcting the myocyte and matrix composition of the failing heart, transplantation of myocytes or progenitor cells into damaged regions of the hearts is an attractive approach to improve cardiac function. Even more fascinating is the possibility to stimulate the terminally differentiated myocyte to proliferate and migrate into damaged regions by interventions that influence cell cycle regulation or to manipulate non-myocyte components of the heart to differentiate into contractile cells.

The present book does not claim to cover the whole gamut of current strategies with the potential to influence failing heart. Nevertheless, we believe that some of the most relevant and appealing possibilities for molecular intervention in the treatment of heart failure are addressed. None of these strategies are ready for clinical application. However, the present knowledge will undoubtedly set the stage for future research from which we may derive a most exciting and beneficial therapeutic armamentarium.

CHAPTER 1

Alterations in excitation-contraction coupling and potential gene therapy targets in failing human hearts

B. PIESKE

Abteilung Kardiologie und Pneumologie,
Zentrum Innere Medizin, Georg-August-Universität
Göttingen, Germany

Introduction

Human heart failure is characterized by both systolic and diastolic contractile dysfunction, related to phenotype alterations of the single myocytes. Substantial progress has been made over the past decade in elucidating the pathophysiology of contractile dysfunction and its various subcellular molecular counterparts. Improved understanding of these molecular phenomena and the rapid development of new methods for gene transfer to the myocardium opens the field for specific gene therapy, targeted to dysregulated or dysfunctional genes and proteins in the failing heart. This review aims at summarizing recent advances in this field by integrating experimental results from our group as well as from other groups to form a more comprehensive picture.

Regular contractions are initiated by depolarizations of the cell membrane, resulting in transsarcolemmal Ca^{2+} influx through L-type Ca^{2+} channels located in the T-tubular regions of the myocytes (Fig. 1). These channels are in close proximity to the Ca^{2+} release channels (ryanodine receptors) of the sarcoplasmic reticulum, the major Ca^{2+} storage organelle of the myocytes. Ca^{2+} entering the cells through a L-type Ca^{2+} channel activates opening of one or a cluster of ryanodine channels, resulting in the local release of Ca^{2+} from the SR (a Ca^{2+} spark). During excitation-contraction coupling, the sum of Ca^{2+} sparks released from the SR results in a pronounced increase in cytosolic Ca^{2+} (the Ca^{2+} transient), which binds to Troponin C, thereby activating the myofilaments and inducing contraction.

Relaxation is brought about by dissociation of Ca^{2+} from the myofilaments and active Ca^{2+} reuptake through SR Ca^{2+}-ATPase pump proteins. SERCA2a, the isoform which is most prevalently expressed in cardiac muscle [108], transports Ca^{2+} back to the luminal space of the SR against a Ca^{2+} gradient by an energy-dependent mechanism (1 mol ATP is hydrolized for transport of 2 moles of Ca^{2+}). SERCA2a activity is regulated by phospholamban, a pentameric protein which inhibits SERCA2a in its unphosphorylated form. Protein kinase A-dependent phosphorylation of phospholamban relieves its inhibitory effects, resulting in increased SERCA2a activity [50], enhanced relaxation, and more powerful contractions due to increased Ca^{2+} release from the SR. For maintaining Ca^{2+} homeostasis during steady-state contractions,

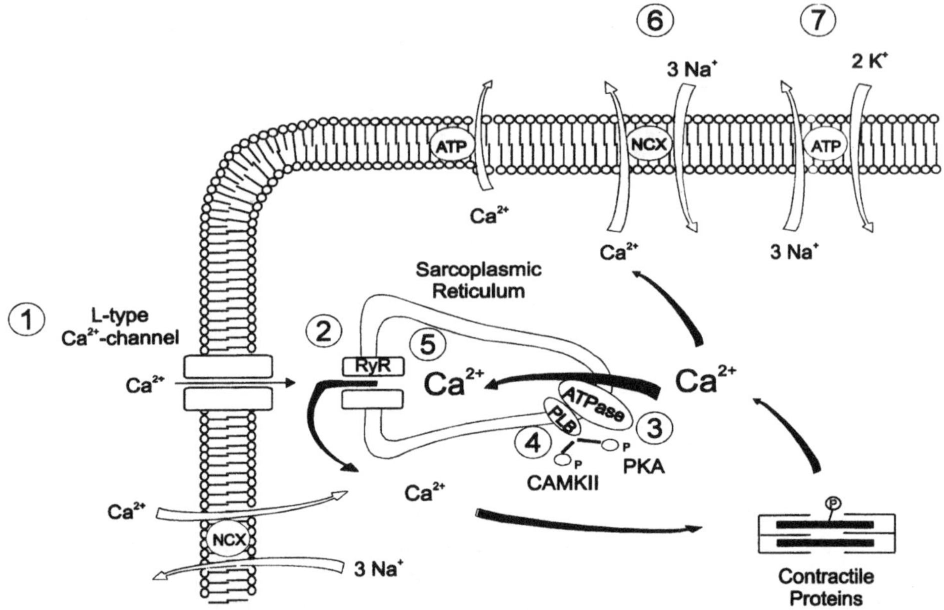

Fig. 1. Electro-mechanical coupling in the human heart. (1) Ca^{2+} enters the cell via L-type Ca^{2+} channels; (2) Ca^{2+} is released from the SR through the ryanodine receptor, thereby inducing contraction; (3) during relaxation, Ca^{2+} is transported to the SR through SERCA2a; (4) phospholamban inhibits SERCA2a activity. PKA- and Ca^{2+}/calmodulin-dependent PLB-phosphorylation relieves this inhibitory effect; (5) Ca^{2+} binds to calsequestrin within the SR; (6) for maintaining Ca^{2+} homeostasis, Ca^{2+} is removed from the myocytes largely via NCX1; (7) Na^+/K^+-ATPase regulates intracellular Na^+ homeostasis and affects NCX1 activity. The corresponding alterations in heart failure are summarized in Table 1.

cytosolic Ca^{2+} that is not transported back to the lumen of the SR (where it binds to calsequestrin, the major Ca^{2+} storage protein of the SR) is eliminated from the cytosol mainly by transsarcolemmal extrusion via the Na^+/Ca^{2+} exchanger. In the nonfailing human heart, it is estimated that ~30% of the Ca^{2+} cycled per beat originates from the extracellular space and is extruded via Na^+/Ca^{2+} exchange under steady-state conditions [92].

The strength of contractions are largely regulated via the β-adrenergic system (see Fig. 2). Circulating or locally released catecholamines bind to myocardial β_1- and β_2-adrenoceptors (AR). β-AR couple to sarcolemmal adenylate cyclase (AC) through stimulatory G-proteins (G_s). Stimulation of adenylate cyclase catalytic activity by $G_{s\alpha}$ results in production of cAMP. cAMP binding to the regulatory subunit of protein kinase (PKA) triggers a conformational change that allows the catalytic subunits of the enzyme to dissociate and phosphorylate protein substrates at serine and threonine subunits [104]. PKA phosphorylates ion channels and proteins involved in Ca^{2+} homeostasis and contraction. Such phosphorylation processes include

- the sarcolemmal L-type Ca^{2+} channels [36],
- phospholamban (at its serine-16 site),

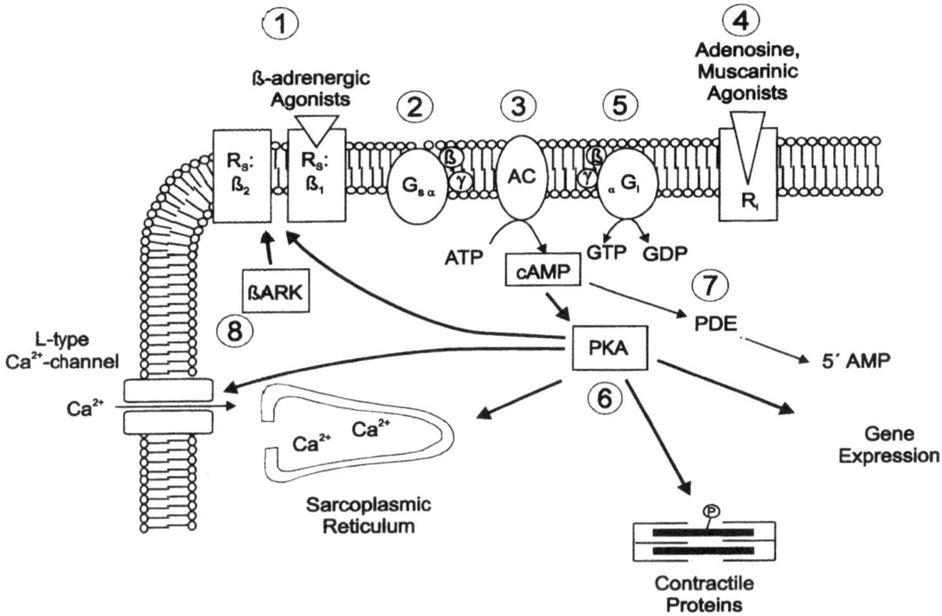

Fig. 2. Adrenergic signaling in the human heart. (1) Catecholamines bind to both β_1- and β_2-adrenoceptors in the cell membrane, which are functionally coupled to adenylate cylcase (3) through a stimulatory G_s-protein (2). AC is under dual control, and inhibitory muscarinergic or adenosin A1-receptors (4) decrease its catalytic activity through an inhibitory G_i protein (5). AC catalyzes the formation of cAMP, which activates protein kinase A (6), thereby inducing phosphorylation processes. cAMP is degenerated by phosphodiesterase type III (7), and phosphorylated proteins are dephosphorylated by phosphatases (8). Adrenoceptor uncoupling results from phosphorylation by β-adrenoceptor kinase at the inner cell membrane (9).

troponin I, the regulatory subunit of the thin filaments [86], and possibly the ryanodine release channel.

As a consequence, cAMP-mediated phosphorylation processes increase force of contraction and fasten relaxation by increasing systolic Ca^{2+} concentrations and Ca^{2+} reuptake to the SR, as well as promoting Ca^{2+} dissociation from its myofilament-binding sites.

Besides β-adrenergic stimulation, heart rate inotropism (the force-frequency relationship) contributes to the regulation of pump function. In men without heart failure, increasing heart rate results in enhanced myocardial contractility [25, 37]. This results from increased transsarcolemmal Ca^{2+} influx due to both high-frequency-induced upregulation of Ca^{2+} currents [80], as well as increased rates of depolarizations per time. As a consequence, more Ca^{2+} is released from the SR [77], and both intracellular Ca^{2+} transients as well as force of contraction increase with higher stimulation rates in isolated nonfailing human myocardium [74, 75].

In addition, length-dependent activation of the myofilaments serves as a largely Ca^{2+}-independent mechanism for short-term regulation of the strength of contractions [76]. However, whether or not this mechanism is blunted in failing human myocardium is still controversial and goes beyond the scope of this review [44, 95].

More or less severe alterations of these mechanisms for regulating the strength of the heart beat have been described in the failing human heart (see Tables 1 and 2), and understanding the molecular basis of these functional alterations may yield a clue for specific therapeutic approaches. Transgenic mice models have greatly improved our understanding of how molecular alterations affect contractile function of the heart. However, this experimental approach is hampered by three major factors:

- the mouse heart differs greatly from the human heart in many aspects,
- knockout or overexpression of a specific gene usually induces widespread phenotype alterations during cardiac development and growth,
- this method has no therapeutic potential.

Table 1. Alterations associated with disturbed excitation-contraction coupling

	mRNA	Protein (or binding sites)	Function	Reference
L-type Ca^{2+} channel	⇔ ⇓	⇔ ⇓	⇔ ⇓	3, 26, 61, 71, 80, 84, 97, 102
Ryanodine receptor	⇔ ⇓	⇔ (⇓)	⇔ (⇓)	7, 15, 31, 42, 62, 70, 90, 91
NCX1	⇑	⇑	⇑	27, 39, 78, 85
SERCA2a	⇓	⇓, ⇔	⇓	38, 41, 56, 57, 60, 62, 66, 74, 77, 78, 93, 96, 98, 103
PLB	(⇓)	(⇓)	⇑	57, 62, 66, 96, 98
Calsequestrin	⇔	⇔	⇔	62, 66, 102

Table 2. Alterations associated with disturbed β-adrenergic signaling

	mRNA	Protein	Function	Reference
β_1-Adrenoceptors	⇓	⇓	⇓	4, 8, 10, 12, 13, 105
β_2-Adrenoceptors	⇔	⇔	⇓	9, 12, 13
G_s	⇔, ⇑	⇔	⇔	20, 22, 94
Adenylate cyclase	⇑	?	⇓	12, 43
G_i	⇑	⇑	⇑	5, 20, 21, 22, 68
Protein kinase A		⇔	⇔[1]	6, 48
Phosphatase I			⇑	69
CaM-kinase	⇑	⇑	⇑	41, 48

[1] = basal PKA activity

Therefore, direct gene transfer using various vectors has been widely tested and applied to mammalian cardiac tissue during the last few years. Adenovirus-mediated gene transfer (see Tables 3 and 4) has evolved as the most commonly applied technique, but again, several concerns need to be addressed:

- the use of potentially infectious and pathogenic agents,
- the need for high virus titer stocks,
- the efficiency and stability of transfection,

Table 3. Adenovirus-mediated gene transfer: EC-coupling

Target	Model	Protein expression	Function	Reference
SERCA2a	Neonatal rat myocytes	⇑ 44-75%	⇑ SR CaATPase act. 4-fold ⇑ peak Ca_i 29% ⇓ resting Ca_i 30%	Hajjar et al., 1997
SERCA2a	Failing rat myocytes	⇑ ~40%	⇑ SR Ca uptake 35% ⇓ τ_{50} Ca 32%	Giordano et al., 1997
SERCA2a	Failing rat *in vivo*			Miyamato et al., 1998
SERCA2a	Rabbit myocytes	⇑ 2.4-fold	⇑ shortening (n.s.) ⇓ RT_{50} 23%	Meyer et al., 1999
SERCA2a	Human failing myocytes	⇑ (n.r.)	⇑ +dS/dt (61%) ⇑ −dS/dt (112%) ⇑ peak Ca_i 18%	Del Monte et al., 1999
SERCA1	Chick embryonic myocytes	⇑ (n.r.)	⇑ SR Ca uptake 4-fold ⇓ TT_{50} 28% ⇓ τ_{50} Ca 40%	Inesi et al., 1998
SERCA1 vs SERCA2a	Chick embryonic myocytes	⇑ 3-fold	⇑ SR Ca uptake (SERCA1 (5-fold)>SERCA2a (2.6-fold)	Sumbilla et al., 1999
PLB	Neonatal rat myocytes	⇑ 280±43%	⇑ τ_{50} Ca 137% ⇓ peak Ca_i 35% ⇑ resting Ca_i 49%	Hajjar et al., 1997
PLB	Rat *in vivo*	⇑ 2–4-fold	⇓ contractility	Hajjar et al., 1998
PLB	Rabbit myocytes	⇑ 3.3-fold	⇓ shortening 47% ⇑ RT_{50} 39%	Meyer et al., 1999
PLB-Antisense	Neonatal rat myocytes	⇓ 24%	⇑ SR Ca uptake ⇓ τ_{50} Ca 38%	Poller et al., 1998
Parvalbumin	Failing rat myocytes	⇑ (n.r.)	⇓ τ_{50} Ca 42% ⇓ RT_{50} 24%	Wahr et al., 1999

Table 4. Adenovirus-mediated gene transfer: β-adrenergic signaling

Target	Model	Protein expression	Function	Reference
β_2 AR	Rat Langendorff heart		⇑ Basal contractility ⇑ ISO-stim. contractility	Kypson et al., 1998
β_2 AR[3]	Rat hypertrophied heart	⇑ ~5-fold	⇑ ISO-stim. contractility	Kawahira et al., 1998
β_2 AR	Rabbit myocytes	⇑ ~20-fold	⇑ ISO-stim. cAMP ~2-fold	Drazner et al., 1997
β_2 AR	Rabbit *in vivo*	⇑ 5–10-fold[1]	⇑ $+dP/dt_{max}$ ⇑ ISO-response	Maurice et al., 1999
β_2 AR	Rabbit *in vivo*	⇑ 9–15-fold[1]	⇑ basal $+dP/dt_{max}$ ⇑ ISO-stim. $+dP/dt_{max}$	Shah et al., 2000
β_2 AR	Failing rabbit myocytes	⇑ ~30-fold[1]	⇑ basal cAMP ⇑ ISO-stim. cAMP	Akhter et al., 1997
βARK inhibitor	Rabbit myocytes	⇑ (n.r.)	Inhibition of ISO-induced desensitization	Drazner et al., 1997
βARK inhibitor	Failing rabbit myocytes	⇑ (n.r.)	⇑ basal cAMP ⇑ ISO-stim. cAMP inhibition of ISO-induced desensitization	Akhter et al., 1997
Adenylate cyclase VI	Pig *in vivo*	n.r.	⇑ ISO-stim. LV +dP/dt ⇑ ISO-stim. C.O.	Lai et al., 1999
Vasopressin V2 receptor	Rat myocytes	⇑ ~3.2-fold[1]	⇑ shortening 300%[2]	Laugwitz et al., 1999

[1] radioligand binding; [2] arginine-vasopressin stimulation; [3] using the hemagglutinating virus of Japan (HVJ); *n.r.* data not reported; RT_{50} time to 50% relaxation; TT_{50} total twitch time at 50% of twitch amplitude; *+dT/dt* maximal rate of tension increase; *–dT/dt* maximal rate of tension decline; *+dS/dt* maximal rate of shortening; *–dS/dt* maximal rate of relaxation; $\tau_{50}Ca$ time to 50% decline of the Ca transient; *ISO* isoproterenol

nonspecific transfection of non-target cells,
the induction of an immune response.

Some of these concerns might be minimized in the future, e.g., by the use of cell-targeted adeno-associated viruses [30]. However, before clinical applications can be considered we must identify and characterize potential gene therapy targets in isolated failing human myocardium.

Alterations in excitation-contraction coupling and potential gene therapy targets

Major alterations in excitation-contraction coupling of the failing human heart have been characterized and related to contractile dysfunction. Contractile dysfunction is described by reduced twitch amplitude, delayed relaxation, and disturbed diastolic function. These alterations are associated with parallel changes in intracellular Ca^{2+} handling. Fig. 3 shows typical tracings of an isometric twitch and the corresponding intracellular Ca^{2+} transient from an isolated muscle strip obtained from a nonfailing and a failing human heart at a basal stimulation rate of 1 Hz. The amplitudes of the signals are normalized to 100%. It becomes evident that both time to maximal contraction as well as relaxation time is prolonged, associated with a prolonged decay time of the Ca^{2+} transient. Reduced systolic $[Ca^{2+}]_i$, delayed decline rates of the Ca^{2+} transient, as well as increased diastolic $[Ca^{2+}]_i$ have also been observed in isolated failing human myocytes [2].

Disturbed contractile function and Ca^{2+} homeostasis becomes more pronounced at higher rates of contraction. While in non-failing human myocardium, force of contraction and the amplitude of the Ca^{2+} transient increase with increasing stimulation rates (positive force-frequency behavior), frequency inotropism is blunted or even inverse in end-stage failing hearts ([67, 74]; Fig. 4, right). This negative force-frequency behavior in diseased human myocardium is associated with a frequency-dependent decline in intracellular Ca^{2+} transients, directly associated with reduced SR Ca^{2+} uptake capacity [74]. In fact, reduced SR Ca^{2+}-ATPase activity has been consistently observed in failing human hearts [56, 93, 96] and was related to decreased SERCA2a mRNA and protein expression [60, 62, 78, 83, 103]. However, since variations in the degree of downregulation of SERCA2a occur, not all groups were able to detect a significant overall reduction in SERCA2a on the protein

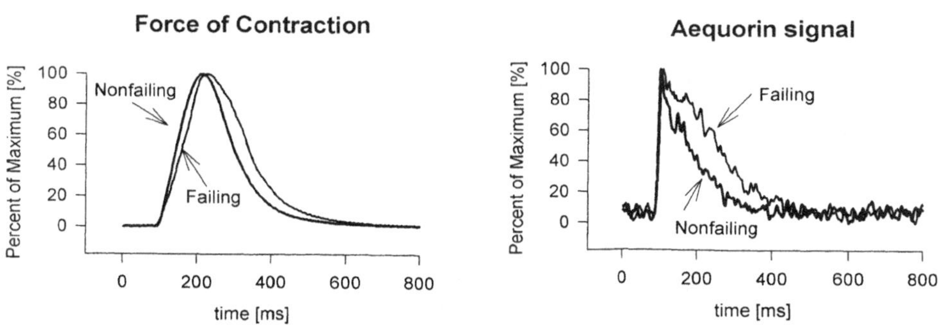

Fig. 3. Time course of contraction and relaxation, as well as the corresponding intracellular Ca^{2+} transient (aequorin method) in human nonfailing and failing myocardium. Typical registrations are superimposed, and their amplitudes are normalized to 100%. Both time to peak tension as well as relaxation times are prolonged in failing myocardium, associated with prolonged decay rates of the Ca^{2+} signal.

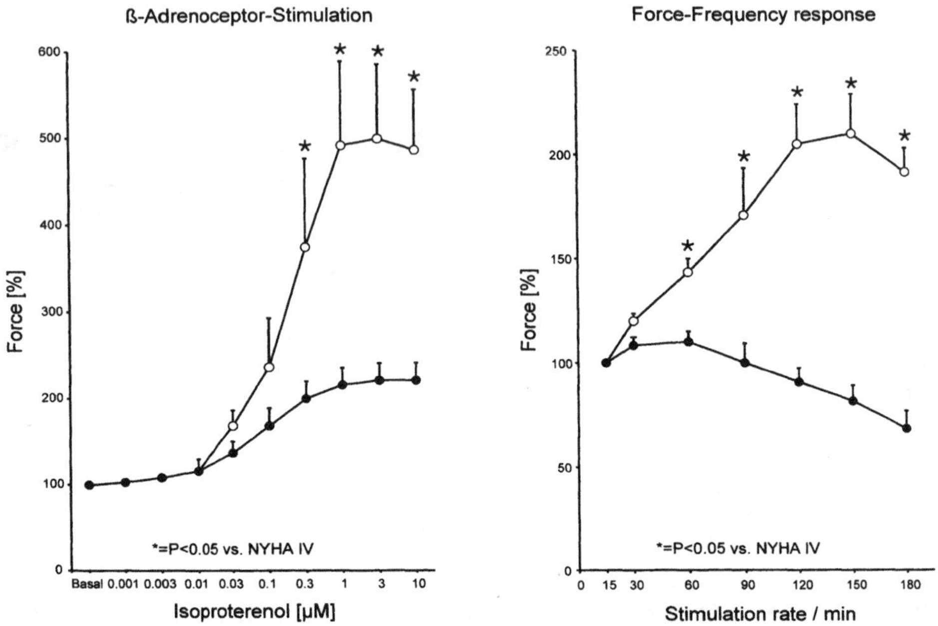

Fig. 4. Responsiveness of isolated human myocardium to β-adrenoceptor stimulation (left) and increases in stimulation rate (right). Nonfailing myocardium is characterized by a positive force-frequency relationship and a pronounced increase in force of contraction upon β-adrenoceptor stimulation with isoproterenol. In contrast, force of contraction declines with increasing stimulation rates in failing myocardium, and the positive inotropic effect of isoproterenol is severely reduced.

level [96]. In this regard, the relation between SERCA2a expression and myocardial function in the individual heart is of greater clinical importance. Hasenfuß et al. [38] demonstrated a direct relationship between the degree of SERCA2a downregulation and the severity of force-frequency negativation in failing human hearts (Fig. 5). These findings demonstrate the relevance of SERCA2a protein levels for contractile function.

Besides reduced expression of SERCA2a, a prominent phenotype change in failing human myocytes is the increased expression of the sarcolemmal Na^+/Ca^{2+}-exchanger (NCX1) on mRNA- and protein levels [27, 100]. The upregulation of NCX1 is associated with increased activity [27, 85] and, accordingly, the fraction of cytosolic Ca^{2+} removed from the cell during each contraction is larger in failing as compared to nonfailing human hearts [77, 92]. Also, the fractional transsarcolemmal Ca^{2+} extrusion via NCX1 (as compared to Ca^{2+} reuptake to the SR) increases with increasing stimulation rates, possibly as a result of exhaustion of SERCA2a transport capacity at shorter diastolic intervals [77]. As a consequence, in the failing human heart, there is reduced SR Ca^{2+} content under basal [58] and frequency-stimulated [77] conditions. Although interindividual variations with respect to the degree of downregulation of SERCA2a, or upregulation

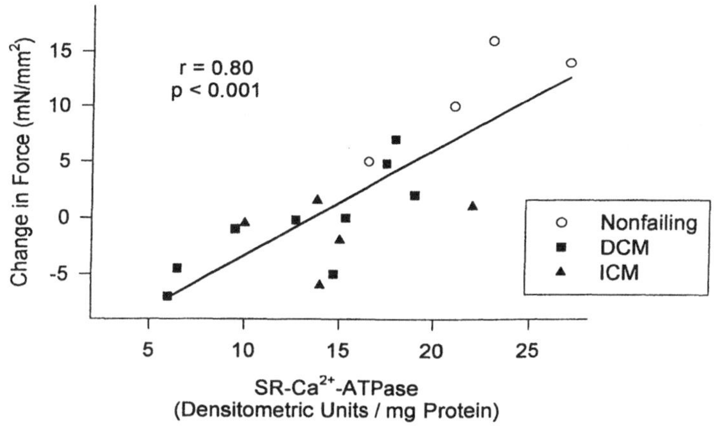

Fig. 5. Relation between SERCA2a protein levels (abscissa) and force-frequency behavior (ordinate) in individual failing and nonfailing human hearts. The change in force of contraction upon an increase in stimulation rate from 0.5 to 2.0 Hz is given. Each point reflects the data from one individual heart. Though variations in SERCA2a expression occur, low SERCA2a levels were associated with severely altered contractile behavior.

of NCX1 may occur [38, 39], the relative stoichiometry of NCX1/SERCA2a is very consistently increased in failing human hearts (Fig. 6; see also [39]).

It is important to consider that these two major transport mechanisms compete for cytosolic Ca^{2+}. As a consequence, either downregulation of SERCA2a or upregulation of NCX1 may decrease intracellular and SR Ca^{2+} content. On the other hand, upregulation of NCX1 in the presence of reduced SERCA2a levels may prevent diastolic Ca^{2+} accumulation and diastolic dysfunction. Accordingly, there was a close inverse correlation between the degree of NCX1 overexpression and the extent of diastolic dysfunction in failing human hearts [39]. However, possibly related to enhanced intracellular Na^{+} accumulation, the increased activity of NCX1 might also have disadvantageous effects on electrical membrane stability [81].

In addition to regulation of SERCA2a, expression of its inhibitory regulatory protein phospholamban may contribute to altered excitation-contraction coupling. There is general agreement that phospholamban protein expression is only marginally affected in heart failure [62, 96]. However, the resulting stoichiometric increase in the PLB to SERCA ratio due to reduced SERCA2a levels, but unchanged or only slightly reduced phospholamban levels, may further increase SERCA2a pump inhibition and Ca^{2+} uptake to the SR. The importance of the PLB to SERCA ratio for the control of the force-frequency relationship has directly been demonstrated in isolated rabbit myocardium [63]. However, frequency potentiation of contractile force is also under control of the adrenergic system and, under normal conditions, β-adrenoceptor stimulation renders the force-frequency relation more positive [88]. Therefore, alterations in the β-adrenergic system will contribute to altered EC coupling and SR Ca^{2+}-ATPase activity.

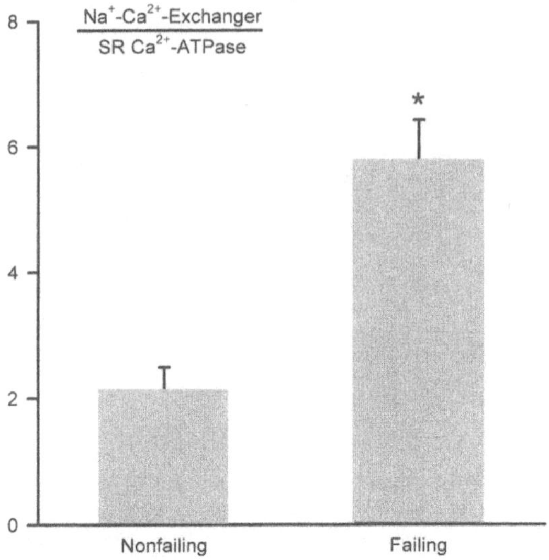

Fig. 6. Stoichiometry of NCX1/SERCA2a protein expression in nonfailing and failing human myocardium. Though variations in the expression levels of these proteins may occur between failing hearts, the protein expression of NCX1 was always increased relative to SERCA2a. Adapted with permission from [39].

Although reports are not completely conclusive, protein expression of L-type Ca^{2+} channels [97], the Ca^{2+} release channel of the SR [62, 91], and calsequestrin, the major Ca^{2+} storage protein of the SR [62], appear to be unaltered in human heart failure. However, altered function of the L-type Ca^{2+} channels, such as reduced frequency-dependent upregulation of L-type Ca^{2+} currents [80] or altered function of ryanodine release channels [15] may contribute to disturbed excitation-contraction coupling processes in diseased myocardium. Expression and function data for these proteins involved in excitation-contraction coupling are summarized in Table 1. However, altered excitation-contraction coupling does not exclusively depend on altered protein expression or function or Ca^{2+} handling proteins [32].

From the pathophysiological and molecular observations described above, several gene therapy targets in heart failure patients can be identified: in patients with primary systolic dysfunction and reduced SERCA2a levels, overexpression of SERCA2a (or SERCA1, its more active skeletal muscle counterpart [45]) might be promising. In patients with predominant diastolic dysfunction and cytosolic Ca^{2+} overload, an increase in NCX1 might improve relaxation. In addition, strategies targeted at reducing phospholamban expression, thereby enhancing SERCA2a pump function, could be considered. Recent work describing adenovirus-mediated gene transfer of Ca^{2+} handling proteins is summarized in Table 3.

Alterations and potential targets for gene therapy in the β-adrenergic system

In 1982, Bristow et al. [8] first described desensitization and downregulation of β-adrenoceptors in end-stage failing as compared to nonfailing human myocardium. Since then, multiple lines of evidence indicate fundamental alterations in the myocardial β-adrenoceptor system (see Fig. 2 and Table 2) that both precede and accompany the development of heart failure [12, 79, 89].

In end-stage failing human myocardium, there is approximately a 50% decrease in β_1-adrenoceptors in radioligand-binding experiments, as well as on the protein- and mRNA levels [10, 105], but no decrease in the number of β_2-adrenoceptors. The remaining receptors (both β_1 and β_2) are functionally uncoupled from adenylate cyclase activation [9]. Functional uncoupling may be related to the increased expression and activity of β-adrenoceptor kinase 1 (βARK-1) in failing myocardium [105]. βARK-1 is a cytosolic enzyme which translocates to the membrane upon agonist-binding to adrenoceptors and phosphorylates both β_1- and β_2-adrenoceptors at cytosolic phosphorylation sites. The phosphorylated receptor is a substrate for β-arrestin which uncouples the βAR from G_s [106].

β-adrenoceptors are linked to adenylate cyclase within the cell membrane through a stimulatory guanine-nucleotide-binding protein (G_s), and G_s expression and function seems to be unaltered in failing hearts. However, adenylate cyclase in the membrane is under dual control of stimulatory (Gs) as well as inhibitory (Gi) proteins. Inhibitory $G_{i\alpha}$ proteins, which couple inhibitory m-cholino- or adenosin A_1-receptors to adenylate cyclase [40], are overexpressed in failing human hearts [21, 22, 68]. As a consequence, both basal as well as isoproterenol-stimulated adenylate cyclase activity [12, 13] as well as cAMP levels [6] are decreased in failing human hearts. In contrast, direct pharmacological activation of the catalytic subunit of adenylate cyclase with forskolin yields unchanged activity and also cAMP levels in failing myocardium [12]. This indicates functional competence of adenylate cyclase (most of which is of the isoform V in the human heart), but altered stimulatory and inhibitory pathways with preponderance of adenylate cyclase inhibition. Unchanged catalytic activity of AC by direct stimulation is also in agreement with recent reports of unchanged isoform expression patterns and expression levels of AC in failing human myocardium.

As a result of these molecular disease-related changes, reduced functional responsiveness to β-adrenergic agonists or cAMP-dependent inotropic agents (such as PDE-III inhibitors) have been repeatedly described in failing human hearts under in vitro (e.g., [4, 24, 76]; see also Fig. 4, left) as well as clinical [11] conditions and represent an important cause of contractile dysfunction.

We have recently addressed the question whether overexpression of $G_{i\alpha}$ may mimic reduced β-adrenoceptor responsiveness in isolated rabbit myocytes. We used adenoviral-mediated gene transfer of a cDNA encoding $G_{i\alpha}$, coupled to a CMV promoter and expressed in a type V adenovirus as a vector. Transfection of the myocardium was performed through coronary perfusion of isolated rabbit hearts in the Langendorff mode with the adenovirus at a MOI of 100 for 10 min, according to the protocol of Donahue [17]. This protocol resulted in a 90% transfection efficiency, as demonstrated by parallel Lac Z transfection and staining of myocytes for β-Gal. After transfection, thin left ventricular trabeculae were transferred to a special long-term organ chamber [46] and kept under culture conditions for 48 hours. $G_{i\alpha}$ overexpression resulted in a significant rightward shift of the concentration-response curve for isoproterenol in rabbit myocardium. This indicated that $G_{i\alpha}$ overexpression in failing human hearts may be of functional relevance, and gene therapy targeted at reducing $G_{i\alpha}$ levels may partly restore β-adrenoceptor responsiveness in these hearts.

"Resensitization" of the β-adrenergic signaling cascade might be used to enhance cardiac function of the failing human heart. This mechanism could in part explain the beneficial effects of some β-blockers, such as metoprolol, in heart failure patients [28]. One approach to simulate this resensitization is the overexpression of the βARK-1 inhibitor protein (βARK_{mini}), consisting of the carboxyl terminus of βARK-1 [49]. Transgenic mice with overexpressed βARK_{mini} showed increased contractility and increased cAMP levels for the duration of their lives without signs of myocardial damage [49], and stable LV contractility after aortic banding in contrast to pronounced cardiac dysfunction in aortic banded wild-type litter mates [14].

In addition, interventions that increase the expression of β-adrenoceptors, $G_{\alpha s}$, or possibly adenylate cyclase type V or type VI might restore β-agonistic responsiveness in heart failure. Though data in animal models of heart failure are limited, Akhter et al. [1] recently demonstrated that adenoviral-mediated β_2-adrenoceptor gene transfer to cultured ventricular myocytes isolated from rabbit hearts paced into heart failure restores β-adrenergic signaling to normal levels. In addition, the same group recently reported enhanced basal and isoproterenol-stimulated contractility after adenoviral-mediated in vivo intracoronary β_2-adrenergic receptor gene delivery [59]. Heart failure patients possessing a β_2-adrenoceptor gene polymorphism resulting in β_2 receptors that couple to adenylate cyclase less efficiently have significantly lower survival rates [55]. Gene therapy using the wild-type β_2-adrenoceptor, which couples efficiently to adenylate cyclase, may be especially useful in this patient group.

In a different approach, Laugwitz et al. [53] transfected the human V2 vasopressin receptor into rat cardiomyocytes. Physiologically, this receptor is exclusively expressed in the kidney where it activates adenylate cyclase through a G_s protein. Rat cardiomyocytes expressing the vasopressin V2 receptor demonstrated marked cAMP production upon stimulation with arginine-vasopressin, a hormone that is highly upregulated in heart failure patients. Therefore, at least under experimental conditions, both normalization of the expression of physiological components of the β-adrenoceptor-adenylate cyclase pathway, or introduction of new functional active proteins might normalize altered function of the β-adrenergic signal transduction cascade. Table 4 summarizes recent reports on adenovirus-mediated regulation of proteins involved in β-adrenoceptor/adenylate cyclase-dependent signaling in mammalian myocardium.

However, in contrast to βARK_{mini} (see above), transgenic mice overexpressing the β_2 adrenoceptor demonstrated mild cardiac fibrosis. In addition, transgenic β_2-adrenergic receptor overexpression exacerbates the development of heart failure after aortic stenosis in mice [19]. Furthermore, overexpression of $G_{\alpha s}$ led to severe cardiac fibrosis and cardiomyopathy [73]. Therefore, some therapeutic interventions aimed at restoring β-adrenoceptor responsiveness might be disadvantageous for heart failure patients. In addition, long-term β-adrenoceptor stimulation or phosphodiesterase-III inhibition increased mortality in patients with heart failure [72], but β-adrenoceptor blockade greatly improves survival in these patients [54].

Can we extrapolate improved contractile function after gene transfer under in vitro conditions to the clinical situation?

None of these potential proteins have been targeted in patients under in vivo conditions. Before considering clinical application, the functional, electrophysiological, and genomic effects of altering the expression of one or several target proteins must be carefully analyzed in mammalian and human isolated cardiac tissue as well as in long-term expression studies. In addition, it is still unclear whether the described alterations in gene expression are etiological for heart failure or simply reflect an adaptive change of the overloaded heart.

There are several caveats that have to be resolved before in vitro techniques can be applied under clinical situations, e.g., safety concerns related to the use of infectious agents, the efficiency and stability of transfection, and immune responses related to the use of adenoviral vectors. Some of these caveats can possibly be overcome in the future by use of new vectors such as the non-pathogenic human adeno-associated viruses (AAV), which might possibly be targeted to the specific cell types of interest [30].

A further aspect is whether positive results of gene regulation in isolated myocytes under specific experimental conditions can be reproduced under more physiological aspects. For example, Meyer et al. [64] observed enhanced contractility and relaxation in SERCA2a-transfected rabbit cardiac myocytes at a low stimulation rate, but the force-frequency relationship in the transfected myocardium became negative.

Therefore, before gene therapy can be considered in heart failure, potential targets must be identified and characterized in isolated failing human myocardium. We have developed a new method for high-yield isolation of ventricular myocytes from failing human hearts which can be kept in cell culture for 48 hours without loss of contractile function. This model allows the care-

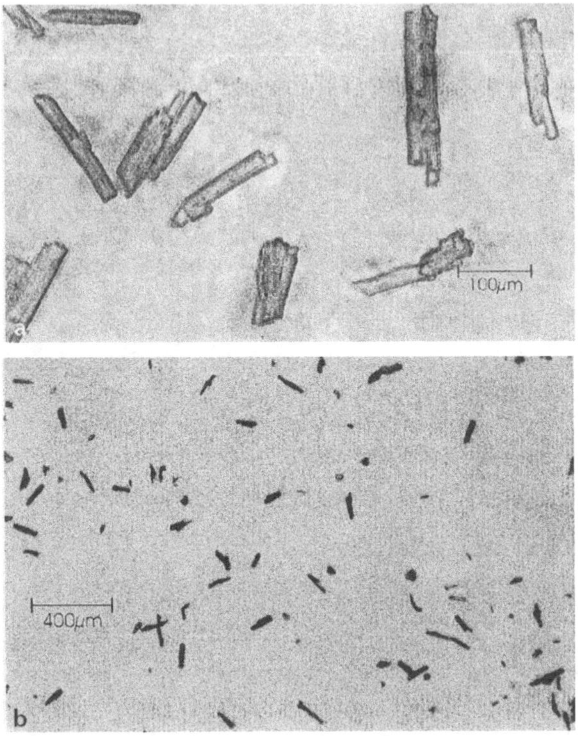

Fig. 7. Gene transfer in isolated human myocardium. **a** Freshly isolated left ventricular cardiomyocytes. **b** Cardiomyocytes after adenovirus-mediated transfer of the LacZ gene and blue staining for β-galactosidase expression (48 hour cell culture).

ful evaluation of functional consequences of adenovirus-mediated gene transfer. Figure 7 shows typical freshly isolated myocytes and myocytes transfected with the LacZ gene after a 48 hour cell culture from a failing human heart. Fractional shortening was 4.6% of resting cell length in the fresh myocytes, and 4.3% in the transfected myocytes, and transfection efficiency was ~70–80% at a MOI of 500 pfu/cell. Recently, Del Monte et al. [16] reported efficient gene transfer of SERCA2a to myocytes from failing human hearts, resulting in improved Ca^{2+} handling. In addition, the first phase I clinical trial using adenovirus-mediated gene transfer of VEGF to the hearts of patients with severe coronary artery disease was reported [87]. However, any gene therapy approach for the treatment of heart failure should be validated before clinical application by demonstrating a hemodynamic and survival benefit in animal models of congestive heart failure.

References

1. Akhter S, Skaer C, Kypson A, McDonald P, Peppel K, Glower D, Lefkowitz R, Koch W (1997) Restoration of β-adrenergic signaling in failing cardiac ventricular myocytes via adenoviral-mediated gene transfer. Proc Natl Acad Sci USA 99:12100–12105
2. Beuckelmann DJ, Näbauer M, Erdmann E (1992) Intracellular Ca^{2+} handling in isolated ventricular myocytes from patients with terminal heart failure. Circulation 85:1046–1055
3. Beuckelmann DJ, Erdmann E (1992) Ca^{2+} currents and intracellular Ca^{2+} transients in single ventricular myocytes isolated from terminally failing human myocardium. Bas Res Cardiol 87:235–243
4. Böhm M, Beuckelmann D, Brown L, Feiler G, Lorenz B, Näbauer M, Kemkes B, Erdmann E (1988) Reduction of beta-adrenoceptor density and evaluation of positive inotropic responses in isolated, diseased human myocardium. Eur Heart J 9:844–852
5. Böhm M, Eschenhagen T, Giershick P et al (1994) Radioimmunochemical quantification of Giα in right and left ventricles from patients with ischemic and dilated cardiomyopathy and predominantly left ventricular failure. J Mol Cell Cardiol 26:133–149
6. Böhm M, Reiger B, Schwinger RHG, Erdmann E (1994) cAMP concentrations, cAMP dependent protein kinase activity and phospholamban in nonfailing and failing myocardium. Cardiovasc Res 26:133–149
7. Brillantes AM, Allen P, Takahashi T, Izumo S, Marks AR (1992) Differences in cardiac calcium release channel (ryanosidine receptor) expression in myocardium from patients with end-stage heart failure caused by ischemic versus dilated cardiomyopathy. Circ Res 71:18–26
8. Bristow MR, Ginsburg R, Minobe W, Cubicciotti RS, Sageman WS, Lurie K, Billingham ME, Harrison DC, Stinson EB (1982) Decreased catecholamine sensitivity and β-adrenergic receptors in failing human hearts. N Engl J Med 307:205–211
9. Bristow MR, Hershberger RE, Port JD, Minobe W, Rasmussen R (1988) β_1 and β_2-adrenergic receptor-mediated adenylyl-cyclase stimulation in nonfailing and failing human myocardium. Mol Pharmacol 35:335–343
10. Bristow MR, Minobe W, Reynolds M, Port D, Rasmussen R, Ray P, Feldman AM (1993) Reduced β_1 receptor messenger RNA abundance in the failing human heart. J Clin Invest 92:2737–2745
11. Bristow MR, Lowes BD (1994) Low-dose inotropic therapy for ambulatory heart failure. Coron Art Dis 5:112–118
12. Brodde OE (1993) Beta-adrenoceptors in cardiac disease. Pharmacol Ther 60:405–430
13. Brodde OE (1991) β_1- and β_2-Adrenoceptors in the human heart: properties, function, and alterations in chronic heart failure. Pharmacol Rev 43:203–242
14. Choi DW, Koch WJ, Hunter JJ, Rockman HA (1997) Mechanism of β-adrenergic receptor desensitization in cardiac hypertrophy is increase β-adrenergic receptor kinase. J Biol Chem 272:17223–17229
15. D'Agnolo A, Luciani GB, Mazzucco A, Gallucci V, Saviati G (1992) Contractile properties and Ca^{2+} release activity of the sarcoplasmic reticulum in dilated cardiomyopathy. Circulation 85:518–525
16. Del Monte F, Harding S, Schmidt U, Matsui T, Kang Z, Dec W, Gwathmey K, Rosenzweig A, Hajjar R (1999) Restoration of contractile function in isolated cardiomyocytes from failing human hearts by gene transfer of SERCA2a. Circulation 100:2308–2311

17. Donahue K, Kikkawa K, Johns D, Marban E, Lawrence J (1997) Ultrarapid, highly efficient viral gene transfer to the heart. Proc Natl Acad Sci USA 94:4664–4668
18. Drazner MH, Peppel KC, Dyer S, Grant AO, Koch WJ, Lefkowitz RJ (1997) Potentiation of β-adrenergic signaling by adenoviral-mediated gene transfer in adult rabbit ventricular myocytes. J Clin Invest 99:288–296
19. Du XJ, Autelitano DJ, Dilley R, Wang B, Dart A, Woodcock E (2000) β_a-adrenergic overexpression exacerbates development of heart failure after aortic stenosis. Circulation 101:71–77
20. Eschenhagen T, Mende U, Nose M, Schmitz W, Scholz H, Haverich A, Hirt S, Döring V, Kalmar P, Höppner W, Seitz HJ (1992) Increased messenger RNA level of the inhibitory G-protein α-subunit Giα2 in human end-stage heart failure. Circ Res 70:688–696
21. Feldman AM, Cates AE, Veazey WB, Hershberger RE, Bristow MR, Baughman KL, Baumgartner WA, Van Dop C (1988) Increase of the 40,000-mol wt pertussis toxin substrate (G-protein) in the failing human heart. J Clin Invest 82:189–197
22. Feldman AM, Cates AE, Bristow MR, Van Dop C (1989) Altered expression of the α-subunits of G-proteins in failing human hearts. J Mol Cell Cardiol 21:359–365
23. Feldman AM, Ray PE, Silan C, Mercer JA, Winobe W, Bristow MR (1991) Selective gene expression in failing human heart. Quantification of steady-state levels of messenger RNA in endomyocardial biopsies using the polymerase chain reaction. Circulation 83:1866–1872
24. Feldmann MD, Copelas L, Gwathmey JK, Phillips P, Warren SE, Schoen FJ, Grossmann W, Morgan JP (1987) Deficient production of cyclic AMP: pharmacologic evidence of an important cause of contractile dysfunction in patients with end-stage heart failure. Circulation 75:331–339
25. Feldmann MD, Aldermann JD, Aroesti JM, Royal HD, Ferguson JJ, Owen RM, Grossmann W, McKay RG (1988) Depression of systolic and diastolic myocardial reserve during atrial pacing tachycardia in patients with dilated cardiomyopathy. J Clin Invest 44(12):2051–2062
26. Finkel MS, Patterson RE, Roberts WC, Smith TD, Keiser HR (1988) Calcium channel binding characteristics in the human heart. Am J Cardiol 62:1281–1284
27. Flesch M, Schwinger RHG, Schiffer F, Frank K, Südkamp M, Kuhn-Regnier F, Arnold G, Böhm M (1996) Evidence for functional relevance of an enhanced Na-Ca exchanger expression in failing human myocardium. Circulation 94:992–1002
28. Gilbert EM, Abraham WT, Olsen S, Hattler B, White M, Mealy P, Larrabee P, Bristow MR (1996) Comparative hemodynamic, LV functional, and antiadrenergic effects of chronic treatment with metoprolol vs. carvedilol in the failing heart. Circulation 94:2817–2825
29. Giordano R, He H, McDonough P, Meyer M, Sayen R, Dillmann W (1997) Adenovirus-mediated gene transfer reconstitutes depressed sarcoplasmic reticulum Ca^{2+}-ATPase levels and shortens prolonged cardiac myocyte Ca^{2+} transients. Circulation 96:400–403
30. Girod A, Ried M, Wobus C, Lahm H, Leike K, Kleinschmidt J, Deléage G, Hallek M (1999) Genetic capsid modifications allow re-targeting of adeno-associated virus type 2. Nature Med 5:1052–1056
31. Go L, Moschella M, Watras J, Handa KK, Fyfe BS, Marks AR (1995) Differential regulation of two types of intracellular calcium release channels during end-stage heart failure. J Clin Invest 95:888–894
32. Gomez AM, Valdivia HH, Cheng H, Lederer MR, Santana LF, Cannell MB, McCune SA, Altschuld RA, Lederer WJ (1997) Defective excitation-contraction coupling in experimental cardiac hypertrophy and heart failure. Science 276:800–806
33. Hajjar RJ, Schmidt U, Kang J, Matsui T, Rosenzweig A (1997) Adenoviral gene transfer of phospholamban in isolated rat cardiomyocytes. Circ Res 81:145–153

34. Hajjar RJ et al (1998) Modulation of ventricular function through gene transfer in vivo. Proc Natl Acad Sci USA 95:534–539
35. Hajjar RJ, Kang JX, Gwathmey JK, Rosenzweig A (1997) Physiological effects of adenoviral gene transfer of sarcoplasmic reticulum calcium ATPase in isolated rat myocytes. Circulation 95:423–429
36. Hartzell HC, Mery PF, Fischmeister R, Szabo G (1991) Sympathetic regulation of cardiac calcium current is due exclusively to cAMP-dependent phosphorylation. Nature 352:573–576
37. Hasenfuß G, Holubarsch C, Hermann HP, Astheimer K, Pieske B, Just H (1994) Influence of the force-frequency relationship on haemodynamics and left ventricular function in patients with non-failing hearts and in patients with dilated cardiomyopathy. Europ Heart J 15:164–170
38. Hasenfuß G, Reinecke H, Studer R, Meyer M, Pieske B, Holtz J, Holubarsch C, Posival H, Just H, Drexler H (1994) Relation between myocardial function and expression of sarcoplasmic reticulum Ca^{2+} ATPase in failing and nonfailing human myocardium. Circ Res 75:434–442
39. Hasenfuß G, Schillinger W, Lehnart SE, Preuss M, Pieske B, Maier LS, Prestle J, Minami K, Just H (1999) Relationship between Na^{+}/Ca^{2+}-exchanger protein levels and diastolic function of failing human myocardium. Circulation 99:641–648
40. Hershberger RE, Feldman AM, Bristow MR (1991) A1-Adenosine receptor inhibition of adenylate cyclase in failing and nonfailing human myocardium. Circulation 83:1343–1351
41. Hoch B, Meyer R, Hetzer R, Krause EG, Karczewski P (1999) Identification and expression of δ-isoforms of the multifunctional Ca^{2+}/calmodulin-dependent protein kinase in failing and nonfailing human myocardium. Circ Res 84:713–721
42. Holmberg S, Williams A (1992) The calcium release channel from cardiac sarcoplasmic reticulum: function in the failing and acutely ischemic heart. Basic Res Cardiol 87(1):255–268
43. Holmer S, Eschenhagen T, Nose M, Rieger G (1996) Expression of adenylyl cyclase and G-protein β subunit in end-stage human heart failure. J Card Failure 2:279–283
44. Holubarsch Ch, Ruf T, Goldstein D, Ashton RC, Nickl W, Pieske B, Pioch K, Lüdemann J, Wiessner S, Hasenfuß G, Posival H, Just H, Burckhoff D (1996) Existence of the Frank-Starling mechanism in the failing human heart. Investigations at the organ, tissue, and sarcomere level. Circulation 94:683–689
45. Inesi G, Lewis D, Sumbilla C, Nandi A, Strock C, Huff KW, Rogers TB, Johns DC, Kessler P, Ordahl C (1998) Cell-specific promoter in adenovirus vector for transgenic expression of SERCA1 ATPase in cardiac myocytes. Am J Physiol 274:C645–C653
46. Janssen PM, Lehnart S, Prestle J, Hasenfuß G (1999) Preservation of contractile characteristics of human myocardium in multi-day cell culture. J Mol Cell Cardiol 31:1419–1427
47. Kawahira Y, Sawa Y, Nishimura M, Sakakida S, Ueda H, Kaneda Y, Matsuda H (1998) In vivo gene transfer of a β_2-adrenergic receptor gene into the pressure-overloaded rat heart enhances cardiac response to β-adrenergic agonist. Circulation 98:II-262–II-268
48. Kirchhefer U, Schmitz W, Scholz H, Neumann J (1999) Activity of cAMP-dependent protein kinase and Ca^{2+}/calmodulin dependent protein kinase in failing and nonfailing human hearts. Cardiovasc Res 42:254–261
49. Koch WJ, Rockman HA, Samama P, Hamilton R, Bond RA, Milano CA, Lefkowitz RJ (1995) Cardiac function in mice overexpressing the β-adrenergic receptor kinase or a βARK inhibitor. Science 268:1350–1353

50. Koss KL, Kranias EG (1996) Phospholamban: a prominent regulator of myocardial contractility. Circ Res 79:1059–1063
51. Kypson AP, Peppel K, Akhter SA, Lilly E, Glower DD, Lefkowitz RJ, Koch WJ (1998) Ex-vivo adenoviral-mediated gene transfer to the transplanted adult rat heart. J Thorac Cardiovasc Surg 115:623–630
52. Lai C, Roth D, Gao M, Head B, Zhu J, Hammond K (1999) Intracoronary delivery of an adenovirus expressing adenylylcyclase VI is associated with marked global changes in LV function and cardiac output in conscious pigs. Circulation 100 (Suppl I):A550
53. Laugwitz KL, Ungerer M, Schöneberg T, Weig HJ, Kronsbein K, Moretti A, Hoffmann K, Seyfarth M, Schultz G, Schömig A (1999) Adenoviral gene transfer of the human V2 vasopressin receptor improves contractile force of rat cardiomyocytes. Circulation 99:925–933
54. The Cardiac Insufficiency Bisoprolol Study II (CIBIS-II) (1999) A randomised trial. Lancet 353:9–13
55. Ligget SB, Wagoner LE, Craft LL, Hornung RW, Hoit BD, McIntosh TC, Walsh RA (1998) The ile164 β_2-adrenergic receptor polymorphism adversely affects the outcome of congestive heart failure. J Clin Invest 102:1534–1539
56. Limas CJ, Olivari MT, Goldenberg IF, Levine TB, Benditt DG, Simon A (1987) Calcium uptake by cardiac sarcoplasmic reticulum in human dilated cardiomyopathy. Cardiovasc Res 21:601–605
57. Linck B, Boknik P, Eschenhagen T, Müller FU, Neumann J, Nose M, Jones LR, Schmitz W, Scholz H (1996) Messenger RNA expression and immunological quantification of phospholamban and SR Ca^{2+}-ATPase in failing and nonfailing human hearts. Cardiovasc Res 31:625–632
58. Lindner M, Erdmann E, Beuckelmann DJ (1998) Calcium content of sarcoplasmic reticulum in isolated ventricular myocytes from patients with terminal heart failure. J Mol Cell Cardiol 30:743–749
59. Maurice JP, Hata J, Shah A, White D, McDonald P, Dolber P, Wilson K, Lefkowitz R, Glower D, Koch W (1999) Enhancement of cardiac function after adenoviral-mediated in vivo intracoronary β_2-adrenergic receptor gene delivery. J Clin Invest 104:21–29
60. Mercadier JJ, Lompre AM, Duc P, Boehler KR, Fraysse JB, Wisnewski C, Allen PD, Komajda M, Schwartz K (1990) Altered sarcoplasmic reticulum CA^{2+}-ATPAse gene expression in the human ventricle during end-stage heart failure. J Clin Invest 85:305–309
61. Mewes T, Ravens U (1994) L-type calcium currents of human myocytes from ventricles of nonfailing and failing hearts and from atrium. J Mol Cell Cardiol 26:1307–1320
62. Meyer M, Schillinger W, Pieske B, Holubarsch C, Heilmann C, Posival H, Kuwajama G, Mikoshiba K, Just H, Hasenfuß G (1995) Alterations of sarcoplasmic reticulum proteins in failing human dilated cardiomyopathy. Circulation 92:778–784
63. Meyer M, Bluhm W, He H, Post S, Giordano F, Lew W, Dillmann W (1999) Phospholamban-to-SERCA2 ratio controls the force-frequency relationship. Am J Physiol 276:H779–H785
64. Meyer M, Dillmann W (1998) Sarcoplasmic reticulum Ca^{2+}-ATPase overexpression by adenovirus mediated gene transfer and in transgenic mice. Cardiovasc Res 37:360–366
65. Miyamato M, Guerrero JL, Schmidt U, Gwathmey J, Dec W, Rosenzweig A, Hajjar R (1998) Adenoviral gene transfer of SERCA2a improves LV function in aortic-banded rats in transition to heart failure. Circulation 98:736 (abstract)

66. Movsesian MA, Karimi M, Green K, Jones LR (1994) Ca^{2+}-transporting ATPase, phospholamban, and calsequestrin levels in nonfailing and failing human myocardium. Circulation 90:653–657
67. Mulieri LA, Hasenfuß G, Leavitt B, Allen PD, Alpert NR (1992) Altered myocardial force-frequency relation in human heart failure. Circulation 85:1743–1750
68. Neumann J, Schmitz W, von Meyerinck I, Scholz H, Döring V, Kalmar P (1988) Increase in myocardial G_i proteins in heart failure. Lancet 2:936–937
69. Neumann J, Eschenhagen T, Jones LR, Linck B, Schmitz W, Scholz H, Zimmermann N (1997) Increased expression of cardiac phosphatases in patients with endstage heart failure. J Mol Cell Cardiol 29:265–272
70. Nimer L, Needleman D, Hamilton S, Krall J, Movsesian M (1995) Effect of ryanodine on sarcoplasmic reticulum Ca^{2+} accumulation in nonfailing and failing human myocardium. Circulation 92:2504–2510
71. Ouadid H, Albat B, Nargeot J (1995) Calcium currents in diseased human cardiac cells. J Cardiovasc Pharmacol 25:282–291
72. Packer M, Carver JR, Rodeheffer RJ (1991) Effects of oral milrinone on mortality in severe chronic heart failure. N Engl J Med 325:1468–1475
73. Peppel K, Koch WJ, Lefkowitz RJ (1997) Gene transfer strategies for augmenting cardiac function. Trends Cardiovasc Med 7:9–14
74. Pieske B, Kretschmann B, Meyer M, Holubarsch C, Weirich J, Posival H, Minami K, Just H, Hasenfuß G (1995) Alterations in intracellular calcium handling associated with the inverse force-frequency relation in human dilated cardiomyopathy. Circulation 92:1169–1178
75. Pieske B, Sütterlin M, Schmidt-Schweda S, Minami K, Meyer M, Olschewski M, Holubarsch C, Just H, Hasenfuß G (1996) Diminished post-rest potentiation of contractile force in human dilated cardiomyopathy. J Clin Invest 98:764–776
76. Pieske B, Schlotthauer K, Schattmann J, Beyersdorf F, Martin J, Just H, Hasenfuß G (1997) Ca^{2+}-dependent and Ca^{2+}-independent regulation of myocardial contractility. Bas Res Cardiol 1997; 92(I):75–86
77. Pieske B, Maier LS, Bers DM, Hasenfuß G (1999) Ca^{2+} handling and sarcoplasmic reticulum Ca^{2+} content in isolated failing and nonfailing human myocardium. Circ Res 85:38–46
78. Pieske B, Schillinger W, Dieterich S, Maier L, Hasenfuß G, Prestle J (2000) Distinct phenotype patterns of Ca handling proteins in end-stage failing human hearts. Bas Res Cardiol 94(I):19–32
79. Ping P, Anzai T, Gao M, Hammond HK (1997) Adenylyl cyclase and G protein receptor kinase expression during development of heart failure. Am J Physiol 273:H707–717
80. Piot C, Lemaire S, Albat B, Seguin J, Nargeot J, Richard S (1996) High frequency-induced upregulation of human cardiac calcium currents. Circulation 93:120–128
81. Pogwidz S, Qi M, Samarel AM, Bers DM (1997) Upregulation of Na^{+}/Ca^{2+}-exchanger gene expression in an arrhythmogenic model of nonischemic cardiomyopathy in the rabbit. Circulation 96 (Suppl I):1–8
82. Poller W, Fechner H, Eizema K, Bezstarosti K, vdLaarse A, Pauschinger M, Wang H, Wang X, Schultheiss HP, Lamers J (1999) Adenovirus-based phospholamban-antisense expression as a novel approach to improve cardiac diastolic dysfunction. Circulation 100 (Suppl I):A2538
83. Prestle J, Dieterich S, Preuss M, Bieligk U, Just H, Hasenfuß G (1999) Differential transmural expression of calcium-handling proteins and natriuretic peptides in the human heart. Cardiovasc Res 43:323–331
84. Rasmussen RP, Minobe W, Bristow MR (1990) Calcium antagonist binding sites in failing and non-failing human ventricular myocardium. Biochem Pharmacol 39:691–696

85. Reinecke H, Studer R, Vetter R, Holtz J, Drexler H (1996) Cardiac Na/Ca exchange activity in patients with end-stage heart failure. Cardiovasc Res 31:48–54
86. Robertson SP, Johnson JD, Holroyde MJ, Kranias EG, Potter JD, Solaro RJ (1982) The effect of troponin I phosphorylation on the Ca^{2+}-regulatory site of bovine troponin. J Biol Chem 257:260–263
87. Rosengart T, Lee L, Patel S, Sanborn T, Parikh M, Bergmann G, Hachamovitch R, Szulc M, Kligfield P, Okin P, Hahn R, Devereux R, Post M, Hackett N, Foster T, Grasso T, Lesser M, Isom W, Crystal R (1999) Angiogenesis gene therapy. Phase I assessment of direct intramyocardial administration of an adenovirus vector expressing VEGF121 cDNA to individuals with clinically significant severe coronary artery disease. Circulation 100:468–474
88. Ross J Jr, Miura T, Kambayashi M, Eising P, Ryu K-H (1995) The adrenergic control of the force-frequency relation. Circulation 92:2327–2332
89. Rundquist B, Elam M, Bergmann-Sverrisdottir Y, Eisenhofer G, Friberg P (1997) Increased cardiac adrenergic drive precedes generalized sympathetic activation in human heart failure. Circulation 95:169–175
90. Sainte Beuve C, Allen PD, Dambin G et al (1997) Cardiac calcium release channel (ryanodine receptor) in control and cardiomyopathic human hearts: mRNA and protein contents are differentially regulated. J Mol Cell Cardiol 29:1237–1246
91. Schillinger W, Meyer M, Kuwajima G, Mikoshiba K, Just H, Hasenfuß G (1996) Unaltered ryanodine receptor protein levels in ischemic cardiomyopathy. Mol Cell Biochem 160/161:297–302
92. Schlotthauer K, Schattmann J, Bers DM, Maier LS, Schütt U, Minami K, Just H, Hasenfuß G, Pieske B (1998) Frequency-dependent changes in contribution of SR Ca^{2+} to Ca^{2+} transients in failing human myocardium assessed with ryanodine. J Mol Cell Cardiol 30:1285–1294
93. Schmidt U, Hajjar R, Helm P, Kim C, Doye A, Gwathmey JK (1998) Contribution of abnormal sarcoplasmic reticulum ATPase activity to systolic and diastolic dysfunction in human heart failure. J Mol Cell Cardiol 30:1929–1937
94. Schnabel P, Böhm M, Gierschik P, Jakobs KH, Erdmann E (1990) Improvement of cholera toxin-catalyzed ADP-ribosylation by endogenous ADP-ribosylation factor from bovine brain provides evidence for unchanged amounts of $Gs\alpha$ in failing human myocardium. J Mol Cell Cardiol 22:73–82
95. Schwinger RHG, Böhm M, Koch A, Schmidt U, Morano I, Eissner HJ, Überfuhr R, Reichart B, Erdmann E (1994) The failing human heart is unable to use the Frank-Starling mechanism. Circ Res 74:959–969
96. Schwinger RHG, Böhm M, Schmidt U, Karczewski P, Bavendick U, Flesch M, Krause EG, Erdmann E (1995) Unchanged protein levels of SERCA II and phospholamban but reduced Ca^{2+} uptake and Ca^{2+}-ATPase activity of cardiac sarcoplasmic reticulum from dilated cardiomyopathy patients compared with patients with nonfailing hearts. Circulation 92:3220–3228
97. Schwinger RHG, Hoischen S, Reuter H, Hullin R (1999) Regional expression and functional characterization of the L-type Ca channel in myocardium from patients with end-stage heart failure and in nonfailing human hearts. J Mol Cell Cardiol 31:283–296
98. Schwinger RHG, Münch G, Bölck B, Karczewski P, Krause EG, Erdmann E (1999) Reduced Ca^{2+} sensitivity of SERCA2a in failing human myocardium due to reduced serin-16 phospholamban phosphorylation. J Mol Cell Cardiol 31:479–491
99. Shah AS, Lilly E, Kypson A, Tai O, Haza J, Pippen A, Silvestri S, Lefkowitz R, Glower D, Koch WJ (2000) Intracoronary adenovirus-mediated delivery and overexpression of the β_2-adrenergic receptor in the heart. Circulation 101:408–414

100. Studer R, Reinecke H, Bilger J, Eschenhagen T, Böhm M, Hasenfuß G, Just H, Holtz J, Drexler H (1994) Gene expression of the cardiac Na^{+}-Ca^{2+} exchanger in end-stage human heart failure. Circ Res 75:443–453
101. Sumbilla C, Cavagna M, Zhong L, Ma H, Lewis D, Farrance I, Inesi G (1999) Comparison of SERCA1 and SERCA2a expressed in COS-1 cells and cardiac myocytes. Am J Physiol 277:H2381–H2391
102. Takahashi T, Allen PD, Larco RV, Marks A, Dennis R, Schoen F, Grossman W, Marsh JD, Izumo S (1992) Expression of dihydropyridine receptor (Ca^{2+} channel) and calsequestrin genes in the myocardium of patients with endstage heart failure. J Clin Invest 90:927–935
103. Takahashi T, Allen PD, Izumo S (1992) Expression of A-, B-, and C-type natriuretic peptide genes in failing and developing human ventricles: correlation with expression of the Ca^{2+}-ATPase gene. Circ Res 71:9–17
104. Taylor SS (1989) cAMP-dependent protein kinase: a model for an enzyme family. J Biol Chem 264:8443–8446
105. Ungerer M, Böhm M, Elce JS, Erdmann E, Lohse MJ (1993) Altered expression of β-adrenergic receptor kinase and β_1-adrenergic receptors in failing human heart. Circulation 87:454–463
106. Ungerer M, Parruti G, Böhm M, Puzicha M, DeBlasi A, Erdmann E, Lohse MJ (1994) Expression of β-arrestins and β-adrenergic receptor kinases in the failing human heart. Circ Res 74:206–213
107. Wahr P, Michele D, Metzger JM (1999) Parvalbumin gene transfer corrects diastolic dysfunction in diseased cardiac myocytes. PNAS 96:11982–11985
108. Zarain-Herzberg A, MacLennan D, Periasamy M (1990) Characterization of rabbit cardiac sarco(endo)plasmic reticulum Ca^{2+}-ATPase gene. J Biol Chem 265:4670–4677

CHAPTER 2

Cardiac overexpression of β-adrenergic receptors

M. J. LOHSE, S. ENGELHARDT
Institute for Pharmacology, University of Würzburg, Würzburg, Germany

Summary

The ability to increase cardiac frequency and contractility is essentially dependent on the stimulation of cardiac β-adrenergic receptors. These receptors are mostly of the β_1-subtype, while the β_2-subtype constitutes only a small fraction. Both receptors are coupled to an increase in the production of cAMP and increased opening of calcium channels. Thus, the consequences of their acute stimulation are similar.

Transgenic models with heart-specific overexpression have been generated for both receptor subtypes. The characterization of these mice has shown marked differences in the respective phenotypes. Overexpression of the β_2-subtype revealed very significant constitutive activity of these receptors, as evident from an increase in basal heart rate and contractility. These effects appeared to be sustained at least for the time periods of investigation. In contrast, the overexpression of the β_1-subtype resulted in only a short-lived improvement of contractility, which was only seen when the receptors were stimulated. There was very little change in basal heart rate, suggesting a low constitutive activity of this receptor subtype. From four months of age onwards, cardiac function and structure deteriorated. Histologically, there was marked myocyte hypertrophy and fibrosis; macroscopically, only minimal hypertrophy was visible. Cardiac catheterization revealed a progressive loss of contractility, which at an age of nine months was reduced by about 50%. In vivo NMR imaging also indicated a massive reduction of the ejection fraction, which was only about 20% at nine months of age, compared to about 60% in wild-type control mice.

Thus, the data available so far suggest strikingly dissimilar phenotypes resulting from the heart-specific overexpression of the two β-adrenergic receptors. Further studies will have to show whether β_2-adrenergic receptor transgenic mice maintain their phenotype at an older age and – if so – will have to elucidate the biochemical basis of these discrepancies. And finally, the usefulness of the β_1-receptor overexpressing mice as a model for heart failure in human patients will have to be evaluated.

Adrenergic receptor pharmacology

Adrenaline and noradrenaline exert their effects via nine subtypes of adrenergic receptors. The development of the current concept of these receptors is depicted in Fig. 1. The first subdivision, introduced by Ahlquist in 1948 [1] was that between α- and β-subtypes; the α-subtype was responsible for mediating the contraction of smooth muscle whereas the β-subtype was mediating the opposite effect, i.e., relaxation of smooth muscle. About 20 years later it became evident that both of these subtypes were heterogeneous. First, Lands et al. [26] discovered pharmacological differences between β-adrenergic receptors in the heart, which mediate positive chronotropic and inotropic effects, and smooth muscle, which cause relaxation. They found that noradrenaline preferentially stimulated the cardiac β-receptors, whereas adrenaline was equipotent in both tissues. Consequently, they named the cardiac receptor subtype β_1 and the smooth muscle subtype β_2.

A few years later, the laboratories of Langer and Starke introduced a subdivision of α-adrenergic receptors which was based on the functional effects of a series of agonists and antagonists on synaptic function. Differences between the effects of compounds on presynaptic function (neurotransmitter release) and postsynaptic function (smooth muscle contraction) led them to name the post-synaptic receptors α_1 and the presynaptic α_2 [46].

Even though further pharmacological studies had already provided hints that there must be further subdivisions, the most significant progress was made by molecular cloning techniques, which entered the field in 1986 with the cloning of the cDNA of the β_2-adrenergic receptor [13]. In the following years, a total of nine distinct cDNAs for adrenergic receptors were isolated which code for three α_1, three α_2 and three β-receptor subtypes (Fig. 1). While these can be clearly distinguished on the basis of their primary sequence, tools for a pharmacological and biochemical distinction are only slowly emerging. Thus, ligands previously thought to be specific for a subtype family have proved to also interact with subtypes of another

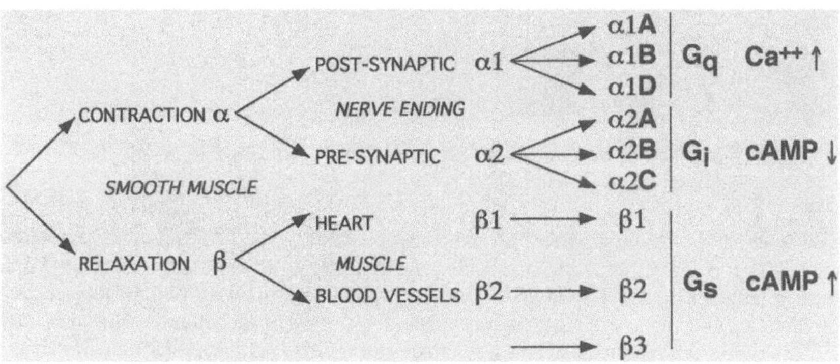

Fig. 1. Adrenergic receptors and their main signaling and effector systems..

family; for example, the classical α_1-receptor antagonist prazosin was found to also have relatively high affinity for the α_{2B}- and α_{2C}-receptor subtypes. Furthermore, the subtype-specific tissue localization is still under investigation, and while a few functions have been unequivocally assigned to defined receptor subtypes, many other effects still need such identification.

Biochemically, the signaling mechanisms for each of the three subfamilies appear to be the same. Coupling occurs to the $G_{q/11}$ family of G-proteins for the α_1-receptors, resulting in activation of phospholipase with subsequent increases in cytosolic free calcium concentrations and activation of protein kinase C. The α_2-receptors couple to the $G_{i/o}$ family of G-proteins, which mediate inhibition of cAMP production (resulting in a reduced activity of protein kinase A) as well as increased opening of K^+ channels (resulting in hyperpolarization). Finally, the β-receptors all couple to G_s-proteins and thereby cause increased cAMP production as well as increased opening of Ca^{++} channels.

Like most other G-protein-coupled receptors, adrenergic receptors are subject to a variety of regulatory mechanisms which can affect both the expression and the function of the receptor proteins. It appears that several of these regulatory mechanisms occur in a subtype-specific manner. This is, for example, quite pronounced for the most important mechanism mediating rapid agonist-dependent desensitization of such receptors, the

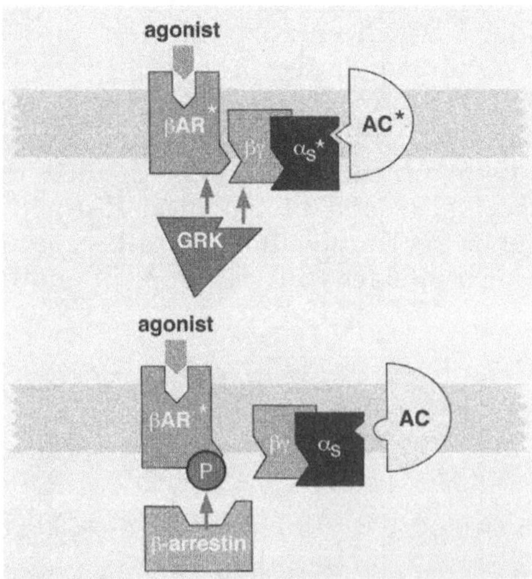

Fig. 2. Schematic of the mechanism of homologous desensitization by G-protein-coupled receptor kinases (GRKs) and β-arrestins. Agonist activated β-adrenergic receptors cause activation of the G-protein G_s and its effector, adenylyl cyclase (AC). This activation also provides two anchoring points for the cytosolic GRKs, i.e., the active receptor and dissociated G-protein $\beta\gamma$-subunits. GRKs phosphorylate serine/threonine residues in the receptor's C-terminus and thereby generate a binding site for the inhibitor protein β-arrestin. β-Arrestin binding to the receptors physically uncouples the receptor from G_s and also appears to provide an adaptor for clathrin, thereby initiating receptor internalisation.

inhibition of receptor function by G-protein-coupled receptor kinases (GRKs) and β-arrestins (Fig. 2). This mechanism is thought to proceed in two steps: first, agonist-occupied, active receptors are phosphorylated by the GRKs; second, β-arrestins bind to the phosphorylated receptors and thereby uncouple them from their G-proteins [32, 33]. Thus, this process which can occur with a half-life of a few seconds [42] results in the formation of signaling-incompetent receptors. Among the subtypes of the β-adrenergic receptor family, it appears that the β_2-subtype is most sensitive to homologous desensitization, whereas the β_1-subtype is less sensitive, and the β_3-subtype essentially resistant [37].

Cardiac β-adrenergic receptors

In most species, the heart contains β-adrenergic receptors with a clear ($\approx$70–80%) predominance of the β_1-subtype (reviewed in [8]). Most of the remainder appear to be of the β_2-subtype. Both subtypes are coupled to G_s-proteins, and the main consequence of their stimulation is an increased production of cAMP. There are also data suggesting the presence of β_3-receptors in the heart of some – including humans – but not all species [21]. These β_3-receptors result in activation of NO synthase and thereby appear to cause negative inotropic effects [20]. However, others have failed to detect the mRNA of the β_3-subtype in the human heart, or have attributed it to periatrial fat rather than cardiomyocytes [47]; furthermore, Harding et al. [22] and Molenaar et al. [36] failed to see negative inotropic effects of the β_3-receptor agonist BRL 37344 in isolated myocytes or atrial and ventricular tissue. A fourth subtype, termed β_4, has been postulated on the basis of functional data showing positive inotropic effects of β-adrenergic receptor antagonists [24], but the distinct molecular nature of this hypothetical new adrenergic receptor subtype remains to be proven.

Cardiac β-adrenergic receptors are the main physiological switch to increase the frequency, electrical conductance, contractile force and speed of relaxation of the heart. Again, these functional effects are mainly mediated via the predominant β_1-subtype. The signaling events responsible for these effects include an increased opening probability of cardiac Ca channels and improved Ca storage in the sarcoplasmic reticulum due to phosphorylation of phospholamban, the regulator of the sarcoplasmic Ca pump.

The ability of β-adrenergic receptors to mediate these effects is subject to a variety of control mechanisms. These correspond to the biochemical mechanisms of receptor regulation mentioned above.

In the context of the cardiac β-adrenergic receptor system there appear to be two predominant regulatory mechanisms:

- decreased receptor function caused by GRK/β-arrestin-mediated desensitization, and
- downregulation of the receptors mainly due to a decrease in the corresponding mRNA.

Chronic heart failure appears to trigger both of these mechanisms, and it may do so essentially via the increased activity of the sympathetic nervous system which is a hallmark of this disease. The increased concentrations of noradrenaline and adrenaline initiate the desensitization mechanisms that have been studied in much detail in isolated cell systems. Downregulation of β-adrenergic receptors in chronic heart failure was first observed by Bristow et al. [5]. It appears to affect predominantly the β_1-subtype which is reduced by about 50% in severe heart failure; some but not all studies have also found smaller reductions in β_2-subtype levels (reviewed in [7]). The reductions in receptor levels are paralleled by similar reductions in the corresponding mRNA levels; again, these are essentially restricted to the β_1-subtype where they amount to about 50% in patients with end-stage heart disease [6, 48]. In a study of biopsies taken from patients with different degrees of heart failure, there was a good correlation between the severity of the disease and the loss of β_1-adrenergic receptor mRNA [16]. Mechanistically, although this has only been shown for isolated cells and not in the heart, the reason for this reduction is likely to be a cAMP-dependent reduced transcription of the corresponding gene [23].

The second change induced in chronic heart failure is an increased expression and activity of G-protein-coupled receptor kinases, the GRKs (reviewed in [31]). Depending on the experimental or clinical situation, the subtype of GRK affected may vary. In human heart failure [48, 49] as well as the development of heart failure in pigs [39, 40], the kinase most elevated is GRK2. It is reasonable to assume that such increased activity of GRKs is involved in reduced contractile function, since in transgenic models overexpression of GRK2 [25] or GRK5 [42] results in impaired contractility.

β_2-Adrenergic receptor overexpression

Overexpression of the β_2-adrenergic receptor subtype in the heart has been achieved in transgenic mice, where the receptor was expressed under the control of the α-myosin heavy chain (α-MHC) promoter. The line used for most studies shows approximately a 200-fold overexpression of ventricular β_2-receptors. In these mice, the basal production of cAMP in cardiac membranes was enhanced to levels seen in wild-type membranes after maximal stimulation with isoprenaline, and an increased left ventricular contractility was observed *in vivo* [35]. Interestingly basal adenylyl cyclase activity and spontaneous beating frequency of isolated right atria showed marked increases in the absence of agonist, thereby supporting the concept of spontaneous, constitutive activity of β_2-adrenergic receptors [4]. This two-state model assumes the existence of two distinct conformational states of G-protein-coupled receptors: an inactive state (R) and an active state (R*) which is able to activate G-proteins. In the absence of agonist, an equilibrium between R and R* is postulated, with a proportion of the receptors being spontaneously in the active conformation and thus initiate downstream signaling in an agonist-free environment. Binding of an agonist shifts this equilibrium to the active conformation while neutral antagonists preserve the "basal" equilibrium and prevent solely the shift towards the active R* conformation by agonists. With this concept, a third class of ligands can be derived: inverse agonists which shift the equilibrium to the inactive R state and thus decrease spontaneous signaling of the receptor. Such inverse agonist effects have been demonstrated using the β_2-adrenergic receptor overexpressing mouse model [4]. The enhanced basal activation of adenylyl cyclase and contractility seen in this animal model could be blocked by ICI-188551, whereas alprenolol did not change the basal activity and thus behaved as a pure (neutral) antagonist. This behavior is very similar to the data obtained in isolated cells expressing wild-type or constitutively active mutants of the β_2-adrenergic receptor [11, 44, 45]. The concept of spontaneous constitutive activity of receptors and, hence, of inverse agonism, has also been validated for other receptors, but it is still a matter of debate whether there is also constitutive activity and inverse agonism at the β_1-adrenergic receptor [27].

Interestingly, stimulation of the overexpressed β_2-adrenergic receptors with agonists did not produce a marked response above the elevated "basal" levels. This lack of responsiveness may in part be due to a saturation of the downstream signaling chain. In addition, β_2-adrenergic receptors have been shown to be capable of coupling efficiently to inhibitory G_i-proteins [9, 29]. Such G_i-coupling has more recently also been demonstrated for β_2-adrenergic receptors in murine cardiomyocytes [50]. In the β_2-receptor transgenic mice, pertussis toxin treatment significantly enhanced agonist-stimulated adenylyl cyclase activity as well as contractility; this would be compatible with the concept that the overexpressed β_2-adrenergic receptors caused significant stimulation of G_i and that this obscured the stimulation of G_s [51]. Whether coupling of β_2-adrenergic receptors to G_i is also relevant at the much lower levels physiologically present in the heart remains to be shown.

Mice overexpressing β_2-adrenergic receptors had not only increased contractility but also markedly enhanced relaxation; this was associated with a decrease of myocardial phospholamban [41]. This is reminiscent of data obtained in mice with a deletion of the phospholamban gene, which showed more rapid calcium uptake into the sarcoplasmic reticulum and enhanced relaxation kinetics [34].

Because of the enhanced inotropy of hearts from β_2-adrenergic receptor transgenic mice, gene therapy with β_2-adrenergic receptors has been proposed [35]. Adenoviral gene transfer of β_2-adrenergic receptors indeed restored contractility of cardiomyocytes from failing hearts of rabbits [2, 15]. However, due to the short expression period achieved so far by adenoviral mediated transfection, these experiments were necessarily restricted to short-term effects. A recent study in β_2-adrenergic receptor transgenic mice found however increased susceptibility to ischemic injury in these animals [12]. This adverse effect was again seen in the mice with ≈200-fold overexpression of these receptors, and it is yet to be determined whether more moderate overexpression would have different effects, as seen in the rescue of the $G_{\alpha q}$ model by Dorn and coworkers [14].

β_1-Adrenergic receptor overexpression

The first successful attempt to overexpress β_1-adrenergic receptors in the heart was reported by Bertin et al. in 1993 [3]. Using the promoter of the human atrial natriuretic factor to direct the expression of the transgenic receptor in mouse heart, these authors achieved a 5 to 10-fold overexpression which was essentially restricted to the atria. The functional consequences of this restricted overexpression were very small.

In analogy to the approach used for the β_2-subtype, two groups subsequently used the α-MHC promoter to overexpress β_1-adrenergic receptors in the mouse heart [17, 38]. The phenotype of mice with ≈15-fold overexpression in the ventricles as measured with radioligand binding at eight weeks of age [18] differs in many respects from that described above for the β_2-subtype. At young age (<4 months), these animals display cardiac function similar to those expected from acute stimulation of cardiac β-adrenergic receptors: *in vivo* frequency, contractility and relaxation were all significantly increased. *In vitro*, the frequency of isolated right atria was only very slightly increased; this is in good agreement with the very low constitutive activity of the β_1-subtype mentioned above [27]. However, the responsiveness of isolated right atria to isoprenaline was markedly increased in transgenic animals, and the extent of this increase correlated with the extent of receptor overexpression [18].

However, at higher age these positive changes disappeared and were replaced by marked functional and structural deficits. Thus, the contractility measured by left ventricular catheterization showed a progressive decline and was only ≈50% of that seen in wild-type animals at nine months of age [18]. At this point, the ejection fraction as seen by imaging NMR was reduced to about 20%, whereas it was about 65% in control wild-type animals, confirming severe left-ventricular systolic dysfunction. At four months of age, left ventricular contractility appeared to be similar to that of wild-type animals under basal conditions. However, in the presence of propranolol (to block endogenous as well as overexpressed β-receptors), a marked contractile deficit became visible. This contractile deficit was apparently masked by the increased β-adrenergic signaling resulting from the overexpression of the receptors.

The most pronounced alterations in the β_1-receptor transgenic were of a structural kind. First, there was marked hypertrophy of the cardiomyocytes in the transgenic mice. Figure 3a shows the average cross-sectional areas of wild-type vs. transgenic mice as a function of age. While these areas increased by about 3-fold in wild-type mice from neonatal to 20 weeks, there was a 8-fold increase in the transgenic mice. In spite of the marked hypertrophy at the level of individual cardiomyocyte, there was virtually no hypertrophy of the heart as a whole, suggesting that the number of cells must have decreased. At higher age, there was also marked fibrosis which could be seen throughout the transgenic hearts (see Fig. 3b).

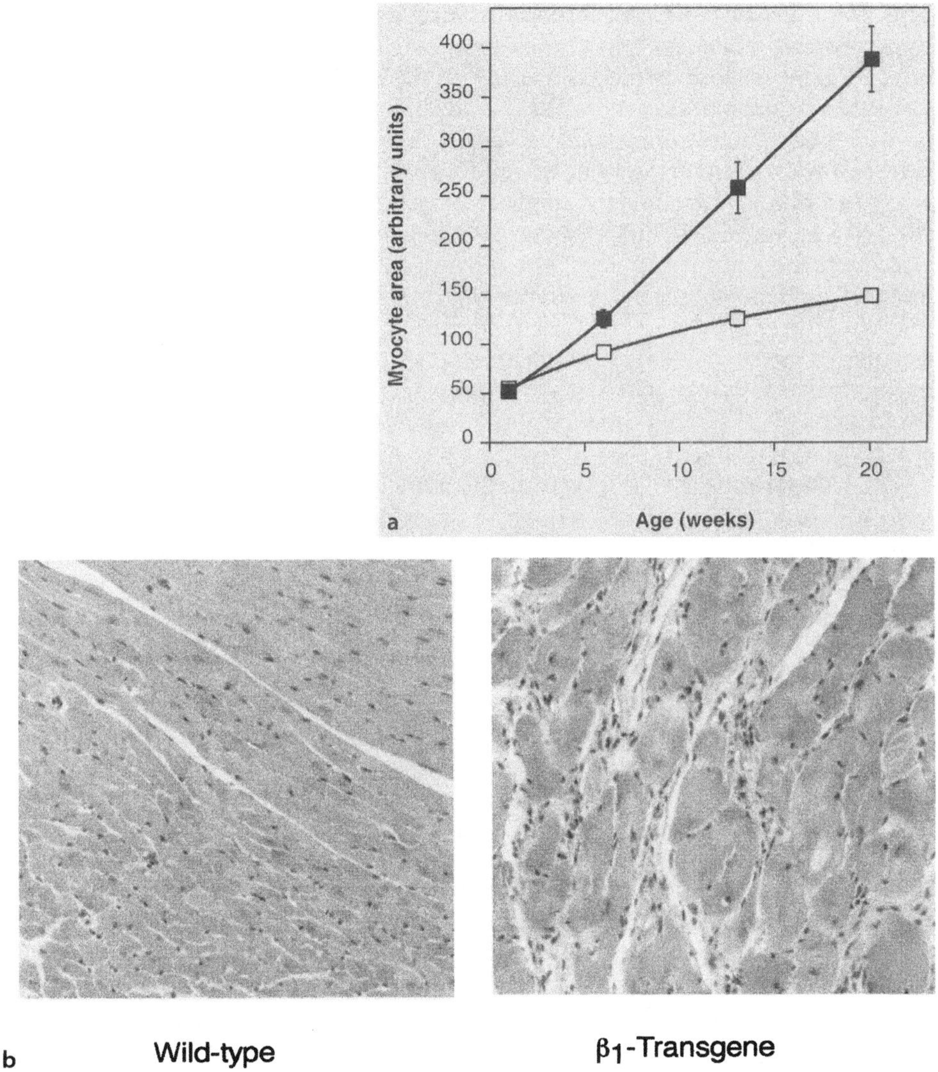

Fig. 3. Histological alterations in mouse hearts overexpressing β_1-adrenergic receptors. **a** The average cardiomyocyte cross-sectional areas (in arbitrary pixel units) of wild-type (open symbols) and β_1-receptor transgenic mice as a function of age are shown. **b** Representative sections from 20-week old wild-type (left) and transgenic (right) hearts are shown.

Differences between cardiac β_1- and β_2-adrenergic receptor overexpression

Comparing the phenotypes of β_1- and β_2-overexpressing mice, striking differences become apparent. While 200-fold overexpression of the β_2-adrenergic receptor did not induce detrimental myocardial changes [35, 51], overexpression of the β_1-adrenergic receptor at relatively low levels (15-fold at young age) led to progressive hypertrophy, fibrosis and heart failure [18]. This phenotypical difference is further underlined by the rescue of a hypertrophic phenotype in $G_{\alpha q}$-overexpressing mice by mating them to β_2-adrenergic receptor transgenic mice [14]. In this model, however, higher (140-fold) overexpression of the β_2-adrenergic receptor was clearly detrimental [14]. Detrimental effects for high β_2-overexpression were also reported in a different murine heart failure model [19]. While it is not clear what the precise mechanism of the rescue effect is, it appears to be plausible that enhanced β_2-signaling via G_i-proteins might be involved. In line with this are recent data that not only show that apoptotic signaling by β-adrenergic receptors occurs exclusively via the β_1-subtype but can also be inhibited by G_i-protein-mediated β_2-stimulation [10]. Whereas these experiments were not carried out *in vivo*, but in hypoxic neonatal cardiomyocytes, this novel mechanism might also be involved in the prominent phenotypical difference between β_1- and β_2-adrenergic receptor transgenic mice.

As a consequence, we interpret the loss of β_1-adrenergic receptor number and function in heart failure as a protective mechanism, which may acutely decrease cardiac performance in response to demand, but which may in the long term help to preserve cardiac function. Similarly, it appears for the same reasons that the upregulation of GRKs in heart failure might be beneficial. Both of these may reduce the danger of structural damage to the heart that would otherwise result from chronic stimulation of β_1-adrenergic receptors.

The changes seen in the β_1-adrenergic receptor overexpressing mice as well as their protracted time-course appear to make these mice a suitable model for the study of heart failure in human patients. However, further studies will have to show whether, in addition to the reported functional and structural deficits, other hallmarks of failure in patients are also reproduced in this model. Furthermore, it remains to be seen whether therapeutic strategies successful in patients will also work in this animal model.

These data suggest that in spite of their very similar acute effects, cardiac β_1- and β_2-adrenergic receptors produce quite different responses upon chronic stimulation. These differences in long-term responses may be the "reason" why cardiomyocytes express two seemingly quite similar isoforms of these receptors. Future studies will have to show whether in the long term any type of overstimulation – via β_1- or β_2-receptors – turns out to be detrimental, as suggested by some [30], or whether indeed there is hope that selective β_2-adrenergic signaling might be beneficial in heart failure.

At any rate these studies show that, in spite of the wealth of knowledge about cardiac β-adrenergic receptors, we are still far from really understanding this system and that a plausible explanation of the mechanism of action of β-adrenergic receptor antagonists in heart failure is still missing.

Acknowledgments. These studies were supported by grants from the Deutsche Forschungsgemeinschaft - SFB 355, the European Commission and the Fonds der Chemischen Industrie.

References

1. Ahlquist RP (1948) A study of adrenotropic receptors. Am J Physiol 153:586-600
2. Akhter SA, Skaer CA, Kypson AP, McDonald PH, Peppel KC, Glower DD, Lefkowitz RJ, Koch WJ (1997) Restoration of β-adrenergic signaling in failing cardiac ventricular myocytes via adenoviral-mediated gene transfer. Proc Natl Acad Sci USA 94:12100-12105
3. Bertin B, Mansier P, Makeh I, Briand P, Rostene W, Swynghedauw B, Strosberg AD (1993) Specific atrial overexpression of G protein coupled human β_1 adrenoceptors in transgenic mice. Cardiovasc Res 27:1606-1612
4. Bond RA, Leff P, Johnson TD, Milano CA, Rockman HA, McMinn TR, Apparsundaram S, Hyek MF, Kenakin TP, Allen LF, Lefkowitz RJ (1995) Physiological effects of inverse agonists in transgenic mice with myocardial overexpression of the β_2-adrenoceptor. Nature 374:272-276
5. Bristow MR, Ginsburg R, Minobe W, Cubiciotti RS, Sageman WS, Lurie K, Billingham ME, Harrison DE, Stinson EB (1982) Decreased catecholamine sensitivity and β-adrenergic receptor density in failing human hearts. N Engl J Med 307: 205-211
6. Bristow MR, Minobe WA, Raynolds MV, Port JD, Rasmussen R, Ray PE, Feldman AM (1993) Reduced β_1 receptor messenger RNA abundance in the failing human heart. J Clin Invest 92:2737-2745
7. Brodde O-E (1993) Beta-adrenoceptors in cardiac disease. Pharmac Ther 60:405-430
8. Brodde O-E, Michel MC (1999) Adrenergic and muscarinic receptors in the human heart. Pharmacol Rev 51:651-689
9. Cerione RA, Staniszewski C, Caron MG, Lefkowitz RJ, Codina J, Birnbaumer L (1985) A role for Ni in the hormonal stimulation of adenylate cyclase. Nature 318:293-295
10. Chesley A, Ohtani S, Asai T, Lundberg M, Xiao RP, Lakatta EG, Crow M (1999) A pertussis toxin-sensitive signalling pathway linked to β_2-adrenergic receptor stimulation blocks apoptosis in hypoxic neonatal cardiomyocytes. Circulation 100:1-64
11. Chidiac P, Hebert TE, Valiquette M, Dennis M, Bouvier M (1994) Inverse agonist activity of beta-adrenergic antagonists. Mol Pharmacol 45:490-499
12. Cross HR, Steenbergen C, Lefkowitz RJ, Koch WJ, Murphy E (1999) Overexpression of the cardiac β_2-adrenergic receptor and expression of a β-adrenergic receptor kinase-1 (βARK1) inhibitor both increase myocardial contractility but have differential effects on susceptibility to ischemic injury. Circ Res 85:1215-1223
13. Dixon RAF, Kobilka BK, Strader DJ, Benovic JL, Dohlman HG, Frielle T, Bolanowski MA, Bennett CD, Rands E, Diehl RE, Mumford RA, Slater EE, Sigal ES, Caron MG, Lefkowitz RJ, Strader CD (1986) Cloning of the gene and cDNA for mammalian β-adrenergic receptor and homology with rhodopsin. Nature 321:75-79

14. Dorn GW, Tepe NM, Lorenz JN, Koch WJ, Liggett SB (1999) Low- and high-level transgenic expression of β_2-adrenergic receptors differentially affect cardiac hypertrophy and function in $G_{\alpha q}$-overexpressing mice. Proc Natl Acad USA 96:6400–6405
15. Drazner MH, Peppel KC, Dyer S, Grant AO, Koch WJ, Lefkowitz RJ (1997) Potentiation of β-adrenergic signalling by adenoviral-mediated gene transfer in adult rabbit ventricular myocytes. J Clin Invest 99:288–296
16. Engelhardt S, Böhm M, Erdmann E, Lohse MJ (1996) Analysis of β-adrenergic receptor mRNA-levels in human ventricular biopsies by RT-PCR: progressive reduction of β_1-adrenergic receptor mRNA in heart failure. J Am Coll Cardiol 27:146–154
17. Engelhardt S, Hein L, Schmitteckert E, Lohse MJ (1998) Transgenic modification of receptor signalling in the mouse heart. Naunyn Schmiedeberg's Arch Pharmacol 357(Suppl):R103
18. Engelhardt S, Hein L, Wiesmann F, Lohse MJ (1999) Progressive hypertrophy and heart failure in β_1-adrenergic receptor transgenic mice. Proc Natl Acad Sci USA 96:7059–7064
19. Freeman K, Iaccarino G, Bohlmeyer T, Leinwand LA (1999) Overexpression of the β_2-adrenergic receptor accelerates heart failure in hypertrophic cardiomyopathy mice. Circulation 100:1–493
20. Gauthier C, Leblais V, Kobzik L, Trochu J-N, Khandoudi N, Bril A, Balligand J-L, Le Marec H (1998) The negative inotropic effect of β_3-adrenoceptor stimulation is mediated by activation of a nitric oxide pathway in human ventricle. J Clin Invest 102:1377–1384
21. Gauthier C, Tavernier G, Trochu J-N, Leblais V, Laurent K, Langin D, Escande D, Le Marec H (1999) Interspecies differences in the cardiac negative inotropic effects of β_3-adrenoceptor agonists. J Pharmacol Exp Ther 290:687–693
22. Harding SE (1997) Lack of evidence for β_3-adrenoceptor modulation of contractile function in human ventricular myocytes. Circulation 96(Suppl 1):1–53
23. Hosoda K, Feussner GK, Rydelek-Fitzgerald L, Fishman PH, Duman RS (1994) Agonist and cyclic AMP-mediated regulation of β_1-adrenergic receptor mRNA and gene transcription in rat C6 glioma cells. J Neurochem 63:1635–1645
24. Kaufmann AJ, Molenaar P (1997) Modulation of human cardiac function through 4 β-adrenoceptor populations. Naunyn-Schmiedeberg's Arch Pharmacol 355:667–681
25. Koch WJ, Rockman H, Samama P, Hamilton RA, Bond RA, Milano CA, Lefkowitz RJ (1995) Cardiac function in mice overexpressing the β-adrenergic receptor kinase or a βARK inhibitor. Science 268:1350–1353
26. Lands AM, Arnold A, McAuliff JP, Luduena FP, Brown TG (1967) Differentiation of receptor systems activated by sympathomimetic amines. Nature 214:597–598
27. Lattion A-L, Abuin L, Nenniger-Tosato M, Cotecchia S (1999) Constitutively active mutants of the β_1-adrenergic receptor. FEBS Lett 457:302–306
28. Lefkowitz RJ, Cotecchia S, Samama P, Costa T (1993) Constitutive activity of receptors coupled to guanine nucleotide regulatory proteins. Trends Pharmacol Sci 14:303–307
29. Liggett SB, Caron MG, Lefkowitz RJ, Hantowich M (1991) Coupling of a mutated form of the human β_2-adrenergic receptor to G_i and G_s. Requirement for multiple cytoplasmic domains in the coupling process. J Biol Chem 266:4816–4821
30. Limbird LE, Vaughan DE (1999) Augmenting β-receptors in the heart: short-term gains offset by long-term pains? Proc Natl Acad Sci USA 96:7125–7127
31. Lohse MJ (1995) G-protein coupled receptor kinases and the heart. Trends Cardiovasc Med 5:63–68

32. Lohse MJ, Benovic JL, Codina J, Caron MG, Lefkowitz RJ (1990) β-Arrestin: a protein that regulates β-adrenergic function. Science 248:1547–1550
33. Lohse MJ, Andexinger S, Pitcher J, Trukawinski S, Codina J, Faure J-P, Caron MG, Lefkowitz RJ (1992) Receptor-specific desensitization with purified proteins: kinase dependence and receptor-specificity of β-arrestin and arrestin in the β_2-adrenergic receptor and rhodopsin systems. J Biol Chem 267:8558–8564
34. Luo W, Grupp IL, Harrer J, Ponniah S, Grupp G, Duffy JJ, Doetschmann T, Kranias EG (1994) Targeted ablation of the phospholamban gene is associated with markedly enhanced myocardial contractility and loss of β-agonist stimulation. Circ Res 75:401–409
35. Milano CA, Allen LF, Rockman HA, Dolber PC, McMinn TR, Chien KR, Johnson TD, Bond RA, Lefkowitz RJ (1994) Enhanced myocardial function in transgenic mice overexpressing the β_2-adrenergic receptor. Science 264:582–586
36. Molenaar P, Sorsero D, Areh JRS, Kelly J, Henson SM, Kaumann AJ (1997) Effects of (-)-RO363 at human atrial β-adrenoceptor subtypes, the human cloned β_3-adrenoceptor and rodent intestinal β_3-adrenoceptors. Brit J Pharmacol 120:165–176
37. Nantel F, Bonin H, Emorine LJ, Zilberfarb V, Strosberg AD, Bouvier M, Marullo S (1993) The human β_3-adrenergic receptor is resistant to short term agonist-promoted desensitization. Mol Pharmacol 43:548–555
38. Port JD, Weinberger HD, Bisognano JD, Knudson OA, Bohlmeyer TJ, Pende A, Bristow MR (1998) Echocardiographic and histopathological characterization of young and old transgenic mice overexpressing the human β_1-adrenergic receptor. J Am Coll Cardiol 31(Suppl A):177A
39. Ping P, Gelzer-Bell R, Roth DA, Kiel D, Insel PA, Hammond HK (1995) Reduced β-adrenergic receptor activation decreases G-protein expression and β-adrenergic receptor kinase activity in porcine heart. J Clin Invest 95:1271–1280
40. Ping P, Anzai T, Gao M, Hammond HK (1997) Adenylyl cyclase and G protein receptor kinase expression during development of heart failure. Am J Physiol 273:H707–H717
41. Rockman HA, Hamilton RA, Jones LR, Milano CA, Mao L, Lefkowitz RJ (1996) Enhanced myocardial relaxation in vivo in transgenic mice overexpressing the β_2-adrenergic receptor is associated with reduced phospholamban protein. J Clin Invest 97:1618–1623
42. Rockman HA, Choi DJ, Rahman NU, Akhter SA, Lefkowitz RJ, Koch WJ (1998) Receptor-specific *in vivo* desensitization by the G protein-coupled receptor kinase-5 in transgenic mice. Proc Natl Acad Sci USA 93:9954–9959
43. Roth N, Campbell PT, Caron MG, Lefkowitz RJ, Lohse MJ (1991) Comparative rates of desensitization of β-adrenergic receptors by the β-adrenergic receptor kinase and the cyclic AMP-dependent protein kinase. Proc Natl Acad Sci USA 88:6201–6204
44. Samama P, Cotecchia S, Costa T, Lefkowitz RJ (1993) A mutation-induced activated state of the β_2-adrenergic receptor. Extending the ternary complex model. J Biol Chem 268:4625–4636
45. Samama P, Pei G, Costa T, Cotecchia S, Lefkowitz RJ (1994) Negative antagonists promote an inactive conformation of the β_2-adrenergic receptor. Mol Pharmacol 45:390–394
46. Starke K (1987) Presynaptic α-autoreceptors. Rev Physiol Biochem Pharmacol 107:73–146
47. Strosberg AD (1997) Structure and function of the β_3-adrenergic receptor. Annu Rev Pharmacol Toxicol 37:421–450
48. Ungerer M, Böhm M, Elce JS, Erdmann E, Lohse MJ (1993) Altered expression of β-adrenergic receptor kinase (βARK) and β_1-adrenergic receptors in the failing human heart. Circulation 87:454–463

49. Ungerer M, Parruti G, Böhm M, Puzicha M, DeBlasi A, Erdmann E, Lohse MJ (1994) Expression of β-arrestins and β-adrenergic receptor kinases in the failing human heart. Circ Res 74:206–213
50. Xiao RP, Ji X, Lakatta EG (1995) Functional coupling of the β_2-adrenoceptor to a pertussis toxin-sensitive G protein in cardiac myocytes. Mol Pharmacol 47:322–329
51. Xiao RP, Avdonin P, Zhou YY, Cheng H, Akther SA, Eschenhagen T, Lefkowitz RJ, Koch WJ, Lakatta EG (1999) Coupling of β_2-adrenoceptor to G_i proteins and its physiological relevance in murine cardiac myocytes. Circ Res 73:286–300

CHAPTER 3

Genetic approaches to elucidate the regulatory role of phospholamban in the heart

A. G. SCHMIDT, E. G. KRANIAS

Department of Pharmacology and Cell Biophysics, University of Cincinnati, College of Medicine, Cincinnati, Ohio, USA

Introduction

In end-stage heart failure, several molecular, biochemical and functional alterations have been described to occur at the cellular level [11, 32]. Evidence indicates that disturbed excitation-contraction coupling processes may underlie disturbed myocardial function in various animal models and human conditions [3, 34]. Specifically, Ca^{2+} uptake and release by the sarcoplasmic reticulum (SR) have been shown to be altered, and the ratio of phospholamban/SR Ca^{2+} ATPase has been suggested to play a key role in the pathophysiology of heart failure [10]. Thus, it becomes important to dissect the molecular mechanisms governing the highly regulated excitation-contraction coupling process and their alterations in heart failure in order to develop new therapeutic approaches for this disease.

The contraction-relaxation cycle in the heart is controlled by the sequential rise and fall of cytosolic Ca^{2+} concentration [2]. Physiological studies at the cellular and subcellular levels have helped to characterize the molecular machinery involved in coupling of electrical excitation of the cell membrane to cardiac contraction and subsequent relaxation of the myofilaments. Ca^{2+} entry into the cell occurs upon cell membrane depolarization via L-type voltage-gated Ca^{2+} channels. This rapid Ca^{2+} influx triggers the release of a much larger amount of activator-Ca^{2+} from the sarcoplasmic reticulum (SR) via the release channels (ryanodine receptors) [8]. Ca^{2+} then binds to troponin C and induces conformational changes, which subsequently allow the globular head of myosin to interact with the actin binding site of the thin filament, resulting in contraction. Relaxation results from the rapid removal of cytosolic Ca^{2+}, which is predominantly resequestered into the SR lumen by the SR Ca^{2+} ATPase. The process of active Ca^{2+} re-uptake by the SR Ca^{2+} ATPase is under reversible regulation by phospholamban, a low molecular weight integral SR membrane phosphoprotein. Dephosphorylated phospholamban is an inhibitor of the apparent affinity of SR Ca^{2+} ATPase for Ca^{2+}, while phosphorylation of phospholamban by protein kinases relieves this inhibition [15]. Perturbations of this finely tuned Ca^{2+} homeostasis are associated with alterations in calcium transients and contractile dysfunction, which are characteristics of heart failure [33].

Extensive *in vitro* studies have shown that phospholamban is a pentamer, composed of 6000 Da subunits, and is located in the sarcoplasmic reticulum of cardiac, slow-twitch skeletal and smooth muscles. Phospholamban is a single copy gene and there are currently no isoforms of phospholamban known. It contains 52 amino acids which are organized into two main domains: domain I is hydrophilic and constitutes the cytoplasmic sector (amino acid residues 1–30), whereas domain II contains the hydrophobic membrane spanning part of the protein (amino acid residues 31–52) [29]. Domain I can be further subdivided into two motifs: domain Ia (residues 1–20), which has been suggested to form an α-helical structure, and domain Ib (residues 21–30), which is likely to exist as a random coil. The transmembrane domain II has also been proposed to have an α-helical structure, which may stabilize the phospholamban pentamer and is capable of modifying the apparent Ca^{2+} affinity of the SR Ca^{2+} ATPase in co-expression studies [36]. Phospholamban can be phosphorylated at distinct sites in domain Ia by different protein kinases: serine 10 by protein kinase C, serine 16 by cAMP-dependent protein kinase and threonine 17 by Ca^{2+}-calmodulin-dependent kinases [29]. Each phosphorylation is associated with stimulation of SR Ca^{2+} transport. Beyond these *in vitro* studies, experiments in intact systems demonstrate that phospholamban is a key regulator of basal contractility and β-adrenergic stimulatory effects [22]. However, until recently, little was known about the functional significance of phospholamban *in vivo*. The development of genetic techniques to modify a specific gene product, and the ability to characterize the functional consequences of such manipulations, greatly improved our understanding of the mechanisms and cellular players regulating contractility under physiological and pathophysiological conditions [16]. This manuscript summarizes recent genetic approaches, undertaken in our laboratory and others, to elucidate the functional properties and physiological role of phospholamban *in vivo*.

The relative phospholamban/SERCA ratio is a critical determinant of myocardial contractility

This section centers on the hypothesis that phospholamban is an important regulator of the basal cardiac contraction-relaxation cycle. Genetically engineered models with diagonally opposed levels of phospholamban have demonstrated the power of using loss-of function and gain-of function approaches in defining the physiological role of this single gene product *in vivo* [17, 27]. Further studies in murine atrial and ventricular myocardia have shown a close correlation between the different expression levels of phospholamban and contractile parameters [13, 20, 21]. Besides cardiac muscle, phospholamban is also present in smooth and slow-twitch skeletal muscle, and recent results suggest that phospholamban is a regulator of contractility in both of these muscles [23, 38]. Taken together, the following data

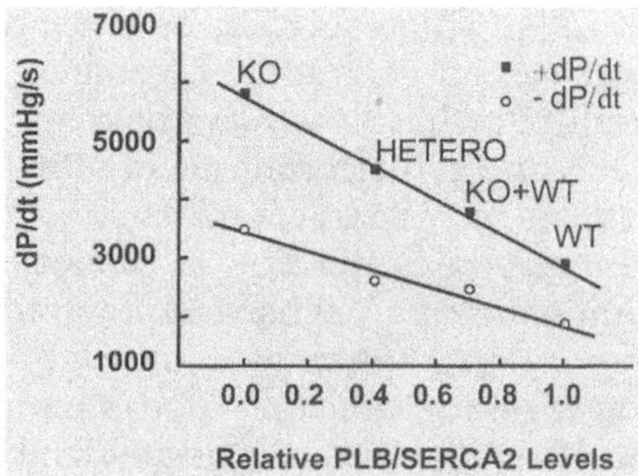

Fig. 1. Effects of phospholamban/SERCA on cardiac contractility. The relative levels of phospholamban/SERCA correlate closely with the rates of contraction (+dP/dt) and relaxation (–dP/dt) in Langendorff-perfused hearts. Wild-type control (WT), phospholamban knockout (PLB-KO), PLB heterozygotes (HETERO), and transgenic mice expressing wild-type PLB in the knock-out background (KO+WT).

suggest that the relative levels of phospholamban:SERCA2 have a determinant function as to the muscle's overall contractility status (Fig. 1) [20].

Phospholamban ablation and cardiac function

In the first model, the murine phospholamban gene was ablated by homologous recombination technology [27]. The endogenous murine phospholamban-coding region was replaced by the neomycin phosphoribosyl transferase (neo) gene, using gene targeting. Ablation of phospholamban was compatible with life in homozygous mice and at the morphological and histological levels, these mice were indistinguishable from their wild-type littermates. Biochemical studies indicated that the affinity of the SR Ca^{2+} ATPase for Ca^{2+} was significantly increased in the phospholamban knockout heart compared to wild-type controls. Physiological measurements in isolated cardiac myocytes revealed enhanced myocyte mechanics (extent of myocyte shortening, rates of shortening and relengthening) and parallel increases in amplitude and kinetics of rising and falling phases of Ca^{2+} transients [24, 41]. The phospholamban-deficient myocytes also exhibited a higher SR Ca^{2+} load (37%) and a reduced Na^+/Ca^{2+} exchange activity [24, 35]. Assessment of the subcellular properties of the Ca^{2+} transients in phospholamban-deficient mice indicated that the spontaneous Ca^{2+} sparks (elementary release events) were three times more frequent and larger than in ventricular cells from wild-type controls [35]. L-type Ca^{2+} channel currents were significantly larger in phospholamban knock-out cells [30, 35]. The fast Ca^{2+}-dependent inactivation component of the L-type channel was also increased, supporting the hypothesis that Ca^{2+} released from the SR regulates Ca^{2+} channel inactivation, by affecting the levels of Ca^{2+} near the channel [30]. The hyperdynamic contractile function of the phospholamban knock-out cardiomyocytes was also observed at the intact organ level, using work-performing heart preparations under identical preload, afterload and heart rate [27]. Again, the rates of contraction and relaxation were significantly increased in the phospholamban knock-out hearts compared to wild types. These findings could also be confirmed in the intact animal, using left ventricular catheter techniques and echocardiography

[12, 25]. Thus, ablation of phospholamban was associated with significant increases in contractile parameters at the cellular, organ, and intact animal levels. Furthermore, isoproterenol stimulation was associated with attenuated contractile responses in either isolated myocytes [41], hearts or intact animals [12, 25]. It is interesting to note that this attenuation of β-agonist stimulation is not due to alterations in the β-adrenergic signal transduction pathway (unchanged β-adrenergic receptor density, adenylyl cyclase activity, and tissue cAMP levels) or the degree of basal phosphorylation of key cardiac regulatory phosphoproteins of the cardiomyocyte [19]. These results indicate that phospholamban is a major regulator of contractility and the β-agonist response in the mammalian heart.

Cardiac specific overexpression of phospholamban

From the phospholamban knock-out studies, the stoichiometric ratio of phospholamban:SR Ca^{2+} ATPase appeared to be a critical determinant of the regulation of the cardiac contraction-relaxation cycle. However, it was not clear whether all the Ca^{2+} pumps in cardiac SR membranes are subject to regulation by phospholamban. In order to determine whether there exist "spare" SR Ca^{2+} pumps, transgenic mice overexpressing phospholamban were generated, using the cardiac specific α-myosin heavy chain promoter [17]. Hearts from transgenic animals and wild-type littermates were analyzed in parallel at the molecular, biochemical and physiological levels. Transgenic mice overexpressing twofold higher levels of phospholamban in the heart showed no morphological abnormalities and no alterations in heart/body weight, heart/lung weight, and cardiomyocyte size remained unchanged compared to their wild-type littermates. However, isolated cardiomyocytes from transgenic animals exhibited a diminished shortening fraction and decreased rates of shortening and relengthening compared with wild-types. The amplitude of the Ca^{2+} signal was decreased and the rate of decay of the Ca^{2+} transient in Fura-2 loaded transgenic myocytes was significantly prolonged, consistent with the decreased Ca^{2+} affinity of the SR Ca^{2+} ATPase for Ca^{2+}. Again, these findings were consistent with depressed contractile parameters at the intact organ and whole animal levels. However, the observed differences in contractile parameters, Ca^{2+} kinetics and depressed left ventricular function *in vivo* were abolished upon isoproterenol stimulation [17, 25]. These results suggest that, in native SR, there exists a fraction of SR Ca^{2+} ATPase molecules which are not subject to regulation by phospholamban.

Previous studies have demonstrated that a) the variation of heart rate is a powerful modulator of cardiac contractility and myocardial function in the anesthetized mouse (force-frequency relation) and b) the biphasic force-frequency relation in the mouse can be characterized by the heart rate at which the peak rate of left ventricular isovolumic contraction is maximal (critical heart rate). In order to determine whether and to what extent phospholamban levels regulate the force-frequency relation *in vivo*, transgenic mice over-

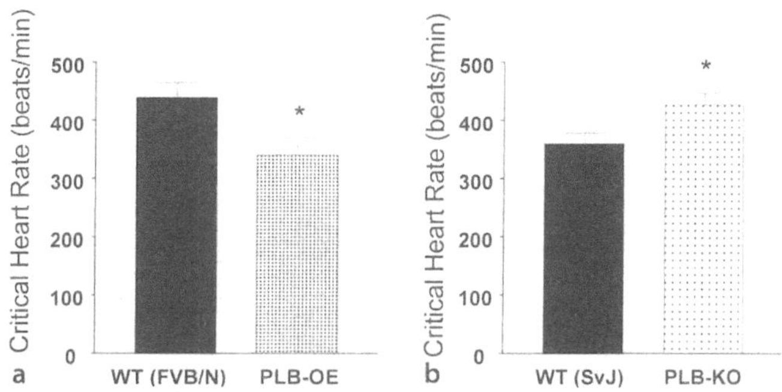

Fig. 2. Effects of phospholamban levels on the critical heart rate. **a** Overexpression of phospholamban (PLB-OE) is associated with a decrease in the critical heart rate (HR_{crit}: 340±30 bpm) compared with isogenic (FVB/N) wild-types (HR_{crit}: 440±25 bpm). **b** Ablation of phospholamban is associated with an increase in the critical heart rate (HR_{crit}: 427±20 bpm) compared with their respective controls (129SvJ) (HR_{crit}: 360±18 bpm).

expressing phospholamban, gene-targeted phospholamban-deficient mice, and their isogenic wild-type controls were studied in parallel [14]. The results indicate that the level of phospholamban is an important negative determinant of the force-frequency relation, such that ablation of phospholamban enhances, whereas overexpression of phospholamban depresses the critical heart rate in anesthetized closed chest mice (Fig. 2) [14].

Based on these studies in genetically engineered phospholamban mouse models, it is interesting to propose that increases in the apparent ratio of phospholamban/SR Ca^{2+} ATPase, such as those observed in human heart failure, may be at least partially responsible for slowed kinetics of Ca^{2+} transients, depressed contractile parameters and functional alterations associated with the disease.

Gene dosage effects and differential gene expression in murine cardiac compartments

Phospholamban ablation or overexpression has been shown to result in parallel changes in cardiac contractile parameters. To determine the effects of a partial reduction in phospholamban levels on cardiac performance and to further examine the sensitivity of the contractile system to alterations in phospholamban levels, phospholamban-heterozygous mice expressing reduced cardiac phospholamban protein (40%) were studied in parallel with wild-type and phospholamban-deficient mice [28].

These experiments demonstrated a close linear correlation between the relative levels of phospholamban in the mouse heart and:

- the affinity of the SR Ca^{2+} pump for Ca^{2+};
- the rates of contraction and relaxation in isolated ventricular myocytes; and
- the contractile parameters in intact beating hearts (Fig. 1).

Again, this phospholamban gene-dosage effect in adult hearts illustrates that physiological and pathophysiological changes in the levels of phospholamban or in the relative phospholamban/SERCA2 ratio may result in parallel changes in sarcoplasmic reticulum function and cardiac contraction.

The stoichiometric ratio of phospholamban/SERCA2 has also been observed to remain constant through murine postnatal development [9]. Our findings in the mouse heart indicate that the SR Ca^{2+} ATPase and phospholamban transcript levels were ~30% of adult levels in newborn mouse hearts and subsequently increased in parallel over the first two weeks of development, approaching adult levels by day 15. Analysis of the initial rates of Ca^{2+} uptake demonstrated that, over the course of development, the upregulation of Ca^{2+} ATPase correlated with increases in the maximal rates of Ca^{2+} uptake. Furthermore, the constant apparent stoichiometric ratio of phospholamban/SERCA2 correlated with a constant affinity of this enzyme for Ca^{2+} [9].

Studies were also designed to test the hypothesis that phospholamban gene expression is differentially regulated in murine atrial and ventricular muscles, and that such differences may reflect alterations in contraction and relaxation rates in these cardiac compartments [21]. The relative transcript ratio of phospholamban to SERCA was found to be four- to fivefold lower in atrial than in ventricular muscle and this was associated with significantly shortened times to half-relaxation, as assessed in isolated superfused atrial tissue preparations. To further define the physiological role of phospholamban in atrial contractility, basal contractile parameters and their responses to β-agonists were studied in atrial muscles, which were either devoid of phospholamban or overexpressed phospholamban [13]. The results, based on the knock-out atria, indicate that phospholamban is a repressor of only basal relaxation in the wild-type atrium, having no significant functional consequence on basal contraction. In contrast, overexpression (threefold) of phospholamban in murine atrial muscle suppresses both the rates of contraction and relaxation, indicating that a critical stoichiometric ratio of phospholamban/SR Ca^{2+} ATPase is necessary for altering both relaxation and contraction rates in cardiac muscle (Fig. 3) [13]. Isoproterenol stimulation resulted in significant increases in the rates of developed tension and relaxation in both phospholamban-deficient and overexpressing atria.

Phospholamban as a regulator of the SR Ca^{2+} pump in smooth muscle and skeletal muscle

Phospholamban is present in the SR of cardiac, smooth, and slow-twitch skeletal muscle. Although the role of phospholamban in the regulation of cardiac contractility has been extensively characterized, the function of phospholamban has been poorly defined (mainly due to the low expression levels of the protein) in smooth and slow-twitch skeletal muscle [15]. Earlier studies even suggested that phospholamban may not be functionally coupled to the SR Ca^{2+} ATPase in the slow-twitch skeletal muscle. However, the availability of the phospholamban-deficient mouse allowed us to exam-

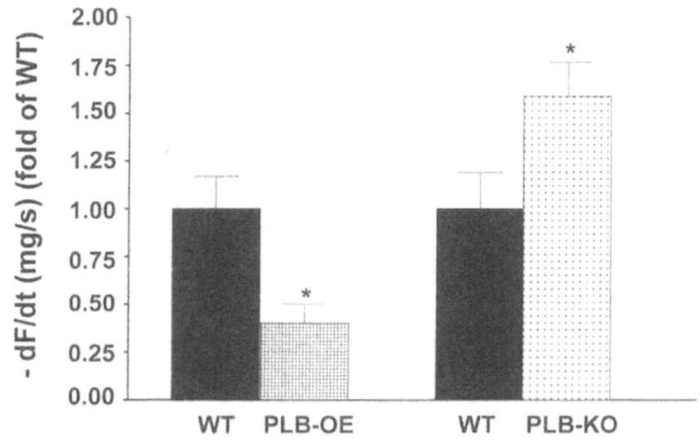

Fig. 3. Effects of phospholamban expression levels on atrial relaxation. Phospholamban overexpression (PLB-OE) results in a decrease in the rate of relaxation (–dF/dt) in left atrial appendages. In contrast, phospholamban knock-out atria exhibit an increase in the rate of relaxation compared to wild-type atria.

ine the functional significance of phospholamban in these muscles. Intact soleus muscle preparations from phospholamban-deficient mice exhibited a significant (25%) decrease in time to half-relaxation with no effects on contraction times compared with wild-type soleus muscle [38]. Furthermore, isoproterenol had no effect on contraction times of either wild-type or phospholamban-deficient mice. However, isoproterenol led to a significant decrease in the half-relaxation time of wild-type soleus muscle, and the maximally stimulated value was similar to the basal value exhibited by phospholamban-deficient muscles, which could not be further stimulated by the β-agonist [38].

As stated above, phospholamban is present in tissues that express the SERCA2 isoform of the sarcoplasmic reticulum Ca^{2+} ATPase and is an inhibitor of the apparent Ca^{2+} affinity of SERCA2. Interestingly, *in vitro* expression studies have shown that phospholamban can also regulate SERCA1, the fast-twitch skeletal muscle isoform. We therefore generated a transgenic mouse model, which ectopically expresses phospholamban exclusively in fast-twitch skeletal muscle under the control of the rat myosin light chain 1 f (MLC 1 f) promoter [37]. Introduction of phospholamban into fast-twitch skeletal muscle resulted in depressed rates of muscle relaxation and a decrease in the affinity of SERCA1 for Ca^{2+} in its native lipid environment. Furthermore, the prolongation of muscle relaxation appeared to correlate with the levels of phospholamban expressed in two transgenic mouse lines. This study presented the first evidence that SERCA1 activity can be regulated by phospholamban *in vivo* [37].

Although previous studies suggested a possible role for phospholamban in vascular smooth muscle Ca^{2+} homeostasis, the importance of phospholamban in regulation of smooth muscle function was only recently established through the availability of the phospholamban-deficient mouse [23, 40]. In mouse aorta, targeted ablation of phospholamban was found to be associated with a marked decrease in sensitivity to both potassium chloride and phenylephrine stimulation. The differences between phospholamban-deficient and wild-type aorta were abolished by SR inhibition [23]. Interestingly, a more recent study demonstrated the existence of phospholamban in vascular endothelium [40]. Vascular endothelial cells regulate vascular smooth muscle tone through Ca^{2+}-dependent production and release of vasoactive molecules. Thus, phospholamban may modulate vascular function through its actions in endothelial cells. These findings may lead to new fields of investigation on Ca^{2+}-regulatory mechanisms in non-muscle tissues, and offer further insights into the regulation of endothelial-vascular interactions.

Transgenic approaches to define the functional unit of phospholamban and the role of dual site phosphorylation of phospholamban

An interesting question is whether a cardiac phenotype, generated by gene ablation, can be reversed by re-introduction of the missing gene in the null background. Thus, the α-myosin heavy chain promoter was used to direct cardiac-specific expression of wild-type phospholamban in the knock-out background [26]. The hyperdynamic function of the phospholamban-deficient hearts was reversed, and the degree of inhibition of the contractile parameters was proportional to the expression levels of phospholamban, in agreement with our previous studies in phospholamban gene-targeted mice. The successful use of phospholamban transgenesis in the genetically altered background offered a unique system for expression of different phospholamban mutants in the murine heart to study structure-function relationships *in vivo*. The following two sections will focus on two specific phospholamban mutants, which were used to

- determine the functional unit of phospholamban and
- elucidate the functional significance of dual site phospholamban phosphorylation *in vivo*.

Monomeric versus pentameric phospholamban: Which is the functional unit *in vivo*?

Based on *in vitro* studies, phospholamban has been proposed to exist as a pentamer in SR membranes [15, 36]. However, in all these studies, pentameric assembly of phospholamban was determined by SDS-PAGE. Thus, it is not clear whether pentameric assembly is essential for its function or whether pentamers arise as a consequence of SDS-PAGE. Towards this end, recent *in vitro* expression experiments, using alanine scanning mutagenesis of phospholamban, suggested that the phospholamban monomer is the active unit, which binds to and inhibits the SR Ca^{2+} ATPase [1, 18]. In this model, the pentamer in the membrane functions as a reservoir for the monomer, and phosphorylation shifts the equilibrium toward pentamers [36]. To elucidate the functional unit of phospholamban *in* vivo, a mutant (Cys^{41} to Phe^{41} (C41F)) form of this protein, which had been shown to form monomers and be an effective inhibitor of SR Ca^{2+} transport in expression systems, or wild-type phospholamban (which contains predominantly pentamers) was expressed in the phospholamban null background [4, 5]. Expression of the monomeric form of phospholamban was associated with inhibition of SR ATPase Ca^{2+} affinity, similar to wild-type or pentameric phospholamban. However, the mutant form was not as effective in depressing relaxation in cardiomyocytes, Langendorff perfused hearts, or intact animals as wild-type or predominantly pentameric phospholamban. These findings support the hypothesis that pentameric assembly of phospholamban may be necessary for optimal regulation of contractility *in vivo*. However, it remains to be elucidated whether the diminished inhibitory effects of the mutated phospholamban *in vivo* are due to its monomeric nature, or perturbations of its interaction with the SR Ca^{2+} ATPase due to the introduced mutation.

Phospholamban phosphorylation *in vivo*

Phosphorylation of phospholamban occurs on both serine^{16} and threonine^{17} during isoproterenol stimulation. Serine^{16} is phosphorylated by cAMP-dependent protein kinase, whereas threonine^{17} is the substrate of Ca^{2+}-calmodulin-dependent protein kinase. *In vitro*, phosphorylation of each site occurs in an independent manner. However, *in vivo* studies indicated that phosphorylation by cAMP-dependent kinase occurs faster than phosphorylation by Ca^{2+}-calmodulin-dependent protein kinase in beating hearts. Therefore, to further examine the physiological role of threonine^{17} phosphorylation in phospholamban, in the absence of serine^{16} phosphorylation, site-specific mutagenesis technology was used to convert serine^{16} to alanine^{16} [26]. Transgenic models expressing either wild-type or the serine^{16} to alanine^{16} mutant phospholamban in the cardiac compartment of the phospholamban knock-out mice were generated, and lines with similar expression levels (0.7-fold) were studied in parallel. Langendorff perfusion indicated that both forms of phospholamban inhibited basal cardiac contractility of the knock-out hearts to the same extent. However, isoproterenol stimulation was associated with much lower responses in the contractile parameters of mutant phospholamban compared with wild-type hearts. Additional ^{32}P-labeling perfusion experiments indicated that this attenuation was due to lack of phosphorylation of mutant phospholamban. The lack of phospholamban threonine^{17} phosphorylation *in vivo* was not due to conversion of the adjacent serine^{16} to alanine^{16} residue, since *in vitro* studies demonstrated that the mutated phospholamban form could still serve as a substrate for Ca^{2+}-calmodulin-dependent protein kinase. Thus, *in vivo* phosphorylation of threonine^{17} requires prior phosphorylation of serine^{16} in phospholamban, and prevention of phosphoserine formation results in attenuation of the β-agonist stimulatory response in the murine heart.

Compensatory mechanisms and exercise capacity in phospholamban-deficient mice

Although the physiological role of phospholamban was highly suggestive from the gene targeting studies, it was not clear whether cardiac compensatory mechanisms accompanied phospholamban ablation and contributed or antagonized the biochemical and physiological effects on SR function and myocardial contractility [7]. Furthermore, working heart preparations of mice lacking phospholamban did not only exhibit increased basal contractility and relaxation, but they were also characterized by lack of a response to β-adrenergic stimulation [27]. This could suggest that the phospholamban deficient hearts were already performing at a maximal level of contractility, and that phospholamban knock-out mice would be unable to further improve cardiac performance during stress. It was therefore interesting to determine the exercise performance of the phospholamban-deficient mice [7].

Phospholamban ablation and compensatory responses

The hyperdynamic cardiac function of the phospholamban knock-out mice was not accompanied by any cytoarchitectural abnormalities [6, 27]. Primary candidates for compensatory changes upon phospholamban ablation are the Ca^{2+} cycling proteins. The cardiac sarcoplasmic reticulum Ca^{2+} ATPase, calsequestrin, Na^{+}/Ca^{2+} exchanger, myosin, actin, troponin I and troponin T levels were not altered. However, the ryanodine receptor levels were significantly reduced (25%) in the phospholamban knock-out hearts. Additionally, ryanodine-binding assays revealed a similar degree of reduction in the maximal number of receptors. This could be interpreted as a cross-talk between SR Ca^{2+} uptake and Ca^{2+} release in an attempt to regulate the observed increase in diastolic SR Ca^{2+} content. Assessment of ATP levels revealed no alterations, although oxygen consumption, determined in work-performing hearts, increased (1.6-fold) to meet the increased ATP utilization in the hyperdynamic phospholamban-deficient heart. However, increases in ATP utilization must then be balanced by increases in ATP synthesis. As a matter of fact, increases in oxygen consumption were associated with a 2.2-fold increase in the active fraction of the mitochondrial pyruvate dehydrogenase, suggesting increased tricarboxylic acid cycle turnover and ATP synthesis. ^{31}P nuclear magnetic resonance studies demonstrated decreases in phosphocreatinine levels and increases in ADP and AMP levels in gene-targeted compared with wild-type hearts. However, the creatinine kinase activity and the creatinine kinase reaction velocity were not different between the groups. Thus, phospholamban ablation is associated with metabolic adaptations to establish a new energetic steady state and meet the increased ATP demand in the hypercontractile phospholamban-deficient hearts [6].

Phospholamban deficiency does not comprise exercise capacity

To determine whether the absence of phospholamban reduces the reserve capacity of the murine cardiovascular system to respond to stress, the cardiovascular performance of awake, active phospholamban-deficient mice and their wild-type control was evaluated during graded treadmill exercise [7]. Phospholamban-deficient mice had slightly higher blood pressure at rest, but had normal tachycardic and hypotensive responses to isoproterenol. Phospholamban knock-out mice could exercise with similar capacity as their wild-type controls, as measured by the duration of exercise and peak oxygen consumption. Since their oxygen pulse curve was normal (peak oxygen consumption/heart rate), these data suggest that compensation may be occurring in the form of improved stroke volumes, possibly via enhanced ventricular filling or reduced ventricular afterload during exercise. Thus, phospholamban ablation does not compromise cardiac performance during maximal cardiovascular stress provided by graded treadmill exercise.

The phospholamban/SR Ca^{2+} complex as a potential therapeutic target

At the cellular level, the pathophysiology of the clinical syndrome *heart failure* is characterized by alterations in calcium homeostasis. Specifically, muscle relaxation and rapid removal of cytosolic Ca^{2+} by the SR Ca^{2+} ATPase are impaired resulting in increased diastolic calcium levels. Consequently, SR Ca^{2+} load is diminished, less Ca^{2+} is available for "Ca^{2+}-induced SR Ca^{2+} release" and this leads to decreased systolic Ca^{2+} levels reflecting impaired contraction.

Although the findings in the mouse provide valuable insights into the mechanisms regulating contractility, it is important to keep in mind that the mouse myocardium is considerably different from human myocardium regarding excitation-contraction coupling and contractile protein isoforms. Nevertheless, genetically altered animal models are critically important for understanding the molecular alterations underlying the pathophysiology of heart failure and are a prerequisite to the development and introduction of new therapeutic strategies. It is therefore interesting to speculate that a phospholamban-inhibitor drug would be beneficial in heart failure, because it would facilitate re-sequestration of diastolic Ca^{2+} through enhanced SR Ca^{2+} uptake capacity. Thereby relaxation would be stimulated, SR Ca^{2+} load enhanced, and systolic E-C coupling and contractility improved. Longitudinal studies in genetically engineered phospholamban knock-out mice have shown no alterations in cardiac morphology and maintenance of exercise endurance as well as life expectancy [7, 39]. Thus, an important therapeutic goal is to stimulate the SR Ca^{2+} ATPase activity through disruption of the phospholamban binding to it [31]. The discovery of a small compound targeted to the phospholamban region, which interacts with the SR Ca^{2+} ATPase, would exhibit high tissue specificity, since phospholamban is mainly present in cardiac tissue. It is expected that such a phospholamban blocking drug may result in increased ATP hydrolysis related to SR Ca^{2+} pump activity, but unlike the cAMP-mediated inotropic interventions, it should not decrease myofilament sensitivity or economy of force generation at the level of the contractile machinery.

Acknowledgments. This work was supported by the National Institutes of Health grants HL26057, HL52318, P40 RR 12358.

References

1. Autry JM, Jones LR (1997) Functional Co-expression of the canine cardiac Ca^{2+} pump and phospholamban in Spodoptera frugiperda (Sf21) cells reveals new insights on ATPase regulation. J Biol Chem 272(25):15872–15880
2. Bers DM, Bassani JW, Bassani RA (1996) Na-Ca exchange and Ca fluxes during contraction and relaxation in mammalian ventricular muscle. Ann N Y Acad Sci 779:430–442
3. Beuckelmann DJ, Nabauer M, Erdmann E (1992) Intracellular calcium handling in isolated ventricular myocytes from patients with terminal heart failure [see comments]. Circulation 85(3):1046–1055
4. Chu G, Dorn GW 2nd, Luo W, Harrer JM, Kadambi VJ, Walsh RA, Kranias EG (1997) Monomeric phospholamban overexpression in transgenic mouse hearts. Circ Res 81(4):485–492
5. Chu G, Li L, Sato Y, Harrer JM, Kadambi VJ, Hoit BD, Bers DM, Kranias EG (1998) Pentameric assembly of phospholamban facilitates inhibition of cardiac function in vivo. J Biol Chem 273(50):33674–33680
6. Chu G, Luo W, Slack JP, Tilgmann C, Sweet WE, Spindler M, Saupe KW, Boivin GP, Moravec CS, Matlib MA, Grupp IL, Ingwall JS, Kranias EG (1996) Compensatory mechanisms associated with the hyperdynamic function of phospholamban-deficient mouse hearts. Circ Res 79(6):1064–1076
7. Desai KH, Schauble E, Luo W, Kranias E, Bernstein D (1999) Phospholamban deficiency does not compromise exercise capacity. Am J Physiol 276(4 Pt 2):H1172–1177
8. Fabiato A (1985) Simulated calcium current can both cause calcium loading in and trigger calcium release from the sarcoplasmic reticulum of a skinned canine cardiac Purkinje cell. J Gen Physiol 85(2):291–320
9. Harrer JM, Haghighi K, Kim HW, Ferguson DG, Kranias EG (1997) Coordinate regulation of SR $Ca^{(2+)}$-ATPase and phospholamban expression in developing murine heart. Am J Physiol 272(1 Pt 2):H57–66
10. Hasenfuss G (1998) Alterations of calcium-regulatory proteins in heart failure. Cardiovasc Res 37(2):279–289
11. Hasenfuss G, Reinecke H, Studer R, Meyer M, Pieske B, Holtz J, Holubarsch C, Posival H, Just H, Drexler H (1994) Relation between myocardial function and expression of sarcoplasmic reticulum $Ca^{(2+)}$-ATPase in failing and nonfailing human myocardium. Circ Res 75(3):434–442
12. Hoit BD, Khoury SF, Kranias EG, Ball N, Walsh RA (1995) In vivo echocardiographic detection of enhanced left ventricular function in gene-targeted mice with phospholamban deficiency. Circ Res 77(3):632–637

13. Kadambi VJ, Koss KL, Grupp IL, Kranias EG (1998) Phospholamban modulates murine atrial contractile parameters and responses to beta-adrenergic agonists. J Mol Cell Cardiol 30(7):1275–1284
14. Kadambi VJ, Ball N, Kranias EG, Walsh RA, Hoit BD (1999) Modulation of force-frequency relation by phospholamban in genetically engineered mice. Am J Physiol 276(6 Pt 2):H2245–2250
15. Kadambi VJ, Kranias EG (1997) Phospholamban: a protein coming of age. Biochem Biophys Res Commun 239(1):1–5
16. Kadambi VJ, Kranias EG (1998) Genetically engineered mice: model systems for left ventricular failure [see comments]. J Card Fail 4(4):349–361
17. Kadambi VJ, Ponniah S, Harrer JM, Hoit BD, Dorn GW 2nd, Walsh RA, Kranias EG (1996) Cardiac-specific overexpression of phospholamban alters calcium kinetics and resultant cardiomyocyte mechanics in transgenic mice. J Clin Invest 97(2):533–539
18. Kimura Y, Kurzydlowski K, Tada M, MacLennan DH (1997) Phospholamban inhibitory function is activated by depolymerization. J Biol Chem 272(24):15061–15064
19. Kiss E, Edes I, Sato Y, Luo W, Liggett SB, Kranias EG (1997) beta-Adrenergic regulation of cAMP and protein phosphorylation in phospholamban-knockout mouse hearts. Am J Physiol 272(2 Pt 2):H785–790
20. Koss KL, Grupp IL, Kranias EG (1997) The relative phospholamban and SERCA2 ratio: a critical determinant of myocardial contractility. Basic Res Cardiol 92(Suppl 1):17–24
21. Koss KL, Ponniah S, Jones WK, Grupp IL, Kranias EG (1995) Differential phospholamban gene expression in murine cardiac compartments. Molecular and physiological analyses [published erratum appears in Circ Res (1995); 77(5):1036]. Circ Res 77(2):342–353
22. Kranias EG, Solaro RJ (1982) Phosphorylation of troponin I and phospholamban during catecholamine stimulation of rabbit heart. Nature 298(5870):182–184
23. Lalli J, Harrer JM, Luo W, Kranias EG, Paul RJ (1997) Targeted ablation of the phospholamban gene is associated with a marked decrease in sensitivity in aortic smooth muscle. Circ Res 80(4):506–513
24. Li L, Chu G, Kranias EG, Bers DM (1998) Cardiac myocyte calcium transport in phospholamban knockout mouse: relaxation and endogenous CaMKII effects. Am J Physiol 274(4 Pt 2):H1335–1347
25. Lorenz JN, Kranias EG (1997) Regulatory effects of phospholamban on cardiac function in intact mice. Am J Physiol 273(6 Pt 2):H2826–2831
26. Luo W, Chu G, Sato Y, Zhou Z, Kadambi VJ, Kranias EG (1998) Transgenic approaches to define the functional role of dual site phospholamban phosphorylation. J Biol Chem 273(8):4734–4739
27. Luo W, Grupp IL, Harrer J, Ponniah S, Grupp G, Duffy JJ, Doetschman T, Kranias EG (1994) Targeted ablation of the phospholamban gene is associated with markedly enhanced myocardial contractility and loss of beta-agonist stimulation. Circ Res 75(3):401–409
28. Luo W, Wolska BM, Grupp IL, Harrer JM, Haghighi K, Ferguson DG, Slack JP, Grupp G, Doetschman T, Solaro RJ, Kranias EG (1996) Phospholamban gene dosage effects in the mammalian heart. Circ Res 78(5):839–847
29. MacLennan DH, Toyofuku T, Kimura Y (1997) Sites of regulatory interaction between calcium ATPases and phospholamban. Basic Res Cardiol 92(Suppl 1):11–15
30. Masaki H, Sato Y, Luo W, Kranias EG, Yatani A (1997) Phospholamban deficiency alters inactivation kinetics of L-type Ca^{2+} channels in mouse ventricular myocytes. Am J Physiol 272(2 Pt 2):H606–612

31. McKenna E, Smith JS, Coll KE, Mazack EK, Mayer EJ, Antanavage J, Wiedmann RT, Johnson RG Jr (1996) Dissociation of phospholamban regulation of cardiac sarcoplasmic reticulum Ca^{2+} ATPase by quercetin. J Biol Chem 271(40):24517–24525
32. Mittmann C, Eschenhagen T, Scholz H (1998) Cellular and molecular aspects of contractile dysfunction in heart failure. Cardiovasc Res 39(2):267–275
33. Morgan JP (1991) Abnormal intracellular modulation of calcium as a major cause of cardiac contractile dysfunction. N Engl J Med 325(9):625–632
34. Pieske B, Kretschmann B, Meyer M, Holubarsch C, Weirich J, Posival H, Minami K, Just H, Hasenfuss G (1995) Alterations in intracellular calcium handling associated with the inverse force-frequency relation in human dilated cardiomyopathy. Circulation 92(5):1169–1178
35. Santana LF, Kranias EG, Lederer WJ (1997) Calcium sparks and excitation-contraction coupling in phospholamban-deficient mouse ventricular myocytes. J Physiol (Lond) 503(Pt 1):21–29
36. Simmerman HK, Jones LR (1998) Phospholamban: protein structure, mechanism of action, and role in cardiac function. Physiol Rev 78(4):921–947
37. Slack JP, Grupp IL, Ferguson DG, Rosenthal N, Kranias EG (1997) Ectopic expression of phospholamban in fast-twitch skeletal muscle alters sarcoplasmic reticulum Ca^{2+} transport and muscle relaxation. J Biol Chem 272(30):18862–18868
38. Slack JP, Grupp IL, Luo W, Kranias EG (1997) Phospholamban ablation enhances relaxation in the murine soleus. Am J Physiol 273(1 Pt 1):C1–6
39. Slack JP, Grupp IL, Tilgmann C, Luo W, Tamura T, Kranias EG (1997) Effects of age on the hyperdynamic cardiac function of phospholamban knockout mice. Circulation (96):1-179 (abstr)
40. Sutliff RL, Hoying JB, Kadambi VJ, Kranias EG, Paul RJ (1999) Phospholamban is present in endothelial cells and modulates endothelium-dependent relaxation. Evidence from phospholamban gene-ablated mice. Circ Res 84(3):360–364
41. Wolska BM, Stojanovic MO, Luo W, Kranias EG, Solaro RJ (1996) Effect of ablation of phospholamban on dynamics of cardiac myocyte contraction and intracellular Ca^{2+}. Am J Physiol 271(1 Pt 1):C391–397

Chapter 4

Manipulation of SERCA2a in the heart by gene transfer

F. del Monte, S.E. Harding[1], R.J. Hajjar
Program in Cardiovascular Gene Therapy,
Cardiovascular Research Center,
Massachusetts General Hospital, Boston, MA and
[1] Cardiac Medicine, National Heart Lung Institute,
Imperial College of Medicine, London, UK

Introduction

In the myopathic heart, a number of abnormalities have been delineated (Fig. 1) at the cellular level [25–33, 35, 38–43]. These include changes at the level of the sarcolemma, sarcoplasmic reticulum, myofilaments, and mitochondria, all of which contribute to depressed contractile function and reserve [25–33, 35, 38–43]. Identifying the mechanisms by which these changes contribute to the observed pathology is frequently confounded by simultaneous alterations in multiple signaling pathways in the complex milieu of the failing heart. Targeting genes to the heart through somatic gene transfer allows us to identify and characterize the molecular changes of diseases as well as to manipulate the targeted pathways [34, 36, 37].

Specific signaling pathways can be perturbed by
- overexpressing either a normal (*wild-type*) form of a specific signaling molecule or
- a mutant that has either no activity (*null mutant*) or
- that actually blocks the endogenous activity of this molecule (*dominant negative mutant*) [14, 15].

By this approach, we can assess the functional relevance of a pathway to the pathogenesis of the cardiomyopathy as well as potentially correct the molecular defect.

To understand efforts at targeting genes to modulate the pathogenesis of cardiomyopathies requires an understanding of both the biology of signal transduction and how it relates to cardiomyopathies and the technology of gene transfer. Dramatic advances have been made in both these areas in recent years. In this chapter we will specifically consider cardiovascular somatic gene transfer and review both the vectors being employed as well as current approaches to *in vivo* delivery of these vectors to the heart as they relate to calcium handling proteins and abnormalities of contractile function, focusing on the changes in excitation-contraction (EC) coupling.

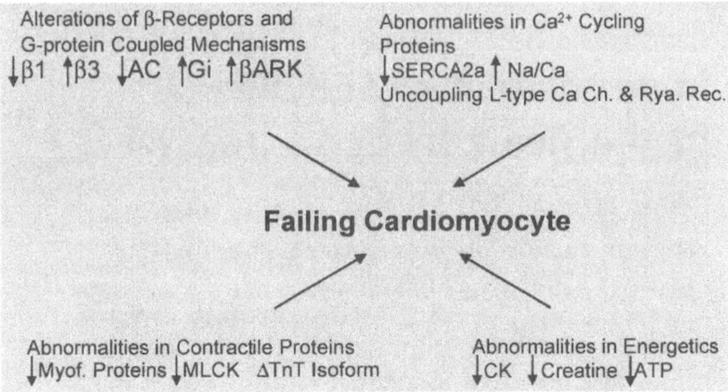

Fig. 1. Abnormalities at the level of the sarcolemma, sarcoplasmic reticulum, myofilaments, and mitochondria all contribute to a dysfunctional cardiac myocyte.

Contractile Function

Cardiac function is classically described as a result of three determinants: preload, afterload and contractility. The intrinsic contractile function of the heart is a feature of the cellular unit of the cardiac muscle and it is controlled at various subcellular levels. These include the neurohormonal receptors, various processes responsible for the EC coupling, and the contractile proteins [25–33, 35, 38–43]. In the setting of heart failure, alterations occur in all three subcellular mechanisms (Fig. 1). This section will review the mechanisms controlling the EC coupling with particular attention to the modulation of the sarcoplasmic reticulum Ca^{2+} ATPase (SERCA2a) pump.

Excitation-Contraction Coupling

In the mammalian heart the intracellular Ca^{2+} movements are tightly regulated at various levels within the cell in order to release Ca^{2+} at the same rate as to remove it from the contractile apparatus (Fig. 2) [9]. Thus, excitation leading to contraction and relaxation occur through a series of coordinated steps whereby electrical excitation across the sarcolemma leads to the opening of voltage-gated Ca^{2+} channels allowing the entry of a small amount of Ca^{2+} into the cell. This triggers the release of a larger amount of calcium from the stores in the sarcoplasmic reticulum (SR) through the ryanodine receptors. This increase in Ca^{2+} activates the myofilaments leading to contraction. The Ca^{2+} pumping activity of SERCA2a is influenced by phospholamban [47]. In the unphosphorylated state, phospholamban inhibits the Ca^{2+}-ATPase, whereas phosphorylation of phospholamban by cAMP-dependent protein kinase and by Ca^{2+}-calmodulin-dependent protein kinase reverses this inhibition (Fig. 2) [47]. This mechanism has been refined by re-

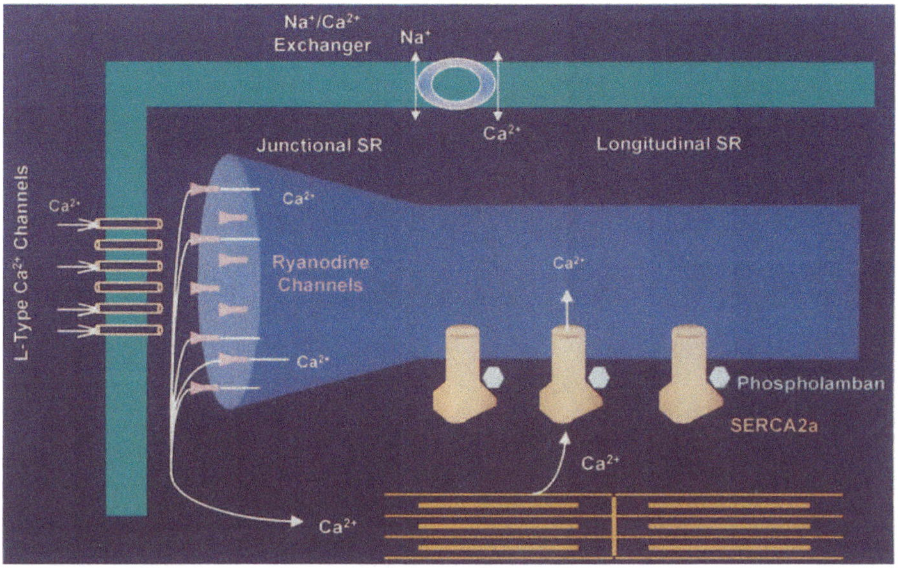

Fig. 2. Excitation-contraction coupling in mammalian myocardium. *SR* Sarcoplasmic reticulum, *SERCA2a* SR Ca^{2+} ATPase pump.

cent data using confocal microscopy which showed the presence of intracellular calcium sparks, arising from a cluster of ryanodine receptors in close proximity to a voltage-dependent calcium channel [2–7, 49–51, 59–64]. In this mechanism labeled "local-control", the coupling of a Ca^{2+} channel with a cluster of ryanodine receptors allows Ca^{2+} influx through a single Ca^{2+} channel to increase the local concentration of Ca^{2+} in the vicinity of the ryanodine receptors, producing a Ca^{2+} spark. When a large number of Ca^{2+} channels are activated, multiple Ca^{2+} sparks combine to increase cytosolic Ca^{2+}, which leads to myofilament activation [2–7, 49–51, 59–64].

At the beginning of relaxation the SR provides the major contribution to the reuptake of Ca^{2+} from the contractile proteins. Further subtraction of Ca^{2+} from the cytoplasm is provided by other mechanisms including mainly the Na^+-Ca^{2+} exchanger, which contribute to the final part of the Ca^{2+} transient to restore diastolic Ca^{2+} levels and, to a lesser extent, by the sarcolemmal Ca^{2+}-ATPase pump, the mitochondria and by binding to intracellular proteins.

Calcium handling is abnormal in failing hearts

The failing myocardium exhibits abnormalities in both the systolic and diastolic phase, and the diastolic changes can appear earlier than systolic. The same feature can be recognized *in vitro* at the tissue as well as cellular level. Muscle strips and single cardiomyocytes from failing hearts show a reduced systolic force, an elevated diastolic force and a slowed relaxation

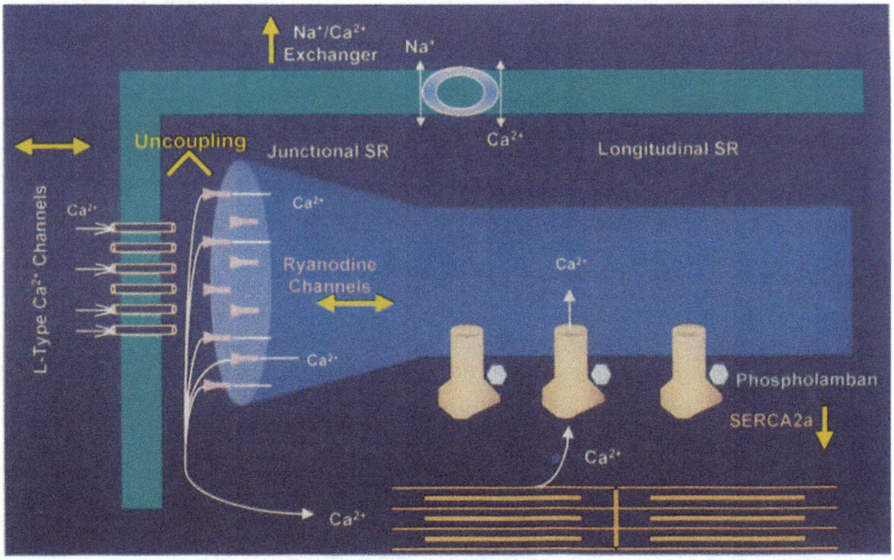

Fig. 3. Abnormalities in excitation-contraction coupling in failing hearts.

(Fig. 3) [25, 26, 28, 30–32]. Ca^{2+} transients recorded from failing human myocardial cells or trabeculae reveal a significantly prolonged Ca^{2+} transient with an elevated end-diastolic intracellular Ca^{2+} [25, 26, 28, 30–32]. At higher levels of stimulation, the amount of Ca^{2+} released from the SR has also been found to be decreased in failing human hearts. Since calcium handling is regulated by the voltage-dependent Ca^{2+} channel, the SR Ca^{2+} release channels ryanodine, the SERCA2a/phospholamban complex, and the Na/Ca exchanger, a number of studies have focused on the relative changes in these proteins between myopathic and normal hearts.

The activities of both the L-type Ca^{2+} channels and the ryanodine release channels from patients with dilated cardiomyopathy, recorded under voltage clamp conditions, are essentially the same as in normal hearts. The mRNA levels of the ryanodine release channels have also been shown not to be significantly different in dilated cardiomyopathy when compared to normal hearts [13]. However, even though the L-type Ca^{2+} channels and the ryanodine release channels may be expressed in normal amounts, their function may be abnormal in failing hearts. It has been recently shown that in failing myocardial cells L-type Ca^{2+} channels have a reduced ability to activate the adjacent ryanodine receptors [6, 7]. These results would point towards impaired coupling between L-type Ca^{2+} channels and adjacent ryanodine receptors. It is still unclear whether all forms of heart failure have this type of coupling abnormality but it would seem that this type of defect in the microenvironment of adjacent channels might be the basis for disease states in the heart.

Functionally, together with the slow relaxation an abnormal force-frequency relationship is observed in the whole muscle as well as in myocytes from failing hearts, both indicating a deficiency in the Ca^{2+} reuptake from the SR. With a pharmacological approach, the failing phenotype can be potentially reproduced in normal cardiomyocytes from both human and animal models of heart failure by exposing contracting cardiac muscle cells to the SERCA inhibitor thapsigargin for a period sufficient to block Ca^{2+} uptake and allow emptying of SR stores [17]. Biochemical measurements also support the functional observations. As described by most investigators, quantification of the steady-state levels of SERCA2a mRNA levels have revealed that they are markedly reduced in both failing human hearts and in experimental models of heart failure [52, 54, 58]. Associated with a decrease in mRNA, there is a decrease in SR Ca^{2+}-ATPase activity and SR Ca^{2+} uptake from SR vesicles and membranes isolated from failing human hearts. However, the protein levels of SR Ca^{2+}-ATPase of failing human hearts have been shown to be significantly reduced by certain investigators while other studies have failed to show significant changes between protein levels of SR Ca^{2+}-ATPase in nonfailing and failing human myocardium [52, 54, 56–58].

An increase in both mRNA and protein levels of the Na/Ca exchanger from the myocardium of failing human hearts have also been described (Fig. 3) [44]. The enhanced expression of the exchanger has been hypothesized to be of functional relevance since the Na/Ca exchanger can operate to bring Ca^{2+} into the cell or extrude it out from the cell. It would be predicted that a transfer of Ca^{2+} removal from SR to Na^+-mediated Ca^{2+} extrusion would have consequences for Na^+ homeostasis within the cell. Several observations are consistent with a change in Na^+ control in failing human myocardium. There is an increase in sensitivity to compounds which produce positive inotropic effects through raised intracellular Na^+, either by inhibiting the Na/K-ATPase or by opening Na^+ channels, in muscle strips from failing human hearts [18, 19]. It has been suggested that the relaxation abnormalities produced by the loss of SERCA2a activity could be, at least partially, compensated by the increase in Na/Ca exchanger [18, 19].

Targeting genes to the heart

Somatic gene transfer

Introduction of genetic material into the cells and tissues of the body is termed *somatic gene transfer* in contradistinction to genetic manipulation of the germline, as in a transgenic mouse model. Despite the nomenclature, the material being transferred is most commonly not the gene itself but rather a cDNA. The cDNA may be delivered in its pure form (so-called "naked DNA") or packaged in association with a variety of vehicles or *vectors* designed to enhance gene transfer. Available vectors are conceptually divided into non-viral vectors employing physical-chemical gene delivery and recombinant viral vectors in which the cDNA of interest has been incorporated into a virus which is then used to infect the target cell and in the process conveys the exogenous cDNA.

Expression of the transferred gene (or transgene) can be quantified in two fundamental ways: the efficiency and level of expression. *Efficiency* refers to the number of cells expressing the transgene divided by total number of cells in the population, and is usually denoted as a percentage. The *level of expression* indicates the total amount of exogenous protein expressed. While these parameters are conceptually distinct, they are often related in practical terms. For example, the determined efficiency of gene transfer critically depends on the sensitivity of the assay employed to detect gene expression. In addition, an increase in the level of expression will usually improve the calculated efficiency since transgene expression will now exceed the threshold necessary for detection in more cells.

As systems for cardiovascular gene transfer are developed, *reporter genes* encoding proteins that are easily identified and/or quantitated are frequently employed. Generally these proteins have either enzymatic activity (e.g., β-galactosidase [β-gal]) (Fig. 4) or fluorescent properties (e.g., green fluorescent protein [GFP]) (Fig. 5). Although reporter genes are imperfect models, they had also been proven extremely useful in establishing and characterizing gene transfer models as well as for biological diagnostics.

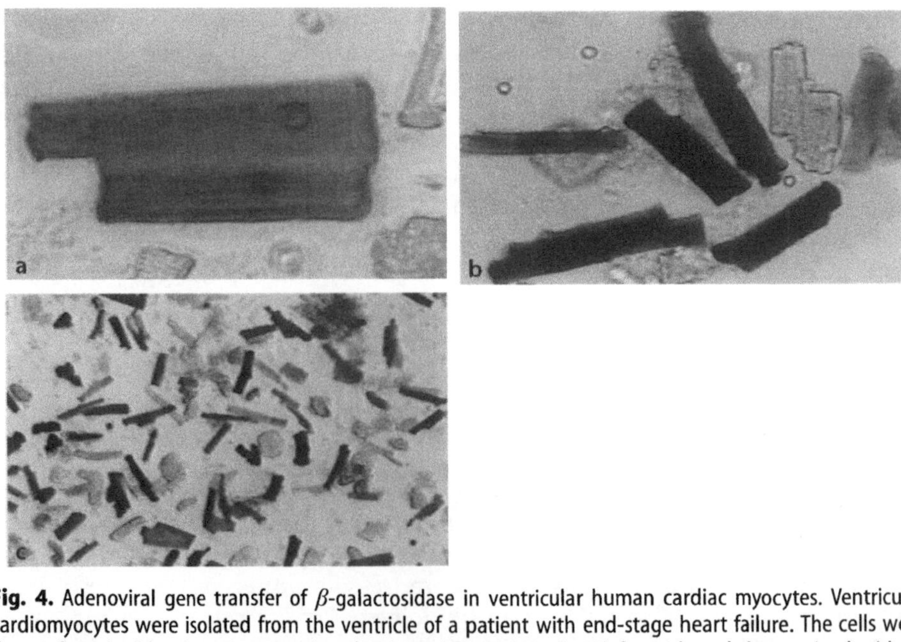

Fig. 4. Adenoviral gene transfer of β-galactosidase in ventricular human cardiac myocytes. Ventricular cardiomyocytes were isolated from the ventricle of a patient with end-stage heart failure. The cells were then infected with adenovirus carrying β-galactosidase (MOI of 100) for 24 h and then stained with X-GAL. A majority of the cells show blue staining reflecting expression of β-galactosidase.

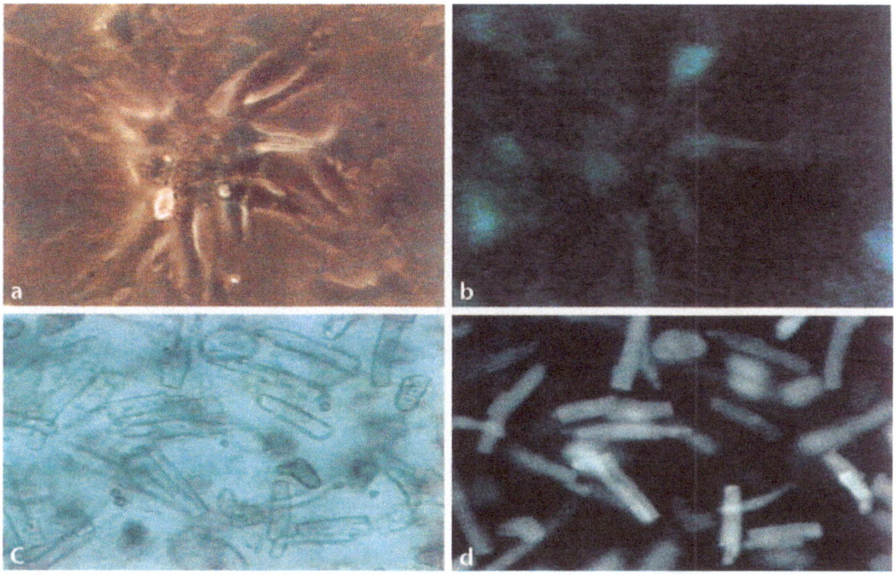

Fig. 5. Adenoviral gene transfer of GFP in neonatal (**a, b**) and ventricular human cardiac myocytes. Ventricular cardiomyocytes were isolated from the ventricle of a patient with end-stage heart failure (**c, d**). The cells were then infected with adenovirus carrying GFP (MOI of 100) for 24 hours. Bright green fluorescence is apparent in all the cells that have been transduced. While background fluorescence in non-infected cells can be clearly distinguished from the infected ones.

Moreover construction of viral vectors [23] encoding for both the interest and the reporter gene had been demonstrated highly useful for targeting individual cells for the physiological evaluation of the functional expression of the gene.

Various viral vectors have been employed for research purposes [23]. Among them, retroviruses have been the most extensively studied and used clinically [1]. Recombinant adenoviral vectors, in contrast, offer several significant advantages [23]. The viruses can be prepared at extremely high titer, infect non-replicating cells, and allow incorporation of relatively large or even multiple cDNAs. They offer the opportunity to investigate the role of local signal transduction pathways in both *in vitro* and *in vivo* model systems.

In vitro and *in vivo* gene transfer

The described vectors confer high-efficiency and high-level transduction of cardiomyocytes *in vitro* (Figs. 4 and 5) [34, 36, 37]. Also *in vivo* cardiac gene transfer has been achieved using recombinant adenoviral vectors [37]. Using an *in vivo* perfusion approach (Fig. 6), we have recently demonstrated the feasibility of modulating ventricular function [37]. In this approach, the viral solution is injected above the aortic valve while the

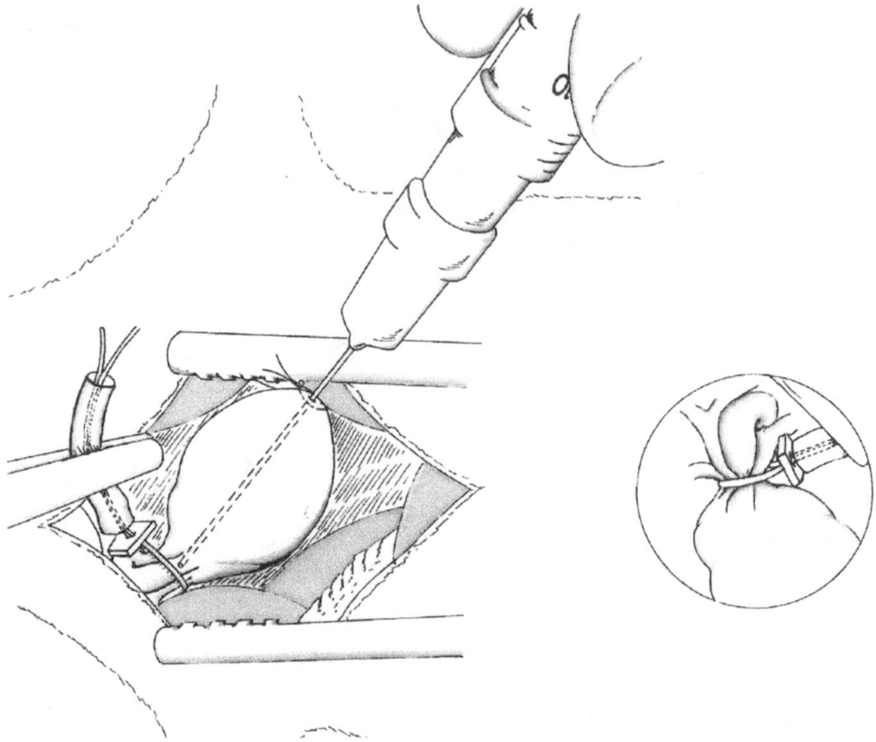

Fig. 6. Delivery of adenoviral vectors to the whole heart. To achieve generalized cardiac gene transfer, viral solution is injected above the aortic valve while the aorta and pulmonary artery are transiently cross-clamped. This method achieves expression of functionally relevant transgenes in proportion of the myocardium sufficient to modulate overall ventricular function.

aorta and pulmonary artery are transiently cross-clamped. The virus is then forced down the coronaries, resulting in relatively diffuse transduction of the myocardium (Fig. 7). Alternative approaches, such as direct myocardial injection and selective coronary cannulation are also actively being pursued, but result in focal transgene expression and may be more applicable to focal diseases such as ischemic heart disease rather than cardiomyopathies which often affect the heart more globally [8, 37]. Nevertheless, these early animal studies establish that *in vivo* adenoviral gene transfer can not only achieve transgene expression in the myocardium, but can also modulate intrinsic functional properties of the intact heart. While expression and functional effects will obviously need to be assessed for each application individually, these data encouragingly suggest that recombinant adenoviral vectors with this transduction technique produce functionally important expression in a substantial proportion of the myocardium.

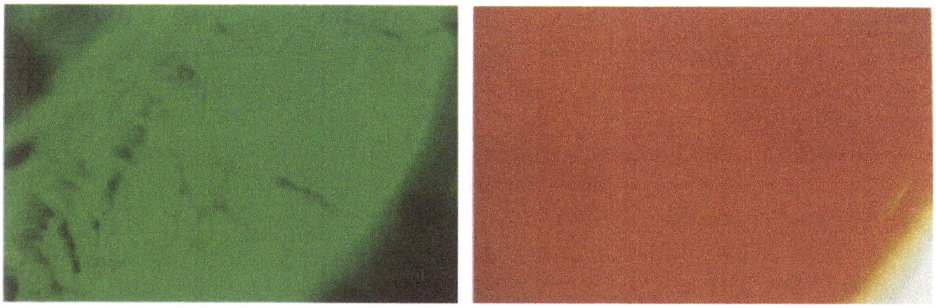

Fig. 7. Transduction of a rat heart with Ad.GFP. A rat heart was transduced with Ad.GFP using the catheter-based technique described in Fig. 6. Forty eight hours after delivery of adenovirus encoding for GFP, the left ventricles of the hearts were removed and visualized with white light (*left panel*), and at 510 nm with single excitation peak at 490 nm of blue light (*right panel*).

Benefits and shortcomings of gene transfer in the cardiovascular system

The transfer of cardiac genes into the heart provides a new approach to treat individuals with acquired cardiac diseases, including ischemic heart disease and congestive heart failure. Recombinant adenoviral vectors hold promise as a vehicle for efficient gene transfer into the heart *in vivo.* Adult cardiac myocytes are terminally differentiated cells that are resistant to genetic modification by conventional means but we and others have shown that adenoviruses readily infect cardiomyocytes with excellent expression of the transgene [8, 37]. This is probably due to the fact that cardiac myocytes have very high levels of the coxsackie b/adenovirus receptor [10]. The virion has an outer protein coat (capsid) in which the subunit capsomeres are arranged in an icosahedral structure containing 12 protruding vertices that are essential for attachment of the virion to cell surface receptors. Adenoviruses, therefore, readily attach to the cell surface. Unlike retroviruses, adenoviruses are capable of transferring foreign genes into post-mitotic cells including adult cardiac myocytes. The insertion of the foreign genes into specific regions of the adenoviral genome renders the adenovirus replication defective thus making it suitable as a gene transfer vehicle for infection of mammalian cells. Recently, we have shown that adenoviral gene transfer can alter ventricular performance *in vivo* by the overexpression of a single excitation-contraction coupling protein, phospholamban [37]. This was the first demonstration of effective gene transfer into the whole heart, resulting in a clear change of ventricular performance.

Adenovirus gene transfer is limited by the transient nature of expression of the transgene *in vivo* [20, 24]. This is the norm for first-generation adenovirus vectors that have deletions in the E1 and E3 region of their gene. The majority of gene transfer experiments into the heart have been obtained using first generation recombinant adenoviral vectors. The deletion of the E1 region disables the replication of the recombinant virus. However, the remaining adenovirus genes (which are still activated) are targeted by the immune system. This leads to antigen presentation of the adenoviral gene products, the subsequent immune response and, ultimately, the destruction of the infected cells.

Prolongation of gene expression *in vivo* has been the target of recent efforts in gene transfer. A number of groups have shown that removing the remaining early genes, such as E4 [11, 12, 46, 48] prolongs expression. These newer generation adenoviral vectors have two main advantages over the first generation vectors. First, transgene expression is prolonged since they produce less adenoviral gene products in the infected cells. Second, they have a larger capacity for carrying DNA fragments [11, 12, 46, 48].

The ultimate goal of adenovirus-mediated gene transfer is to cause a direct and specific modification in cardiac muscle contractile function. Overexpression of SERCA2a by adenoviral gene transfer has been shown to increase contractility in single isolated myocytes and more recently has been shown to enhance contractile function *in vivo* [21, 34, 36].

The immune response to adenoviruses has been shown to follow a specific time course. The initial component is evident at 4 days postinfection, and arises from:

- toxic effects of the delivered adenovirus capsomeres present in the muscle fibers,
- toxic effects of newly synthesized adenovirus gene products after infection, including potential suppression of host protein synthesis or effects of cytokines released by infected cells,
- direct toxic effects resulting from overexpression of the delivered transgene,
- indirect effects of the strong promoters regulating transgene expression which could monopolize available cellular transcriptional machinery, and/or
- specific or non-specific effects of capsids proteins, adenovirus gene expression of transgene overexpression on muscle contraction via alterations in excitation-contraction coupling, or alterations in the interactions between actin and myosin [20, 24].

A second feature of adenovirus gene transfer is a time-delayed, immune-based component culminating in the elimination of the infected muscle cells by $CD8^+$-cytotoxic T lymphocytes [20, 24]. This immune-based component is related to the initial delivery of the virus and/or an immune response directed against either adenovirus gene products or the protein product of the transgene.

Transgenic approaches to these questions are also possible. However, adenoviral transduction offers multiple advantages over transgenic approaches to address these issues. First, developmental issues can be removed from consideration by working in adult animals and *in vitro* systems. For example, mice overexpressing the sarcoplasmic reticulum Ca^{2+} ATPase (SERCA2a) have been generated [45]. However, along with an increase in SERCA2a in the transgenic mice, there was a change in the expression of the ryanodine receptors and the sodium-calcium exchanger. In addition, in mice lacking phospholamban engineered through homologous recombination, there was also an increase in the expression of the ryanodine receptors [16]. These results show that developmental changes can alter the expression of other important cellular proteins which can confound the phenotype. Somatic gene transfer will enable us to overexpress excitation-contraction coupling proteins directly without the influence of developmental confounders. Second, significant expression can be restricted to sites of interest by local delivery of constructs. Third, the high efficiency of adenoviral transduction makes feasible expression of multiple exogenous cDNAs which is difficult to achieve in transgenic systems. Fourth, adenoviral vectors can be used in multiple species thus providing optimal flexibility in selecting a model. By overexpressing genes in fully differentiated adult rodent myocytes, it is less likely that other expression systems will be affected.

Altering the sarcoplasmic reticulum Ca^{2+} ATPase pump/phospholamban ratio by gene transfer

Three different genes (SERCA 1, 2, 3) encode for five distinct SERCA isoforms in the mammalian skeletal, smooth and cardiac muscle. SERCA2 gene encodes for two distinct isoforms for the cardiac (SERCA2a) or the smooth muscle (SERCA2b), both being modulated by the phosphoprotein phospholamban [47]. The relative ratio of phospholamban/SERCA2a is an important determinant of SR function in cardiac myocytes and an increased ratio of phospholamban/SERCA2a is characteristic of heart failure in animal models and particularly in human myocytes which mainly rely on the on SERCA2a function for the removal of Ca^{2+} from the cytoplasm^{+} [34, 36, 53].

Increasing levels of phospholamban relative to SERCA2a in isolated cardiac myocytes significantly altered intracellular calcium handling by prolonging the relaxation phase of the Ca^{2+} transient, decreasing Ca^{2+} release, and increasing resting Ca^{2+} [34, 36, 53]. These results supported the hypothesis that altering the relative ratio of phospholamban to SERCA2a can account for the abnormalities in calcium handling observed in failing ventricular myocardium. On the other hand, overexpressing SERCA2a can largely "rescue" the phenotype created by increasing the phospholamban to SERCA2a ratio. These results could be reproduced *in vitro* and *in vivo* in animal models of heart failure as well as in myocytes from failing human hearts where cells overexpressing SERCA2a could recover the functional characteristics of normal cardiac myocytes. Dilmann et al. have shown that adenovirus-mediated expression of a SERCA2 transgene cultured neonatal myocytes treated with phorbol-12-myristate-13-acetate (PMA), a compound that decreases endogenous SERCA2 expression and results in prolongation of Ca^{2+} transients, can reconstitute depressed endogenous SERCA2 levels, shorten prolonged Ca^{2+} transients, and augment SR Ca^{2+} uptake [21]. In animal models of pressure overload hypertrophy and heart failure *in vivo* overexpressing SERCA2a improved LV systolic and diastolic function indicating that enhancing contractility at the cellular level can be translated into improved ventricular function [55]. It is conceivable that such an approach might be used *in vivo* to normalize altered Ca^{2+} regulation in human heart failure. It is also conceivable that, by decreasing levels of phospholamban using antisense strategies, the SERCA2a/phospholamban ratio can be reconstituted back to normal.

This rescue effect by SERCA2a is especially encouraging since it suggests that restoring the normal phospholamban/SERCA2a ratio through somatic gene transfer could correct the abnormalities of calcium handling and contraction seen in failing hearts.

Conclusion

Gene therapy for cardiovascular diseases is still at the early stages of both basic and clinical applications. There are many hurdles to overcome including better vectors, cardiac specific transgene expression, and prolonged high level expression. Moreover, gene therapy needs to be founded on solid understanding of disease pathogenesis. Targeting genes and signaling pathways by gene transfer represents an important aspect of dissecting the various mechanisms involved in heart failure. By using somatic gene transfer as an experimental tool, we can help elucidate the pathophysiology of heart failure and explore the functional and clinical aspect of modulating specific targets.

Acknowledgments. This work was supported in part by grants from NIH: HL 50361 & HL 57623 (RJH), a Doris Duke Charitable Foundation Clinician Scientist Award, American Federation of Aging Research Grant (RJH), British Heart Foundation Crants PG 97064 and PG 98043.

References

1. Askari F, Hitomi E, Thiney M, Wilson JM (1995) Retrovirus-mediated expression of HUG Br1 in Crigler-Najjar syndrome type I human fibroblasts and correction of the genetic defect in Gunn rat hepatocytes. Gene Therapy 2:203–208
2. Balke CW (1996) Spontaneous Ca^{2+} oscillations and waves in pulmonary vascular endothelial cells [editorial; comment]. Circ Res 79:909–910
3. Balke CW, Egan TM, Wier WG (1994) Processes that remove calcium from the cytoplasm during excitation-contraction coupling in intact rat heart cells. J Physiol 474:447–462
4. Balke CW, Gold MR (1992) Calcium channels in the heart: an overview. Heart Dis Stroke 1:398–403
5. Balke CW, Gold MR (1993) Excitation-contraction-relaxation coupling in the normal and failing heart. Heart Dis Stroke 2:150–155

6. Balke CW, Rose WC, Marban E, Wier WG (1992) Macroscopic and unitary properties of physiological ion flux through T-type Ca^{2+} channels in guinea-pig heart cells. J Physiol 456:247–265
7. Balke CW, Shorofsky SR (1998) Alterations in calcium handling in cardiac hypertrophy and heart failure. Cardiovasc Res 37:290–299
8. Barr E, Carroll J, Kalynych AM, Tripathy SK, Kozarsky K, Wilson JM, Leiden JM (1994) Efficient catheter-mediated gene transfer into the heart using replication-defective adenovirus. Gene Therapy 1:51–58
9. Barry WH, Bridge JHB (1993) Intracellular calcium homeostasis in cardiac myocytes. Circulation 87:1806–1815
10. Bergelson JM, Cunningham JA, Droguett G, Kurt-Jones EA, Krithivas A, Hong JS, Horwitz MS, Crowell R (1997) Isolation of a common receptor for coxsackie B viruses and adenoviruses 2 and 5. Science 275:1320–1324
11. Bett AJ, Haddara W, Prevec L, Graham FL (1994) An efficient and flexible system for construction of adenovirus vectors with insertions or deletions in early regions 1 and 3. Proc Natl Acad Sci USA 91:8802–8806
12. Bett AJ, Prevec L, Graham FL (1993) Packaging capacity and stability of human adenovirus type 5 vectors. J Virol 67:5911-5921
13. Brillantes AM, Allen P, Takahashi T, Izumo S, Marks AR (1992) Differences in cardiac calcium release channel (ryanodine receptor) expression in myocardium from patients with end-stage heart failure caused by ischemic versus dilated cardiomyopathy [published erratum appears in Circ Res (1992) 71(6):1538]. Circ Res 71:18–26
14. Choukroun G, Hajjar R, Frye S, Del Monte F, Guerrero JL, Picard M, Rosenzweig A, Force T (1999) Regulation of cardiac hypertrophy in vivo by the stress-activated protein kinases/c-jun NH_2 terminal kinases. J Clin Invest 104:391–398
15. Choukroun G, Hajjar R, Kyriakis JM, Bonventre JV, Rosenzweig A, Force T (1998) Role of the stress-activated protein kinases in endothelin-induced cardiomyocyte hypertrophy. J Clin Invest 102:1311–1320
16. Chu G, Luo W, Slack JP, Tilgmann C, Sweet WE, Spindler M, Saupe KW, Boivin GP, Moravec CS, Matlib MA, Grupp IL, Ingwall JS, Kranias EG (1996) Compensatory mechanisms associated with the hyperdynamic function of phospholamban-deficient mouse hearts. Circ Res 79:1064–1076
17. Davia K, Davies CH, Harding SE (1997) Effects of inhibition of sarcoplasmic reticulum calcium uptake on contraction in myocytes isolated from failing human ventricle. Cardiovasc Res 33:88–97
18. Flesch M, Putz F, Schwinger RH, Bohm M (1996) Functional relevance of an enhanced expression of the $Na^{(+)}$-Ca^{2+} exchanger in the failing human heart. Ann NY Acad Sci 779:539–542
19. Flesch M, Schwinger RH, Schiffer F, Frank K, Sudkamp M, Kuhn-Regnier F, Arnold G, Bohm M (1996) Evidence for functional relevance of an enhanced expression of the $Na^{(+)}$-Ca^{2+} exchanger in failing human myocardium. Circulation 94:992–1002
20. French BA, Mazur W, Geske RS, Bolli R (1994) Direct in vivo gene transfer into porcine myocardium using replication-deficient adenoviral vectors. Circulation 90:2414–2424
21. Giordano FJ, He H, McDonough P, Meyer M, Sayen MR, Dillmann WH (1997) Adenovirus-mediated gene transfer reconstitutes depressed sarcoplasmic reticulum Ca^{2+}-ATPase levels and shortens prolonged cardiac myocyte Ca^{2+} transients. Circulation 96:400–403
22. Gomez AM, Valdivia HH, Cheng H, Lederer MR, Santana LF, Cannell MB, McCune SA, Altschuld RA, Lederer WJ (1997) Defective excitation-contraction coupling in experimental cardiac hypertrophy and heart failure [see comments]. Science 276:800–806

23. Graham FL, Prevec L (1995) Methods for construction of adenovirus vectors. Mole Biotech 3:207–220
24. Guzman RJ, Lemarchand P, Crystal RG, Epstein SE, Finkel T (1993) Efficient gene transfer into myocardium by direct injection of adenovirus vectors. Circ Res 73:1202–1207
25. Gwathmey JK, Bentivegna LA, Ransil BJ, Grossman W, Morgan JP (1993) Relationship of abnormal intracellular calcium mobilisation to myocyte hypertrophy in human ventricular myocardium. Cardiovasc Res 27:199–203
26. Gwathmey JK, Copelas L, MacKinnon R, Schoen FJ, Feldman MD, Grossman W, Morgan JP (1987) Abnormal intracellular calcium handling in myocardium from patients with end-stage heart failure. Circ Res 61:70–76
27. Gwathmey JK, Davidoff AJ (1994) Pathophysiology of cardiomyopathies: Part II. Drug-induced and other interventions [review] [46 refs]. Curr Opin Cardiol 9:369–378
28. Gwathmey JK, Hajjar RJ (1990) Relation between steady-state force and intracellular [Ca^{2+}] in intact human myocardium. Index of myofibrillar responsiveness to Ca^{2+}. Circulation 82:1266–1278
29. Gwathmey JK, Liao R, Helm PA, Thaiyananthan G, Hajjar RJ (1995) Is contractility depressed in the failing human heart? [Review] [40 refs]. Cardiovasc Drugs Ther 9:581–587
30. Gwathmey JK, Morgan JP (1985) Altered calcium handling in experimental pressure-overload hypertrophy in the ferret. Circ Res 57:836–843
31. Gwathmey JK, Morgan JP (1993) Sarcoplasmic reticulum calcium mobilization in right ventricular pressure-overload hypertrophy in the ferret: relationships to diastolic dysfunction and a negative treppe. Pflugers Arch 422:599–608
32. Gwathmey JK, Slawsky MT, Hajjar RJ, Briggs GM, Morgan JP (1990) Role of intracellular calcium handling in force-interval relationships of human ventricular myocardium. J Clin Invest 85:1599–1613
33. Hajjar RJ, DiSalvo TG, Schmidt U, Thaiyananthan G, Semigran MJ, Dec GW, Gwathmey JK (1997) Clinical correlates of the myocardial force-frequency relationship in patients with end-stage heart failure. J Heart Lung Transplant 16:1157–1167
34. Hajjar RJ, Kang JX, Gwathmey JK, Rosenzweig A (1997) Physiological effects of adenoviral gene transfer of sarcoplasmic reticulum calcium ATPase in isolated rat myocytes. Circulation 95:423–429
35. Harding SE, Jones SM, O'Gara P, del Monte F, Vescovo G, Poole-Wilson PA (1992) Isolated ventricular myocytes from failing and non-failing human heart; the relation of age and clinical status of patients to isoproterenol response. J Mol Cell Cardiol 24:549–564
36. Hajjar RJ, Schmidt U, Kang JX, Matsui T, Rosenzweig A (1997) Adenoviral gene transfer of phospholamban in isolated rat cardiomyocytes. Rescue effects by concomitant gene transfer of sarcoplasmic reticulum Ca^{2+} ATPase. Circ Res 81:145–153
37. Hajjar RJ, Schmidt U, Matsui T, Guerrero JL, Lee KH, Gwathmey JK, Dec GW, Semigran MJ, Rosenzweig A (1998) Modulation of ventricular function through gene transfer in vivo. Proc Natll Acad Sci USA 95:5251–5256
38. Hasenfuss G (1998) Calcium pump overexpression and myocardial function. Implications for gene therapy of myocardial failure [editorial; comment]. Circ Res 83:966–968
39. Hasenfuss G, Holubarsch C, Hermann HP, Astheimer K, Pieske B, Just H (1994) Influence of the force-frequency relationship on haemodynamics and left ventricular function in patients with non-failing hearts and in patients with dilated cardiomyopathy. Eur Heart J 15:164–170

40. Harding SE, MacLeod KT, Jones SM, Vescovo G, Poole-Wilson PA (1991) Contractile responses of myocytes isolated from patients with cardiomyopathy. Eur Heart J 12(Suppl D):44–48
41. Hasenfuss G, Pieske B, Holubarsch C, Alpert NR, Just H (1993) Excitation-contraction coupling and contractile protein function in failing and nonfailing human myocardium. Adv Exp Med Biol 346:91–100
42. Hasenfuss G, Reinecke H, Studer R, Pieske B, Meyer M, Drexler H, Just H (1996) Calcium cycling proteins and force-frequency relationship in heart failure. Basic Res Cardiol 91(Suppl 2):17–22
43. Hasenfuss G, Reinecke H, Studer R, Meyer M, Pieske B, Holtz J, Holubarsch C, Posival H, Just H, Drexler H (1994) Relation between myocardial function and expression of sarcoplasmic reticulum $Ca^{(2+)}$-ATPase in failing and nonfailing human myocardium. Circ Res 75:434–442
44. Hasenfuss G, Schillinger W, Lehnart SE, Preuss M, Pieske B, Maier LS, Prestle J, Minami K, Just H (1999) Relationship between Na^{+}-Ca^{2+}-exchanger protein levels and diastolic function of failing human myocardium. Circulation 99:641–648
45. He H, Giordano FJ, Hilal-Dandan R, Choi DJ, Rockman HA, McDonough PM, Bluhm WF, Meyer M, Sayen MR, Swanson E, Dillmann WH (1997) Overexpression of the rat sarcoplasmic reticulum Ca^{2+} ATPase gene in the heart of transgenic mice accelerates calcium transients and cardiac relaxation. J Clin Invest 100:380–389
46. Hitt MM, Addison CL, Graham FL (1997) Human adenovirus vectors for gene transfer into mammalian cells [Review] [445 refs]. Adv Pharmacol 40:137–206
47. Koss KL, Kranias EG (1996) Phospholamban: a prominent regulator of myocardial contractility. Circ Res 79:1059–1063
48. Krougliak V, Graham FL (1995) Development of cell lines capable of complementing E1, E4, and protein IX defective adenovirus type 5 mutants. Hum Gene Ther 6:1575–1586
49. Lamont C, Luther PW, Balke CW, Wier WG (1998) Intercellular Ca^{2+} waves in rat heart muscle. J Physiol 512:669–676
50. Lopez-Lopez JR, Shacklock PS, Balke CW, Wier WG (1994) Local, stochastic release of Ca^{2+} in voltage-clamped rat heart cells: visualization with confocal microscopy. J Physiol 480:21–29
51. Lopez-Lopez JR, Shacklock PS, Balke CW, Wier WG (1995) Local calcium transients triggered by single L-type calcium channel currents in cardiac cells. Science 268:1042–1045
52. Mercadier JJ, Lompre AM, Duc P, Boheler KR, Fraysse JB, Wisnewsky C, Allen PD, Komajda M, Schwartz K (1990) Altered sarcoplasmic reticulum $Ca^{2(+)}$-ATPase gene expression in the human ventricle during end-stage heart failure. J Clin Invest 85:305–309
53. Meyer M, Bluhm WF, He H, Post SR, Giordano FJ, Lew WY, Dillmann WH (1999) Phospholamban-to-SERCA2 ratio controls the force-frequency relationship. Am J Physiol 276:H779–785
54. Meyer M, Schillinger W, Pieske B, Holubarsch C, Heilmann C, Posival H, Kuwajima G, Mikoshiba K, Just H, Hasenfuss G (1995) Alterations of sarcoplasmic reticulum proteins in failing human dilated cardiomyopathy. Circulation 92:778–784
55. Miyamoto MI, Guerrero JL, Schmidt U, Gwathmey JK, Dec GW, Rosenzweig A, Hajjar RJ (1998) Adenoviral gene transfer of SERCA2a improves LV function in aortic-banded rats in transition to heart failure. Circulation 98:736
56. Schmidt U, Hajjar RJ, Helm PA, Kim CS, Doye AA, Gwathmey JK (1998) Contribution of abnormal sarcoplasmic reticulum ATPase activity to systolic and diastolic dysfunction in human heart failure. J Mol Cell Cardiol 30:1929–1937

57. Schmidt U, Hajjar RJ, Kim CS, Lebeche D, Doye AA, Gwathmey JK (1999) Human heart failure: cAMP stimulation of SR Ca^{2+}-ATPase activity and phosphorylation level of phospholamban. Am J Physiol 277:H474–H480
58. Schwinger RH, Bohm M, Schmidt U, Karczewski P, Bavendiek U, Flesch M, Krause EG, Erdmann E (1995) Unchanged protein levels of SERCA II and phospholamban but reduced Ca^{2+} uptake and $Ca^{(2+)}$-ATPase activity of cardiac sarcoplasmic reticulum from dilated cardiomyopathy patients compared with patients with nonfailing hearts. Circulation 92:3220–3228
59. Shacklock PS, Wier WG, Balke CW (1995) Local Ca^{2+} transients (Ca^{2+} sparks) originate at transverse tubules in rat heart cells. J Physiol 487:601–608
60. Shorofsky SR, Aggarwal R, Corretti M, Baffa JM, Strum JM, Al-Seikhan BA, Kobayashi YM, Jones LR, Wier WG, Balke CW (1999) Cellular mechanisms of altered contractility in the hypertrophied heart: big hearts, big sparks. Circ Res 84:424–434
61. Shorofsky SR, Izu L, Wier WG, Balke CW (1998) Ca^{2+} sparks triggered by patch depolarization in rat heart cells. Circ Res 82:424–429
62. Wier WG, Egan TM, Lopez-Lopez JR, Balke CW (1994) Local control of excitation-contraction coupling in rat heart cells. J Physiol 474:463–471
63. Wier WG, Lopez-Lopez JR, Shacklock PS, Balke CW (1995) Calcium signalling in cardiac muscle cells. Ciba Foundation Symposium 188:146–160; discussion 160–164
64. Wier WG, ter Keurs HE, Marban E, Gao WD, Balke CW (1997) Ca^{2+} 'sparks' and waves in intact ventricular muscle resolved by confocal imaging [see comments] [published erratum appears in Circ Res (1997) 81(5):893]. Circ Res 81:462–469

CHAPTER 5

Changing the cardiac calcium transient: SERCA2 overexpression versus phospholamban inhibition

W. H. DILLMANN
University of California, San Diego, California, USA

Summary

Congestive heart failure is a significant medical problem, and abnormalities in calcium handling leading to a delayed decline in the calcium transient have been identified in failing hearts. Calcium lowering during diastole in cardiac myocytes is markedly influenced by the activity of the calcium ATPase of the sarcoplasmic reticulum which pumps 2 moles of calcium per mole of ATP split from the cytosol into the vesicle of the sarcoplasmic reticulum. In patients with end-stage heart failure, decreases in the level of the SERCA pump have been identified in some reports, however, have not been found by other investigators. To determine if the SERCA2 pump could be overexpressed in the hearts of transgenic mice and what contractile alterations would result, such mice were constructed. No detrimental effects were identified in those animals and a 20% increase in SERCA pump protein lead to an increase in contractile behavior under *in vivo* conditions and to an accelerated calcium transient and contraction in isolated myocytes under not hemodynamically loaded conditions. Compensatory functions for a hypothyroidism-induced decrease in SERCA pump activity were identified in transgenic SERCA mice. The SERCA2 transgene lead to a functional improvement by compensating for the prolonged relaxation of papillary muscle identified in wild-type hypothyroid mice. Similarly, a compensatory effect could be identified using adenoviral vectors expressing a SERCA transgene upon infection of cardiac myocytes exposed to the phorbol ester PMA which leads to a decrease in endogenous SERCA levels. In addition to improving the calcium transient by increasing the expression of SERCA2 protein levels, diminishing the inhibitory effects of phospholamban should also lead to increased SERCA activity and corresponding improvements in calcium handling and in contractile function. To explore this in further detail a dominant negative mutant of phospholamban was constructed by changing the lysine of position 3 to glutamic acid and the arginine of position 14 to glutamic acid. Adenoviral vectors expressing antisense RNA to phospholamban were also used. Infecting neonatal and adult cardiac myocytes with dominant negative mutants of phospholamban or phospholamban antisense constructs lead to a significant increase in SERCA activity, acceleration of the calcium transient, and increased myocyte contractility. The decreased calcium transient occurring in end-stage congestive heart failure may therefore be improved in the future using viral vector-based increases in SERCA transgene expression or in increasing SERCA activity by using phospholamban mutants or antisense constructs.

Introduction

Congestive heart failure presents a very significant medical problem [15], and abnormalities in the calcium transient in the failing heart were identified over ten years ago [10]. Pioneering studies performed in J. Morgan's laboratory indicated that in muscle strips obtained from control hearts, hearts with cardiac hypertrophy, and failing hearts an aequorin-traced calcium signal showed a marked delay in returning to baseline level during muscle relaxation indicating abnormalities in calcium handling in the failing heart [10]. Calcium lowering in mammalian cardiac myocytes is primarily mediated by the reuptake of calcium into the sarcoplasmic reticulum [5, 7]. An ATP-consuming calcium pump, the calcium ATPase of the sarcoplasmic reticulum lowers systolic calcium levels during diastole by actively pumping two moles of calcium into the sarcoplasmic reticulum (SR) which requires the consumption of one mole of ATP. In addition, the sodium calcium exchanger makes a significant contribution to lowering diastolic calcium levels [7]. The contribution of the sodium calcium exchanger is somewhat species dependent. The exchanger plays a minor role only contributing to about 10% of calcium handling in rodent hearts but contributes 20% to 30% in larger mammalian species like rabbits, dogs, and human beings [4]. Some investigators have documented decreased levels of SERCA protein using Western blotting techniques in cardiac species obtained from failing human hearts [18]. In contrast, other investigators observed abnormalities in calcium handling which were however not accompanied by a lowering of the amount of SERCA pump protein [19]. Abnormalities in calcium handling in the face of unchanged SERCA pump levels could, for example, be mediated by alterations of the phosphorylation status of phospholamban, a protein which markedly inhibits in its unphosphorylated state the SERCA pump [16]. Phospholamban is phosphorylated by calcium calmodulin kinase and protein kinase A and phosphorylation of phospholamban decreases the inhibitory action which phospholamban exerts on SERCA-pumping activity. In view of the abnormal calcium transients in the failing heart, it would appear desirable to increase SERCA2 activity in failing hearts. This could be accomplished by increasing the expression of SERCA pump protein. More SERCA pump protein could be produced by enhancing the expression of the endogenous gene or by expressing a SERCA2 transgene using a viral vector-based gene therapy type of approach. In addition, SERCA2 activity could theoretically be enhanced through small pharmacological compounds which bind to SERCA2 itself like the compound jasmone [1]. In addition, decreasing phospholamban amounts or activity would also lead to increased SERCA2 activity as discussed above.

Calcium handling and contractile function in SERCA2 transgenic mice

In order to explore influences of increased SERCA2 expression on cardiac function we constructed transgenic mice overexpressing a SERCA transgene in their heart [11]. Recently SERCA2 overexpressing mice were generated by Dr. Periasamy's group showing contractile changes similar to those described below [3]. Characterization of a heterozygous transgenic mouse line showed that the amount of SERCA2 mRNA increased 2.6-fold. In addition, phospholamban mRNA increased 1.5-fold and the sodium calcium exchanger RNA increased 1.8-fold. However, at the protein level phospholamban and sodium calcium exchanger levels were not altered and sodium calcium exchanger function was not changed in the myocytes from the transgenic mice [21]. In spite of a more than 2-fold increase in SERCA2 mRNA levels, protein levels for SERCA only increased 1.2-fold. To determine the discrepancy for the difference in marked changes in mRNA levels and much lower increases in protein levels, we determined the relative synthesis rate of the SERCA2 protein, which was increased by 82%. One could therefore speculate that the longitudinal SR, which is the site of SERCA2 incorporation, is already filled with SERCA pumps not leaving much room for additional incorporation of SERCA protein. SERCA protein being expressed in the cytoplasm and not finding its proper site of incorporation is probably rapidly degraded. To determine the consequences of increased SERCA activity, we determined contractile parameters in the heart from the SERCA mice under *in vivo* conditions, in papillary muscle strips, and in isolated myocytes. One would predict from increased expression of SERCA2 pump protein that an accelerated decline of the calcium transient occurs leading to an increasing rate of diastolic relaxation. Furthermore, one could postulate that increase SERCA pump activity leads to increased filling of the sarcoplasmic reticulum and increased release of calcium during the next systolic cycle. We determined cardiac function *in vivo* using a 1.8 French Milar micromanometer-tipped catheter and showed a 20% to 25% increase in dP/dt max and a similar decrease in dP/dt min leading to an acceleration of τ by 20% in SERCA2 transgenic mice. Calcium transients determined in isolated myocytes indicated that the intracellular calcium decline and myocyte relengthening were accelerated by 23% and 22%, respectively. These findings demonstrate that the *in vivo* contractile parameters and load- indepedent contractile function determined in myocytes show similar increases. In addition, in collaboration with Dr. Barry, the calcium content of the sarcoplasmic reticulum was determined in voltage-clamped myocytes with a rapid solution switcher by determining the sodium calcium exchanger-mediated current. These data showed that the SR calcium content is increased by 29% in SERCA transgenic mice [21]. We would also like to note that overexpression of SERCA2 leading to enhanced lusitrophy did not result in altered energetics in the mouse hearts. In particular, overexpression of SERCA2 did not lead to changes in myocardial high energy phosphate contents either at baseline levels or at high work loads. One can therefore conclude from these studies that overexpression of SERCA2 in normal hearts enhances cardiac lusitrophy while maintaining normal pressure development and myocardial high energy phosphate content [20].

To determine if the increased expression of SERCA2 would have a compensatory effect towards diminished SERCA2 expression under *in vivo* conditions, we determined the effects of hypothyroidism on cardiac function. In hypothyroid rodent models SERCA2 mRNA protein and SERCA2 activity is significantly decreased [6]. When mice-overexpressing SERCA2 were made hypothyroid and their contractile behavior was studied using isolated papillary muscle obtained from wild-type euthyroid and hypothyroid mice and SERCA2 transgenic euthyroid and hypothyroid mice, a significant compensatory effect occurred [6]. The prolonged contraction and relaxation of papillary muscle which occurred in muscle obtained from hypothyroid wild-type mice was significantly improved in muscle from hypothyroid SERCA2 transgenic mice.

Using adenoviral vectors expressing calcium-handling proteins

In subsequent studies, we wanted to determine whether adenovirus-mediated expression of proteins related to calcium handling like SERCA and phospholamban and mutants of phospholamban could normalize prolonged calcium transients associated with downregulation of SERCA2 levels. Conventional human adenovirus 5 vectors with E1 deletion were used for this purpose [17]. A transgene consisting of SV 40 enhances TK promoters and a rat SERCA2 gene were cloned into the E1 region of an adenovirus-related shuttle plasmid, adenoviral particles which are infectious but replication deficient of titers at 10^9 to 10^{10} plaque forming units were obtained. Exposure of neonatal myocytes to the phorbol ester phorbol-12-myristate-13-acetate (PMA) leads to a significant decrease in the expression of the endogenous SERCA gene product and results in prolongation of the calcium transient [9]. SERCA2 adenovirus infection increases SERCA2 mRNA levels 2.5-fold and reconstitutes SERCA2 protein levels from PMA-treated myocytes. This reconstitution is associated with a 32% reduction in the time of decline of an indol-tracked calcium transient to the half maximal decline of the calcium levels. A 34% augmentation of calcium oxalate-facilitated SR calcium uptake was also documented in SERCA2 adenovirus-infected cells.

Interfering with phospholamban action

An alternate mechanism to increase SERCA2 activity is by inhibiting phospholamban activity. This can be achieved by diminishing phospholamban protein levels using an antisense or anti-phospholamban ribozyme approach. Furthermore, phospholamban action can be diminished by using phospholamban mutants which have decreased SERCA2 interaction. The detailed mechanisms of phospholamban to SERCA interaction are currently somewhat speculative and it is currently unclear if the monomer of phospholamban or phospholamban as multimers, for example, as a pentameter, exerts the inhibitory effects on SERCA2 action [8, 14]. The interaction sites in the cytoplasmic region of phospholamban with SERCA were mapped to amino acid 1 to 20 and to amino acids 30 to 52 in the intermembrane region of phospholamban [2]. The cytoplasmic region of phospholamban forms a helical loop in which positively and negatively charged amino acids of phospholamban and SERCA strongly interact with each other. It could be postulated that phosphorylation of threonine in the phospholamban-cytoplasmic region might, for example, lead to an awakening of the electrostatic-based phospholamban SERCA interacting. To explore the possibility of increasing SERCA2 action by construction dominant negative phospholamban, a mutant was explored in further detail. We constructed mutants in which the lysine at amino acid position 3 of phospholamban was replaced by glutamic acid and the arginine at position 14 was also replaced by glutamic acid [12]. In addition, phospholamban in the antisense orientation was cloned into an adenoviral vector [12]. Cardiac myocytes were infected with phospholamban antisense and mutant constructs, and 3 days later calcium handling was determined using oxalate-facilitated calcium uptake in neonatal myocytes. Indo calcium flux was determined, and contractility measurements using an edge detection approach were performed in adult rabbit cardiac myocytes. In an alternate approach, expression plasmids were constructed with phospholamban-antisense or phospholamban-mutant constructs and myocytes were co-transfected with such plasmids and myocytes expressing the green fluorescent protein. In this way transfected plasmids could be idenified and calcium transients could be determined on such myocytes [13]. Calcium uptake measurements in neonatal rat cardiac myocytes infected with the double phospholamban mutant or the phospholamban antisense indicated that a significant increase in SERCA activity occurs. The phospholamban double mutant K3E/R14E increased SERCA activity by 35% and the phospholamban antisense construct increased SERCA activity by 25%. Similarly calcium transients were markedly accelerated using the phospholamban double mutant in neonatal myocytes [12]. Furthermore, adult rabbit myocytes were infected with the phospholamban double mutant or antisense constructs using adenoviral vectors, and contractile behavior was determined by an edge detection type of approach. The rate of relengthening measured as -DL/-DT was significantly increased in adult rabbit myocytes infected with the phospholamban double mutant. Infection with a phospholamban antisense construct also lead to an increase in the rate of relengthening but to a lesser extent than that obtained with the phospholamban double mutant. To assure that the phospholamban mutant is part of the phospholamban complex, Western blots were performed with a specific chicken-raised phospholamban antibody which recognized the phospholamban mutant [12].

Conclusion

In summary, our results using increased expression of the SERCA pump in transgenic mice or using an adenoviral vector-based approach increases the calcium transient and contractile behavior. Similar results were obtained by inhibiting phospholamban action using the dominant negative phospholamban mutant or decreasing phospholamban levels by phospholamban antisense construct. These results may indicate that increased SERCA2 activity has a beneficial effect on cardiac function. Furthermore, preliminary results indicate that increased SERCA2 activity is not combined with decreased ATP levels. Approaches to increase SERCA2 activity may be useful in the future for the treatment of congestive heart failure using a viral vector-based approach.

References

1. Antipenko QY, Spielman AL, Kirchberger MA (1997) Comparison of the effects of phospholamban and jasmone on the calcium pump of cardiac sarcoplasmic reticulum. J Biol Chem 272:2852–2860
2. ATPase of cardiac sarcoplasmic reticulum are critical for functional association with phospholamban. J Biol Chem 269:22929–22932
3. Baker DL, Hashimoto K, Grupp IL, Ji Y, Reed T, Loukianov E, Grupp G, Bhagwhat A, Hoit B, Walsh R et al (1998) Targeted overexpression of the sarcoplasmic reticulum Ca^{2+} ATPase increases cardiac contractility in transgenic mouse hearts. Circulation Research 83(12):1205–1214
4. Bassani RA, Bassani JW, Bers DM (1992] Mitochondrial and sarcolemmal Ca^{2+} transport reduce $[Ca^{2+}]_i$ during caffeine contractures in rabbit cardiac myocytes. Journal of Physiology 453:591–608
5. Bers DM, Berlin JR (1995) Kinetics of [Ca]i decline in cardiac myocytes depend on peak [Ca]i. American Journal of Physiology 268 (Pt 1):C271–C277
6. Bluhm WF, Meyer M, Sayen MR, Swanson EA, Dillmann WH (1999) Overexpression of sarcoplasmic reticulum Ca^{2+}-ATPase improves cardiac contractile function in hypothyroid mice. Cardiovascular Research 43:382–388
7. Carafoli E (1987) Intracellular calcium homeostasis. Annu Rev Biochem 56:395–433
8. Chu G, Dorn GW, Luo W, Harrer M, Kadambi VJ, Walsh RA, Kranias EG (1997) Monomeric phospholamban overexpression in transgenic mouse hearts. Circ Res 91:485–492
9. Giordano FJ, He H, McDonough P, Meyer M, Sayen MR, Dillmann WH (1997) Adenovirus-mediated gene transfer reconstitutes depressed sarcoplasmic reticulum Ca^{2+} ATPase levels and shortens prolonged cardiac myocyte Ca^{2+} transients. Circulation 96:400–403

10. Gwathmey JK, Copolas L, MacKinnon R, Schoen FJ, Feldman MD, Grossman W, Morgan JP (1987) Abnormal intracellular calcium handling in myocardium from patients with end-stage heart failure. Circ Res 61:70–76
11. He H, Giordano FJ, Hilal-Dandan R, Rockman HA, McDonough PM, Sayen MR, Swanson E, Dillmann WH (1997) Overexpression of the rat sarcoplasmic reticulum (SR) Ca^{2+} ATPase gene in the heart of transgenic mice accelerates calcium transients and cardiac relaxation. J Clin Invest 100:380–389
12. He H, Meyer M, Martin JL, McDonough PM, Ho P, Xiaojing L, Wilbur YW, Hilal-Dandan R, Dillmann WH (1999) Effects of mutant and antisense RNA of phospholamban on SR Ca^{2+}-ATPase activity and cardiac myocyte contractility. Circulation 100:974–980
13. Ho PD, Zechner DK, He H, Dillmann WH, Glembotski CG, McDonough PM (1998) The Raf-MEK-ERK cascade represents a common pathway for alteration of intracellular calcium by ras and protein kinase C in cardiac myocytes. Journal of Biological Chemistry 273(34):21730–21735
14. Kimura Y, Kurzydlowski K, Tada M, MacLennan DH (1997) Phospholamban inhibitory function is activated by depolymerization. J Biol Chem 272:15061–15064
15. Lenfant C (1994) Report of the task force on research in heart failure. Circulation 90:1118–1123
16. Luo W, Grupp IL, Harrer J, Ponniah S, Grupp G, Duffy JJ, Doetschman T, Kranias EG (1994) Targeted ablation of the phospholamban gene is associated with markedly enhanced myocardial contractility and loss of β-agonist stimulation. Circ Res 75:401–409
17. Mestril R, Giordano FJ, Conde AG, Dillmann WH (1996) Adenovirus-mediated gene transfer of a heat shock protein 70 (hsp 70i) protects against simulated ischemia. Journal of Molecular and Cellular Cardiology 28(12):2351–2358
18. Meyer M, Schillinger W, Pieske B, Holubarsch C, Heilmann C, Posival H, Kuwajima G, Mikoshiba K, Just H, Hasenfuß G (1995) Alterations of sarcoplasmic reticulum proteins in failing human dilated cardiomyopathy. Circulation 92:778–784
19. Movsesian MA, Karimi M, Green K, Jones LR (1994) Ca^{2+}-transporting ATPase, phospholamban, and calsequestrin levels in nonfailing and failing human myocardium. Circulation 90:653–657
20. Tian R, Shen W, Dillmann WH, Ingwall JS (1998) Enhanced lusitrophy with unaltered energetics in mouse hearts overexpressing SERCA2. Circulation (Suppl) 98(17):727 (abstract)
21. Yao A, Su Z, Dillmann WH, Barry WH (1998) Sarcoplasmic reticulum function in murine ventricular myocytes overexpressing SR CaATPase. Journal of Molecular and Cellular Cardiology 30(12):2711–2718

CHAPTER 6

Adenovirus-mediated gene transfer of SERCA isoforms

G. INESI, M. CAVAGNA, J.M. O'DONNELL, C. SUMBILLA, L. ZHONG, H. MA, M.G. KLEIN

Department of Biochemistry and Molecular Biology, University of Maryland School of Medicine, Baltimore, MD, USA

Summary

Cultured chicken embryonic or neonatal rat cardiac myocytes were infected with recombinant adenovirus vectors carrying slow muscle SERCA2a or fast muscle SERCA1a cDNA, under control of muscle-specific or constitutive viral promoters. Under optimal conditions, exogenous SERCA expression was obtained in all myocytes in culture, yielding approximately a threefold increase in the level of SERCA protein, and a three- to sixfold increase in the Ca^{2+} transport activity depending on whether SERCA2a or SERCA1a cDNA was used. The kinetics of cytosolic Ca^{2+} transients upon membrane excitation were also affected, with a prominent increase in the rate of decline due to faster Ca^{2+} sequestration by the sarcoplasmic reticulum.

Introduction

Intracellular Ca^{2+} stores play a very important role in several cellular functions by providing signaling Ca^{2+} through their release channels, and in turn serving as a sink for cytosolic Ca^{2+} which is sequestered by active transport. The Ca^{2+}-dependent ATPase (SERCA) associated with sarco- and endoplasmic reticulum membranes is the operator of active transport whereby Ca^{2+} is removed from the cytosol and stored in membrane-bound intracellular compartments. Three SERCA isoforms have been cloned and their splice variants identified in various tissues [6, 12, 32, 33]. Of these, SERCA1a is specifically associated with the sarcoplasmic reticulum (SR) of fast skeletal muscle [3, 4, 34], and SERCA2a is associated with the SR of cardiac muscle and slow skeletal muscle [1]. In muscle, SERCA is involved in excitation-contraction coupling by filling the SR stores with Ca^{2+} to be released for activation of myofibrils [9]. In turn, sequestration of cytosolic Ca^{2+} by SERCA initiates relaxation and determines its kinetics. Consistent with a prominent role of SR in excitation-contraction coupling, it was reported that thapsigargin, a specific inhibitor of SERCA, drastically reduces cytosolic Ca^{2+} transients and tension development in rat cardiac myocytes, without significant effects on membrane action potentials [27]. Reduced expression and/or inadequate function of endogenous SERCA2a may contribute to alterations of Ca^{2+}

homeostasis and contractile function in cardiac muscle [16, 37, 40]. Impaired cardiac performance has been demonstrated in heterozygous mice with a null mutation in the SERCA2a gene [39].

Transfer of SERCA cDNA into cultured cells

SERCA gene transfer and heterologous expression in cultured cells has been used to carry out extensive mutational analyses of the Ca^{2+} ATPase catalytic and transport cycle [36]. The technology of gene transfer has also opened the way for modulation of SERCA expression and studies of its effects on cell functions [10, 13, 14, 17, 22, 23, 29]. For this purpose, stable expression of exogenous SERCA can be obtained by co-transfection of immortalized cell lines with SERCA cDNA and a selectable gene [19]. The resulting cell lines have been quite useful in studies of the effect of thapsigargin on cell proliferation, and the development of resistance to thapsigargin [20]. Transient expression, on the other hand, is in many respects more convenient since it requires shorter times of induction and yields higher levels of recombinant protein. We find that adenovirus vectors [25, 28] provide a very efficient

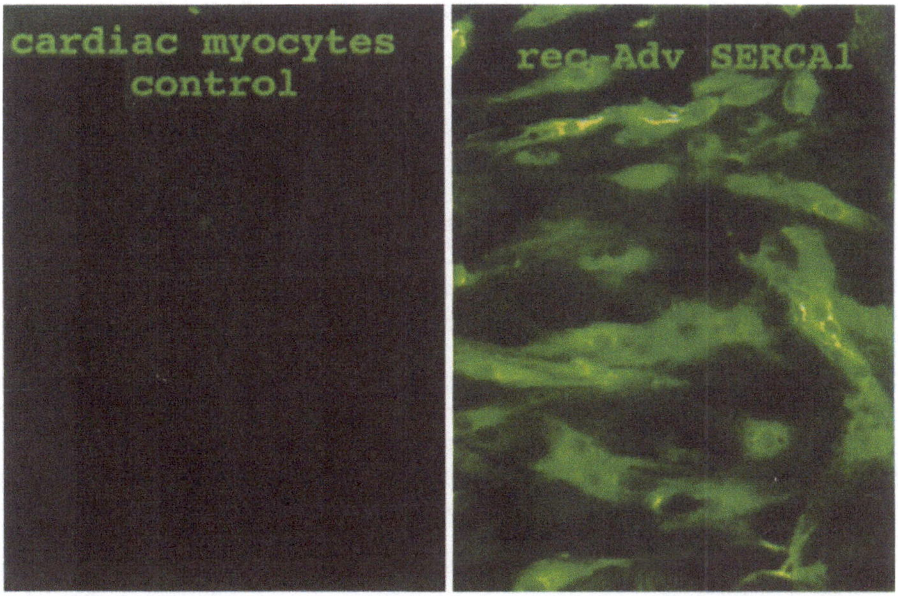

Fig. 1. Efficiency of SERCA1a adenovirus-mediated gene transfer. Chicken embryonic cardiac myocytes were infected with recombinant adenovirus vectors carrying the SERCA1a cDNA under control of the cTnT promoter (*right*), or without SERCA cDNA (*left*). The myocytes were fixed 48 h after infection, and stained with primary SERCA1a mAb and secondary fluorescent Ab. Note the high density of myocytes expressing the SERCA1a protein on the right panel and the lack of any signal in the control panel (from [22]).

method for gene delivery and transient expression in cultured cells, when compared to conventional methods using liposomes, calcium phosphate or DEAE-dextran. In fact, it is possible to efficiently transfect 100% of the cells in culture by the use of adenovirus vectors (Fig. 1), as opposed to 5–10% by other methods. Such high efficiency has the advantage of yielding larger amounts of recombinant protein for biochemical studies, and providing homogeneous overexpression of SERCA for studies of cell functions.

Adenovirus vectors are produced by co-transfecting HEK293 cells with an unpackageable adenovirus DNA plasmid and a shuttle plasmid containing the gene and promoter of interest [11]. Homologous recombination between these plasmids generates a packageable virus containing the gene of interest. While a deletion in the virus genome makes it replication-defective in most cells, the virus can replicate in HEK293 cells because they have been transformed with viral gene elements complementing the deletion present in the recombinant virus. Alternative methods of recombination utilize viral DNA with prokaryotic recombination sites transfected in cell lines derived from HEK293 lines [15], or recombination in bacteria followed by packaging in HEK293 cells [18]. We constructed our shuttle vectors with either SERCA1a or SERCA2a cDNA followed by a c-myc immunogenic tag at the carboxyl terminus [22]. Alternatively, we use a reporter gene such as the enhanced green fluorescence protein (EGFP). These genes can be placed under control of a strong constitutive promoter such as the cytomegalovirus (CMV) promoter, or a muscle-specific promoter (Fig. 2).

Overexpression of SERCA isoforms in cardiac myocytes

Expression of a foreign SERCA gene in cardiac myocytes can be visualized by fluorescence microscopy (Fig. 3) after staining with primary monoclonal and fluorescent secondary antibodies. Foreign SERCA1a and endogenous SERCA2a can be easily detected by the use of isoform-specific antibodies [7, 24]. On the other hand, foreign SERCA2a can be visualized by detecting an immunogenic tag that distinguishes the foreign SERCA2a from the endogenous SERCA2a. Microscopic studies show that the protein encoded by the foreign SERCA is targeted to the sarcoplasmic reticulum membrane with a pattern very similar to endogenous SERCA2a (Fig. 3).

A useful transfection expedient is the use of cell-specific promoters. In fact, we found (Fig. 4) that SERCA expression can be limited to myocytes, without detectable expression in fibroblasts, by placing the SERCA gene under control of the cTnT minimal promoter [35]. Although cell-specific promoters tend to be weaker than constitutive viral promoters, equivalent levels of expression can be obtained in myocytes by increasing adequately the adenovirus vector titer and, thereby, the gene copy number and transcriptional level [22, 42].

Expression of exogenous SERCA gene in chicken embryonic and rat neonatal cardiac myocytes can be assessed by Western blots, using either

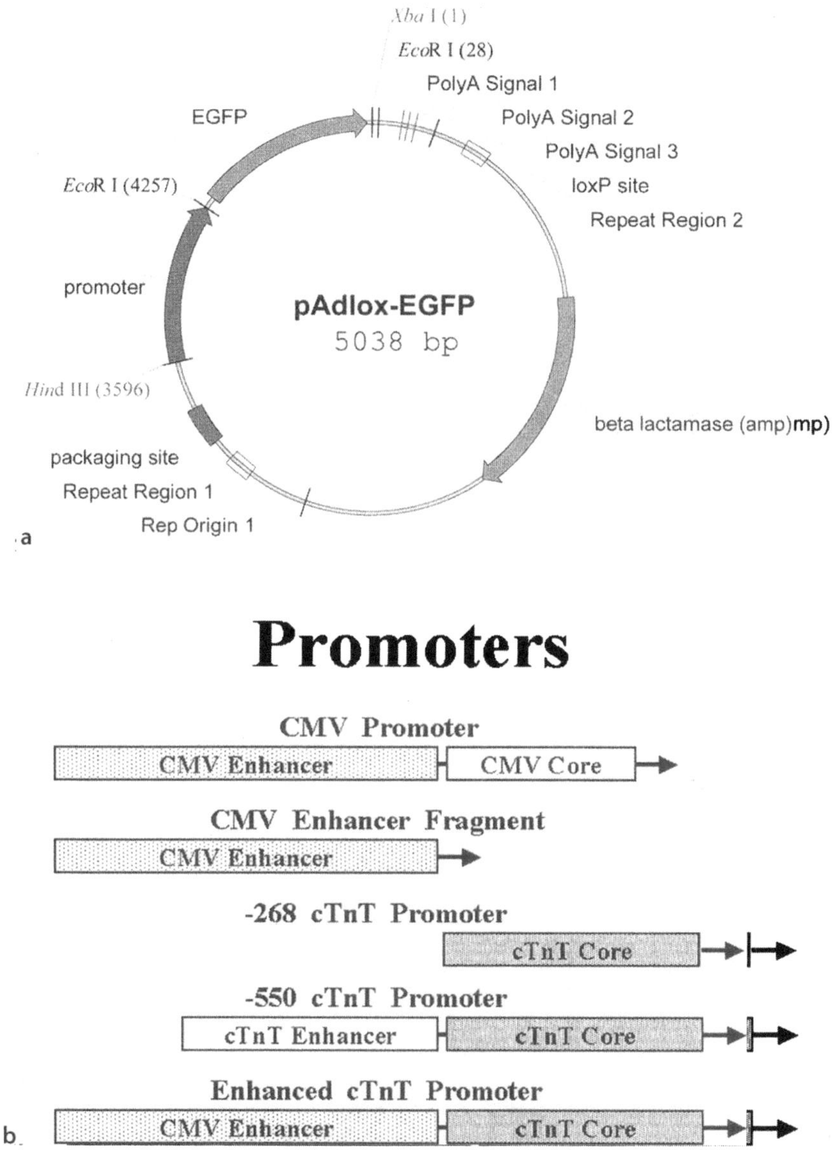

Fig. 2. Construction of shuttle plasmids for generation of adenovirus vectors by homologous recombination. **a** The cDNA-encoding EGFP (reporter gene) or SERCA isoforms were inserted between EcoR I and Xba I sites downstream of the promoter region. **b** Various promoters used in our studies include the constitutive promoter of cytomegalovirus (CMV), the CMV enhancer, the muscle-specific cardiac troponin T minimal promoter segment (–268 cTnT), a longer cTnT promoter segment including its homologous enhancer (–550 cTnT), and a CMV-enhanced cTnT promoter (from [42]).

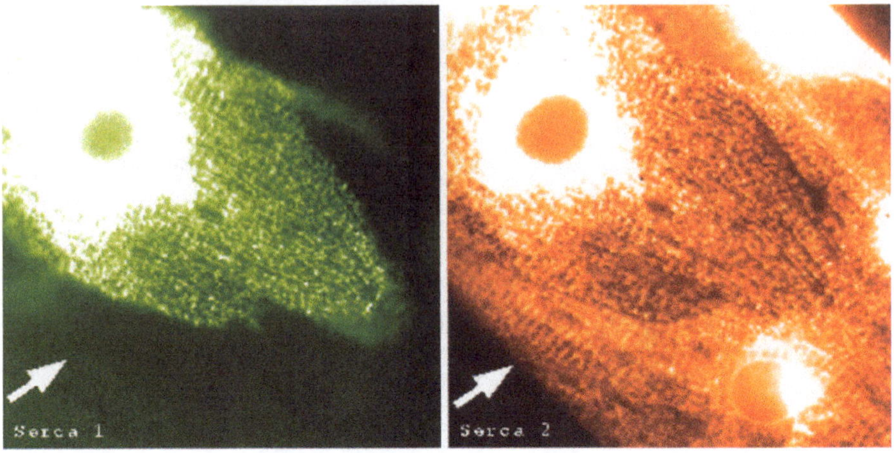

Fig. 3. Intracellular targeting of recombinant SERCA1a. Chicken embryonic cardiac myocytes were infected with recombinant adenovirus vector carrying chicken SERCA1a cDNA under control of the CMV promoter. Two days after infection the myocytes were fixed and stained, first with chicken SERCA1a mAb and FITC-conjugated secondary Ab, then with chicken SERCA2a mAb and Texas red-conjugated secondary Ab. Due to non-specific secondary Ab reactivity, a rigorous comparison of targeting can only be made between the myocyte on the *left panel*, and the lower (non-infected with SERCA1a) myocyte on the *right panel*. The figure shows a similar targeting pattern for the recombinant SERCA1a and the endogenous SERCA2a.

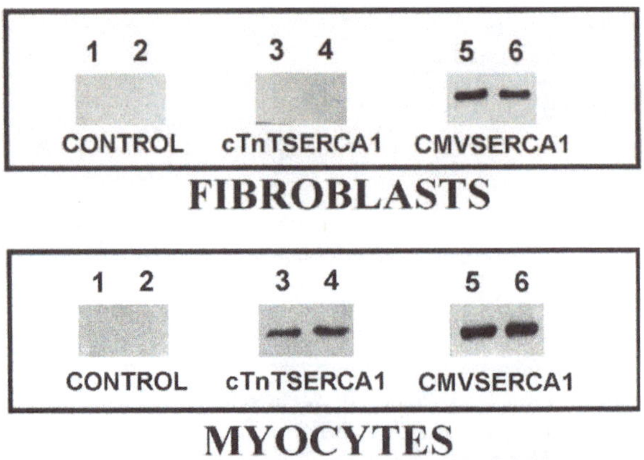

Fig. 4. Western blots showing promoter specificity. Chicken embryonic skin fibroblasts or cardiac myocytes were infected with recombinant adenovirus vector carrying SERCA1a cDNA under control of either the muscle-specific cTnT promoter or the constitutive CMV promoter. The cells were harvested 48 h following infection, and homogenized samples were subjected to Western blotting by the use of SERCA1a-specific mAb. Note that no SERCA1a expression is demonstrated in control cells and in fibroblasts in which the SERCA1a cDNA was under control of the cell-specific cTnT promoter (from [22]).

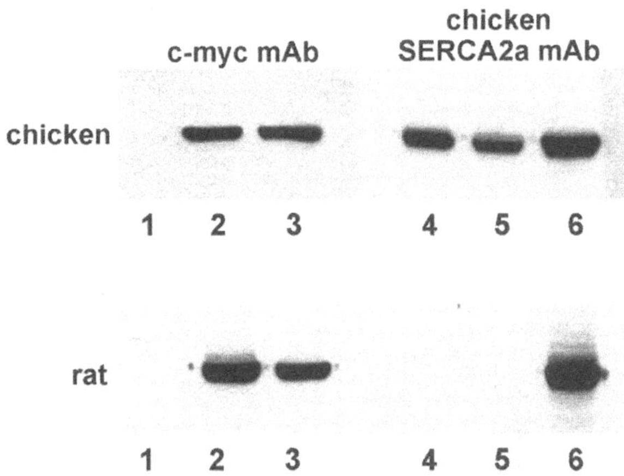

Fig. 5. SERCA isoform expression in chicken and rat cardiac myocytes. Western blots were used to detect the expression of endogenous SERCA2a (lanes 1 and 4), recombinant SERCA1a (lanes 2 and 5), and recombinant SERCA2a (lanes 3 and 6). Immunodetection was obtained using either a c-myc mAb (reactive with a tag in both recombinant enzymes), or a chicken SERCA2a mAb (reactive with endogenous SERCA2a of chicken myocytes, and with recombinant chicken SERCA2a). Note that the c-myc mAb detects both recombinant SERCA1a and SERCA2a, but not endogenous SERCA in chicken and rat myocytes. Note also that the chicken SERCA2a mAb does not cross-react with endogenous SERCA2a of rat myocytes. In the chicken myocyte samples, it is shown that endogenous SERCA2a (lane 4) decreases to about half upon infection with SERCA1a (lane 5). Infection with SERCA2a (lane 6) shows the increase over and above the endogenous level (lane 4).

antibodies reactive to a common immunogenic tag, or isoform-specific antibodies (Fig. 5). It is of interest that when the adenovirus vector titer is raised above the level required to infect 100% of the myocytes in culture, protein expression is further increased due to a higher gene copy number in each cell. However, while expression of soluble proteins such as EGFP continues to increase in proportion to the gene copy number, SERCA expression reaches a maximal level after which no further expression can be obtained (Fig. 6 A). Because Northern blots reveal a rise in mRNA-outpacing protein levels, we conclude that the asymptotic character of SERCA protein expression is not due to a transcriptional block, but rather to post-transcriptional events possibly related to membrane assembly (Fig. 6 B). Our observations explain some discrepancies in mRNA and protein expression levels that have been reported in previous articles [2].

It is then important to define the ratio between the maximal level of foreign SERCA gene expression and the level of endogenous SERCA2a in the cardiac myocytes. In previous studies on isolated myocytes [10, 13, 14] and in transgenic animals [17, 23, 29], exogenous SERCA2a or SERCA1a gene expression produced a 1.5–2.5 fold increase relative to the endogenous SERCA level. By careful titration with increasing titers of adenovirus vectors, we demonstrated that it is possible to obtain SERCA1a levels approximately three times higher than the endogenous SERCA2a level of con-

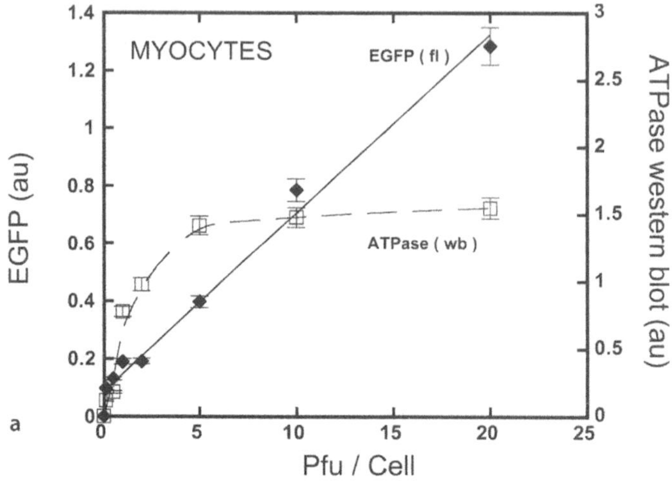

a

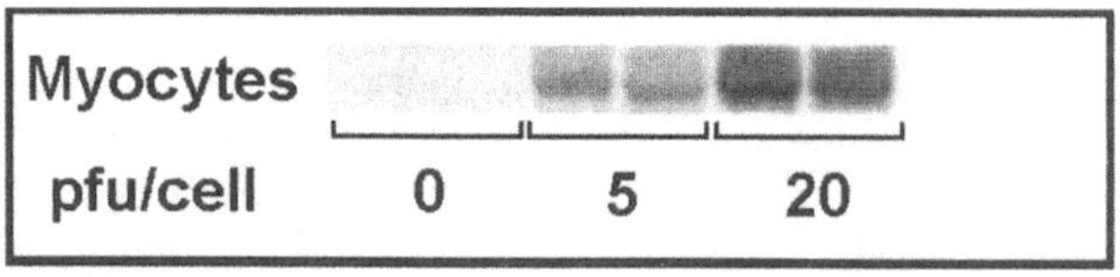

b

Fig. 6. a Expression of EGFP and SERCA1a in chicken embryonic cardiac myocytes following infections with various levels of adenovirus vectors. The EGFP expression was quantitated by fluorescence measurements, and SERCA expression by Western blotting. Note that while SERCA1a expression reaches 100% of maximum at 5–10 pfu/cell ratios, EGFP titer is increased to 20 pfu/cell. **b** Northern blots showing transcription efficiency of SERCA1a as a function of recombinant adenovirus pfu level. For each pfu level, duplicate experiments are shown indicating a continuously increasing level of mRNA produced with increasing amount of adenovirus pfu/cell ratio (from [42]).

trol myocytes [42]. We also observed that, under these conditions, the endogenous SERCA2a expression is reduced to about half; therefore the exogenous SERCA expression level is actually seven times higher than the residual endogenous SERCA2a. These experiments define the maximal level of alternative isoform expression that can be reached, and indicate that optimal expression requires careful manipulation of the gene transfer parameters.

Comparative function of recombinant SERCA isoforms

When SERCA1a or SERCA2a gene copies are increased to yield maximal expression, equivalent levels of either SERCA1a or SERCA2a protein are obtained, as revealed by Western blots. Yet, the Ca^{2+} transport activity is nearly twice higher for the SERCA1a enzyme, as compared with SERCA2a (Fig. 7A). The higher turnover of the SERCA1a enzyme can be further

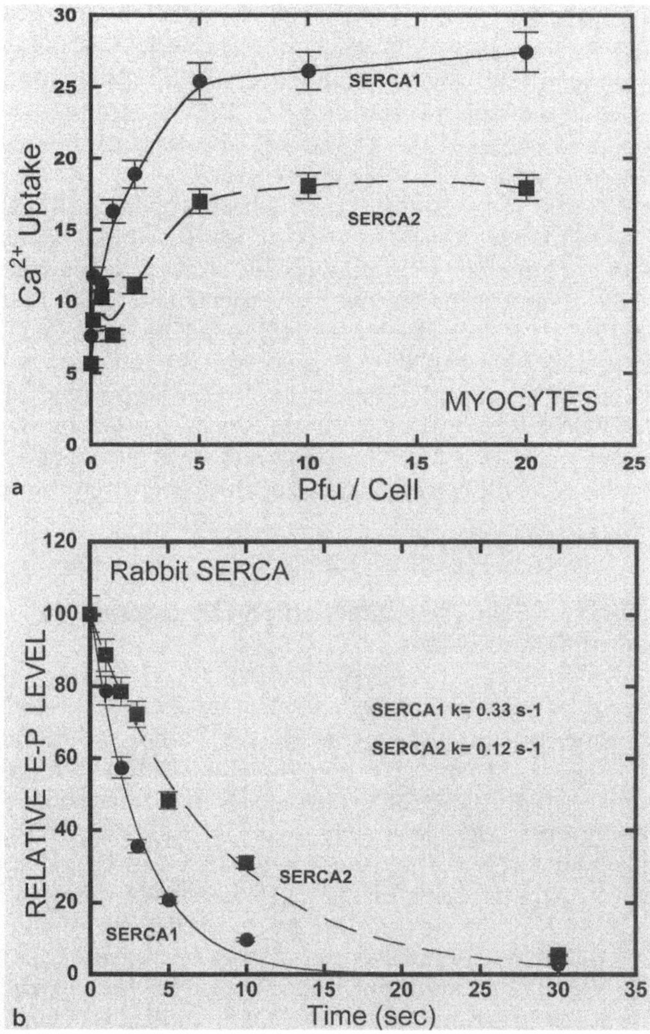

Fig. 7. Comparative activities of recombinant SERCA1a and SERCA2b. **a** Ca^{2+} transport velocities of chicken embryonic cardiac myocyte lysates infected with increasing levels of recombinant adenovirus vector carrying either SERCA1a or SERCA2a cDNA. Note that, under conditions of maximal expression, the myocytes infected with SERCA1a sustain approximately twofold higher activity than myocytes infected with SERCA2a. The activity of control myocytes (0 pfu) corresponds to the endogenous SERCA2a. **b** Exponential decay of radioactive phosphorylated enzyme intermediate following a chase with non-radioactive ATP. Recombinant SERCA1a and SERCA2a samples were microsomes from COS-1 cells infected with adenovirus vectors. Note that the rate constant is approximately twice faster for the SERCA1a enzyme (from [42]).

demonstrated by measuring the decay of radioactive phosphorylated enzyme intermediate, following a chase with non-radioactive ATP [42]. The observed decay (Fig. 7 B), which corresponds to the rate-limiting step for the catalytic and transport cycle [22], is exponential and independent of protein concentration. Therefore, ambiguities related to the accuracy of SERCA1a and SERCA2a concentrations in the experiment, shown in Fig. 7 B, are not in question. It is then apparent that the Ca^{2+} transport activity of myocytes can actually be increased significantly more if SERCA1a cDNA, rather than SERCA2a cDNA, is used in the transfection procedure.

SERCA activation by Ca^{2+} is expected to be influenced by phospholamban [5, 7, 26, 30, 31, 38, 41, 43, 44]. On the other hand, in our experiments, recombinant SERCA isoforms did not display the characteristics of regulation by phospholamban. It should be pointed out that overexpression of SERCA by gene transfer is not accompanied by overexpression of phospholamban [29, 42]. This suggests that endogenous phospholamban is present at limiting concentrations and is entirely bound to the endogenous SERCA.

Effect of SERCA1a expression on the cytosolic Ca^{2+} transients of cardiac myocytes

Release of Ca^{2+} from intracellular stores upon membrane excitation, and subsequent removal of cytosolic Ca^{2+} upon membrane repolarization, results in a transient rise in cytosolic Ca^{2+} which serves as the signaling mechanism for coupling contraction and relaxation of myofibrils to membrane events. The basic role of the sarcoplasmic reticulum is to provide intracellular Ca^{2+} stores from which Ca^{2+} can be released. With specific reference to the kinetics of the Ca^{2+} transients, one may intuitively infer that the SERCA pump has an influence on the rate of Ca^{2+} return from the cytosol to the SR lumen. We previously observed [22] Ca^{2+} transients following repetitive stimulation of chicken embryonic cardiac myocytes by monitoring the fluorescence of the Ca^{2+} indicator Fluo-3. In agreement with other investigators [10, 14, 17, 29, 45], we found that the decay phase of the transients was accelerated in myocytes infected with recombinant adenovirus carrying SERCA1a cDNA. The infected myocytes also exhibited faster contraction-relaxation cycles. We have now monitored Ca^{2+} transients both in chicken embryonic and neonatal rat cardiac myocytes, using dual-wavelength measurements of Fura-2 fluorescence emission. It is shown in Fig. 8 that, in both chicken and rat myocytes, the Ca^{2+} transients of infected myocytes exhibit much faster decays and narrower half-widths. As the Fura-2 measurements allow estimates of Ca^{2+} concentrations, we were able to determine that resting and peak Ca^{2+} were not significantly affected. This is in agreement with the observations by Yao et al. [45], but in apparent disagreement with those by Loukianov et al. [29], who found a 71% increase in the amplitude of the Ca^{2+} transients. It is possible that

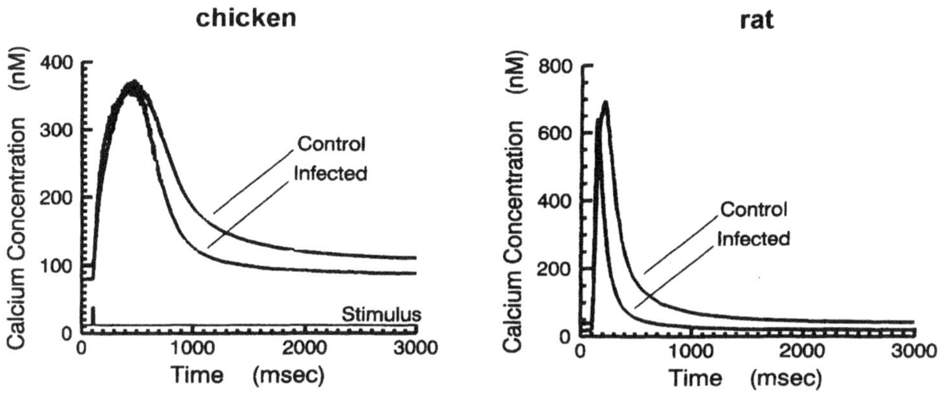

Fig. 8. Cytosolic Ca^{2+} transients in single cells. Chicken embryonic (*left*) and neonatal rat (*right*) cardiac myocytes were infected with recombinant adenovirus vector carrying SERCA1a cDNA under control of the CMV promoter. The Ca^{2+} transients were monitored by measuring FURA2 fluorescence, following single field stimuli. Relative Ca^{2+} concentrations are similar in all experimental groups. Half-widths and decay constants are significantly reduced in infected, as compared with non-infected myocytes.

this difference is due to experimental conditions that may or may not limit the Ca^{2+} filling of sarcoplasmic reticulum by the endogenous SERCA. At any rate, we conclude that the Ca^{2+} signaling mechanism of cardiac myocytes is most significantly affected by overexpression of exogenous fast muscle SERCA1a isoform, under optimal conditions of gene transfer by recombinant adenovirus vectors.

References

1. Arai M, Otsu K, MacLennan DH, Periasamy M (1992) Regulation of sarcoplasmic reticulum gene expression during cardiac and skeletal muscle development. Am J Physiol Cell Physiol 262:C614–C620
2. Baker DL, Hashimoto K, Grupp IL, Ji Y, Reed T, Loukianov E, Grupp G, Bhagwhat A, Hoit B, Walsh R, Marban E, Periasamy M (1998) Targeted overexpression of the sarcoplasmic reticulum Ca^{2+}-ATPase increases cardiac contractility in transgenic mouse hearts. Circ Res 83(12):1205–1214
3. Brandl CJ, Green NM, Korczak B, MacLennan DH (1986) Two Ca^{2+}-ATPase genes: homologies and mechanistic implications of deduced amino acid sequences. Cell 44:597–607
4. Brandl CJ, DeLeon S, Martin DR, MacLennan DH (1987) Adult forms of the Ca^{2+} ATPase of sarcoplasmic reticulum. Expression in developing skeletal muscle. J Biol Chem 262:3768–3774
5. Briggs FN, Lee KF, Wechsler AW, Jones LR (1992) Phospholamban expressed in slow-twitch and chronically stimulated fast-twitch muscles minimally affects calcium affinity of sarcoplasmic reticulum Ca^{2+}-ATPase. J Biol Chem 267:26056–26061
6. Burk SE, Lytton J, MacLennan DH, Shull GE (1989) cDNA cloning, functional expression, and mRNA tissue distribution of a third organellar Ca^{2+} pump. J Biol Chem 264:18561–18568

7. Campbell AM, Kessler PD, Sagara Y, Inesi G, Fambrough DM (1991) Nucleotide sequences of avian cardiac and brain SR/ER Ca^{2+}-ATPases and functional comparisons with fast twitch Ca^{2+}-ATPase. Calcium affinities and inhibitor effects. J Biol Chem 266:16050–16055
8. Cantilina T, Sagara Y, Inesi G, Jones LR (1993) Comparative studies of cardiac and skeletal sarcoplasmic reticulum ATPases. J Biol Chem 268(23):17018–17025
9. Fabiato A (1985) Time and calcium dependence of activation and inactivation of calcium-induced release of calcium from the sarcoplasmic reticulum of a skinned canine cardiac Purkinje cell. J Gen Physiol 85:247–289
10. Giordano FJ, He HP, McDonough P, Meyer M, Sayen MR, Dillmann WH (1997) Adenovirus-mediated gene transfer reconstitutes depressed sarcoplasmic reticulum Ca^{2+}-ATPase levels and shortens prolonged cardiac myocyte Ca^{2+} transients. Circulation 96:400–403
11. Graham FL, Prevec L (1992) Adenovirus based expression vectors and recombinant vaccines. In: Ellis RW (ed) Vaccines: New Approaches to Immunological Problems, Vol 1. Butterworth-Heinemann, Boston, pp 363–390
12. Gunteski-Hamblin A-M, Greeb J, Shull GE (1988) A novel Ca^{2+} pump expressed in brain, kidney, and stomach is encoded by an alternative transcript of the slow-twitch muscle sarcoplasmic reticulum Ca-ATPase gene. Identification of cDNAs encoding Ca^{2+} and other cation-transporting ATPases using an oligonucleotide probe derived from the ATP-binding site. J Biol Chem 263:15032–15040
13. Hajjar RJ, Schmidt U, Kang JX, Matsui T, Rosenzweig A (1997) Adenoviral gene transfer of phospholamban in isolated rat cardiomyocytes – Rescue effects by concomitant gene transfer of sarcoplasmic reticulum Ca^{2+}-ATPase. Circ Res 81(2):145–153
14. Hajjar RJ, Kang JX, Gwathmey JK, Rosenzweig A (1997) Physiological effects of adenoviral gene transfer of sarcoplasmic reticulum calcium ATPase in isolated rat myocytes. Circulation 95:423–429
15. Hardy S, Kitamura M, Harris-Stansil T, Dai Y, Phipps ML (1997) Construction of adenovirus vectors through Cre-lox recombination. J Virol 71(3):1842–1849
16. Hasenfuss G, Reinecke H, Studer R, Meyer M, Pieske B, Holtz J, Holubarsch C, Posival HJ, Drexler H (1994) Relation between myocardial function and expression of sarcoplasmic reticulum Ca^{2+}-ATPase in failing and nonfailing human myocardium. Circ Res 75:434–442
17. He HP, Giordano FJ, Hilal-Dandan R, Choi DJ, Rockman HA, McDonough PM, Bluhm WF, Meyer M, Sayen MR, Swanson E, Dillmann WH (1997) Overexpression of the rat sarcoplasmic reticulum Ca^{2+} ATPase gene in the heart of transgenic mice accelerates calcium transients and cardiac relaxation. J Clin Invest 100(2):380–389
18. He TC, Zhou S, DaCosta LT, Yu J, Kinzler KW, Vogelstein B (1998) A simplified system for generating recombinant adenoviruses. Proc Natl Acad Sci USA 95: 2509–2514
19. Hussain A, Lewis D, Sumbilla C, Lai LC, Melera PW, Inesi G (1992) Coupled expression of Ca^{2+} transport ATPase and a dihydrofolate reductase selectable marker in a mammalian cell system. Arch Biochem Biophys 296:539–546
20. Hussain A, Garnett C, Klein MG, Tsai-Wu J-J, Schneider MF, Inesi G (1995) Direct involvement of intracellular Ca^{2+}-transport ATPase in the development of thapsigargin resistance by Chinese hamster lung fibroblasts. J Biol Chem 270:12140–12146
21. Inesi G, Kurzmack M, Lewis D (1988) Kinetic and equilibrium characterization of an energy-transducing enzyme and its partial reactions. Methods Enzymol 157:154–190

22. Inesi G, Lewis D, Sumbilla C, Nandi A, Strock C, Huff KW, Rogers TB, Johns DC, Kessler PD, Ordahl CP (1998) Cell-specific promoter in adenovirus vector for transgenic expression of SERCA1 ATPase in cardiac myocytes. Am J Physiol 274:C645–C653
23. Ji Y, Loukianov E, Loukianova T, Jones LR, Periasamy M (1999) SERCA1a can functionally substitute for SERCA2a in the heart. Am J Physiol 276:H89–H97
24. Kaprielian Z, Fambrough DM (1987) Expression of fast and slow isoforms of the Ca^{2+}-ATPase in developing chick skeletal muscle. Dev Biol 124:490–503
25. Kass-Eisler A, Falick-Pedersen E, Alvira M, Rivera J, Buttrick PM, Wittenberg BA, Cipriani L, Leinwand LA (1993) Quantitative determination of adenovirus-mediated gene delivery to rat cardiac myocytes in vitro and in vivo. Proc Natl Acad Sci USA 90:11498–11502
26. Kimura Y, Inui M, Kadoma M, Kijima Y, Sasaki T, Tada M (1991) Effects of monoclonal antibody against phospholamban on calcium pump ATPase of cardiac sarcoplasmic reticulum. J Mol Cell Cardiol 23:1223–1230
27. Kirby MS, Sagara Y, Gaa ST, Inesi G, Lederer WJ, Rogers TB (1992) Thapsigargin inhibits contraction and Ca^{2+} transients in cardiac cells by specific inhibition of the sarcoplasmic reticulum Ca^{2+} pump. J Biol Chem 267(18):12545–12551
28. Kirschenbaum LA, MacLennan WR, Mazur W, French BA, Schneider MD (1993) Highly efficient gene transfer into adult ventricular myocytes by recombinant adenovirus. J Clin Invest 92:381–387
29. Loukianov E, Ji Y, Grupp IL, Kirkpatrick DL, Baker DL, Loukianova T, Grupp G, Lytton J, Walsh RA, Periasamy M (1998) Enhanced myocardial contractility and increased Ca^{2+} transport function in transgenic hearts expressing the fast-twitch skeletal muscle sarcoplasmic reticulum Ca^{2+}-ATPase. Circ Res 83(9):889–897
30. Luo W, Grupp IL, Harrer J, Ponniah S, Grupp G, Duffy JJ, Doetschman T, Kranias EG (1994) Targeted ablation of the phospholamban gene is associated with markedly enhanced myocardial contractility and loss of beta-agonist stimulation. Circ Res 75:401–409
31. Luo W, Wolska BM, Grupp IL, Harrer JM, Haghighi K, Ferguson DG, Slack JP, Grupp G, Doetschman T, Solaro RJ, Kranias EG (1996) Phospholamban gene dosage effects in the mammalian heart. Circ Res 78(No 5):839–847
32. Lytton J, MacLennan DH (1988) Molecular cloning of cDNAs from human kidney coding for two alternatively spliced products of the cardiac Ca^{2+}-ATPase gene. J Biol Chem 263:15024–15031
33. Lytton J, Zarain-Herzberg A, Periasamy M, MacLennan DH (1989) Molecular cloning of the mammalian smooth muscle sarco(endo)plasmic reticulum Ca^{2+}-ATPase. J Biol Chem 264:7059–7065
34. MacLennan DH, Brandl CJ, Korczak B, Green NM (1985) Amino-acid sequence of a Ca^{2+}+Mg^{2+} dependent ATPase from rabbit muscle sarcoplasmic reticulum, deduced from its complementary DNA sequence. Nature 316:696–700
35. Mar JH, Antin PB, Cooper TA, Ordahl CP (1988) Analysis of the upstream regions governing expression of the chicken cardiac troponin T gene in embryonic cardiac and skeletal muscle cells. J Cell Biol 107:573–585
36. Maruyama K, MacLennan DH (1988) Mutation of aspartic acid-35, lysine-352 and lysine-515 alters the Ca^{2+} transport activity of the Ca^{2+}-ATPase expressed in COS-1 cells. Proc Natl Acad Sci USA 85:3314–3318
37. Morgan JP, Erny RE, Allen PD, Grossman W, Gwathmey JK (1990) Abnormal intracellular calcium handling, a major cause of systolic and diastolic dysfunction in ventricular myocardium from patients with heart failure. Circulation 81 (Suppl)2:III21–III32

38. Morris GL, Cheng HC, Colyer J, Wang JH (1991) Phospholamban regulation of cardiac sarcoplasmic reticulum (Ca^{2+}+Mg^{2+})-ATPase. Mechanism of regulation and site of monoclonal antibody interaction. J Biol Chem 266(17):11270–11275
39. Periasamy M, Reed TD, Liu LH, Ji Y, Loukianov E, Paul RJ, Nieman ML, Riddle T, Duffy JJ, Doetschman T, Lorenz JN, Shull GE (1999) Impaired cardiac performance in heterozygous mice with a null mutation in sarco(endo)plasmic reticulum Ca^{2+}-ATPase isoform 2 (SERCA2) gene. J Biol Chem 274:2556–2562
40. Schmidt U, Hajjar RJ, Helm PA, Kim CS, Doye AA, Gwathmey JK (1998) Contribution of abnormal sarcoplasmic reticulum ATPase activity to systolic and diastolic dysfunction in human heart failure. J Mol Cell Cardiol 30(10):1929-1937
41. Sham JS, Jones LR, Morad M (1991) Phospholamban mediates the beta-adrenergic-enhanced Ca^{2+} uptake in mammalian ventricular myocytes. Am J Physiol 261(4 Pt 2):H1344–H1349
42. Sumbilla C, Cavagna M, Zhong L, Ma H, Lewis D, Farrance I, Inesi G (1999) Comparison of Ca^{2+}-ATPase isoforms (SERCA1 and SERCA2a) expressed in COS-1 cells and cardiac myocytes. Am J Physiol Heart Circ Physiol (in press)
43. Tada M, Yamada M, Kadoma M, Inui M, Ohmori F (1982) Calcium transport by cardiac sarcoplasmic reticulum and phosphorylation of phospholamban. Mol Cell Biochem 46(2):73–95
44. Toyofuku T, Kurzydlowski K, Tada M, MacLennan DH (1994) Amino acids Lys-Asp-Asp-Lys-Pro-Val^{402} in the Ca^{2+}-ATPase of cardiac sarcoplasmic reticulum are critical for functional association with phospholamban. J Biol Chem 269:22929–22932
45. Yao A, Su Z, Dillmann WH, Barry WH (1998) Sarcoplasmic reticulum function in murine ventricular myocytes overexpressing SR CaATPase. J Mol Cell Cardiol 30(12):2711–2718

CHAPTER 7

Overexpression of FKBP12.6 to influence SR function

J. PRESTLE, P. M. L. JANSSEN, A. JANSSEN, G. HASENFUSS
Georg-August University Goettingen,
Dept. Cardiology and Pneumology, Goettingen, Germany

Summary

Contractile capacity of the heart is critically dependent on sarcoplasmic reticulum (SR) function. Ca^{2+}-handling proteins of the SR may therefore represent promising molecular targets for genetic approaches to improve cardiac function. The ryanodine receptor (RyR) is the primary intracellular Ca^{2+}-release channel in striated muscles mediating muscle contraction by regulating the release of Ca^{2+} from the SR. The skeletal muscle RyR isoform (RyR1) is tightly associated with the FK506-binding protein 12 (FKBP12), whereas the cardiac RyR (RyR2) is known to bind the homologous isoform FKBP12.6. Recent studies indicate that FKBP12 modulates channel function by increasing conductivity and by stabilizing its closed conformation state. However, the precise role of FKBP12.6 in cardiac excitation-contraction coupling (E-C coupling) is not clear.

We used adenovirus-mediated gene transfer to overexpress FKBP12.6 in adult rabbit ventricular myocytes. Contractile function of transfected myocytes was analyzed by a video edge-detection system. We observed an increase in contractility of up to 22% in FKBP12.6-overexpressing myocytes compared with control-transfected myocytes, indicating that FKBP12.6 possesses important regulatory function in cardiac myocytes.

Introduction

E-C coupling in cardiomyocytes, as we know it, involves depolarization of the plasma membrane to open voltage-sensitive Ca^{2+} channels (known as dihydropyridine receptors, DHPR) resulting in a small influx of extracellular Ca^{2+} which in turn triggers the release of a larger amount of Ca^{2+} from the SR to initiate muscle contraction. This phenomenon is referred to as Ca^{2+}-induced Ca^{2+} release (CICR) [10]. Whereas the mechanism of Ca^{2+} reuptake into the SR by the action of the SR Ca^{2+}-ATPase (SERCA) and its accessory protein phospholamban is well understood, we are only beginning to realize that Ca^{2+} release from the SR is a process which involves not only the Ca^{2+}-release channel (ryanodine receptor, RyR) itself, but also a number of regulatory proteins associated with the RyR. This review focuses on a recently identified protein, FKBP12.6 (FK506-binding protein with an apparent MW of 12.6 kDa), and its putative role in cardiac E-C coupling.

SR Ca^{2+}-release channels (RyRs) and associated proteins

cDNA cloning revealed the existence of three different subtypes of RyRs: the skeletal muscle isoform RyR1, the cardiac isoform RyR2, and the brain and smooth muscle isoform RyR3. Structurally related to 1,4,5-triphosphate receptors (IP_3Rs) which are intracellular Ca^{2+}-release channels expressed in most cell types, RyRs are tetramers comprised of four identical subunits with a MW_r of 565 kDa each. The three isoforms share ~66% sequence homology at the amino acid level and are the largest ion channels currently known. Several proteins are physically associated or interact with the RyR subunits to regulate channel activity (see Fig. 1). It should be kept in mind, however, that the skeletal muscle RyR1 and the cardiac muscle RyR2 do have different modes of action: in cardiac cells depolarization-dependent Ca^{2+} influx through DHPR triggers Ca^{2+}-induced Ca^{2+} release via

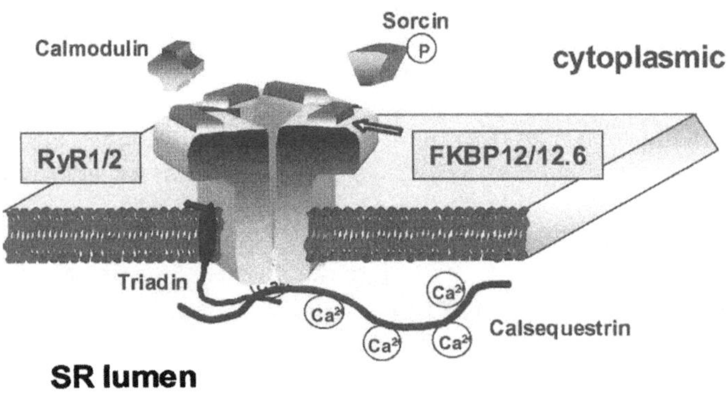

Fig. 1. Schematic representation of the hypothetical molecular architecture of SR Ca^{2+}-release channel (RyR) and associated proteins (for detailed review see [35]). Each RyR is comprised of four identical subunits with a large cytoplasmic domain, forming the "foot" structure of the channel. It is still a matter of debate whether the channel complex has four separate pores, or whether the four subunits form a single large pore. Each subunit of the skeletal muscle RyR (RyR1) binds one molecule FKBP12, while FKBP12.6 is supposed to be associated with the cardiac muscle RyR (RyR2). Several other proteins are known to be involved in the process of SR Ca^{2+} release. It has been suggested that triadin, a transmembrane protein, is involved in the functional coupling between calsequestrin, the Ca^{2+}-binding protein in the SR lumen, and the RyR [4]. Sorcin, a 22 kDa Ca^{2+}-binding protein, is localized at the dyadic junctions of T-tubules and the SR and can be co-immunoprecipitated with the RyR [5]. In single channel recording experiments, the addition of sorcin to the cytoplasmic side of the channel significantly reduced the open probability of the RyR and this inhibition could be relieved by protein kinase A (PKA)-catalyzed phosphorylation of sorcin [6]. Each RyR subunit also contains a calmodulin (CaM)-binding site. Depending on the Ca^{2+} concentration, CaM may either activate or inhibit Ca^{2+}-release channel activity [32].

RyR (CICR). In contrast, in skeletal muscle cells a voltage-induced change in DHPR is believed to be mechanically coupled to the RyR to cause it to open, without the requirement of Ca^{2+} influx. Structural differences and/or different interaction with accessory proteins of the RyR subtypes may underly this functional diversity [39].

The FKBP family includes several proteins of different MW between 12 and 56 kDa, all of them exerting *cis-trans* peptidyl-proly isomerase activity (PPIase activity) which is thought to be essential for protein folding during protein synthesis. They bind the immunosuppressant drugs FK506 (hence their name) and rapamycin with high affinity. Yet, the immunophilins FKBP12 and FKBP12.6 are the only members that have relevance to the immunosuppressive effects of FK506. They are the only ones discovered so far that, in a complex with the drug, bind to and inhibit the Ca^{2+}-dependent serine-threonine phosphatase calcineurin (CaN) in T-lymphocytes, thereby disrupting lymphokine gene induction and consequent immune response [33]. FKBP12 is ubiquitously expressed and phylogenetically well conserved. FKBP12.6 was first cloned in 1994 and found to be closely related to FKBP12 [3, 26]. FKBP12.6 differs from FKBP12 by only 18 of 108 amino acid residues (see Fig. 2) and is also expressed in a wide range of tissues, although less abundant than FKBP12 [3, 14]. From a pharmacological point of view, FKBP12 and FKBP12.6 are virtually indistinguishable. Both immunophilins bind FK506 with comparable affinity and are equipotent to one another as CaN inhibitors [14, 26]. Until recently the physiological function of these

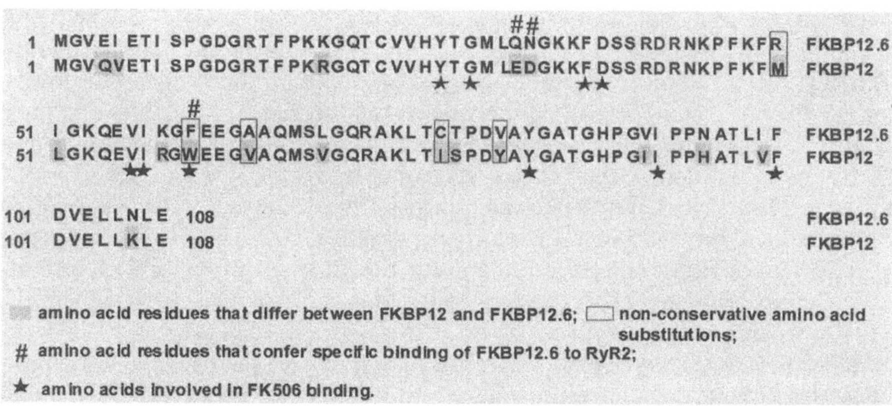

Fig. 2. Alignment of amino acid sequences of human FKBP12.6 and FKBP12. Both proteins share 85% amino acid sequence homology (18 of 108 amino acid residues differ). Based on the three-dimensional structure of FKBP12 determined by NMR [20, 21], structure-modeling studies suggested a similar three-dimensional structure for FKBP12.6 [38]. By site-directed mutagenesis, three out of the 18 amino acid residues that differ between FKBP12 and FKBP12.6 were found to be critical for selective binding of FKBP12.6 to the cardiac RyR2. Vice versa, mutation of these three residues in FKBP12 to that of FKBP12.6 conferred selective binding to RyR2 [38]. Amino acids involved in FK506 binding are conserved between FKBP12 and FKBP12.6 except for Phe^{60} in FKBP12.6, which replaces Trp^{60} in FKBP12 [34].

proteins was completely unknown. Besides their role in regulating the gating of the Ca^{2+}-release channel in striated muscles (see below), other putative cellular functions have been described, such as modulation of Ca^{2+} flux through IP_3Rs, anchoring calcineurin to the IP_3R [6, 7], and inhibition of type I transforming growth factor β family receptors (TGF-β receptors) [36]. FKBP12.6 is thought to be involved in regulation of insulin secretion from pancreatic islets. In islet microsome preparations, the second messenger cyclic ADP-ribose binds to FKBP12.6, causing it to dissociate from the islet RyR to release Ca^{2+} [22]. Furthermore, anti-FKBP12 autoantibodies were found in patients with autoimmune diseases [27].

Modulation of RyRs activity by FKBPs

The first indication of interaction of RyR with FKBP12 was documented by Collins in 1991, who found, by sequence comparison, a 15-mer peptide from a proteolytic digest of the purified rabbit skeletal muscle RyR to be identical to the N-terminus of FKBP12 [8]. By co-purification and co-immunoprecipitation, Jayaraman *et al.* thereafter demonstrated that FKBP12 is indeed tightly associated with the skeletal muscle RyR [12]. Numerous studies illustrated a significant role of FKBP12 in regulating skeletal muscle RyR activity. In purified RyR1 preparations, one FKBP12 molecule is associated with each subunit of the RyR1 such that the channel tetramer complex binds four FKBP12 molecules [30]. Using a baculovirus expression system, Brilliantes *et al.* showed that recombinant RyR1, expressed in Sf9 cells which do not express detectable amounts of either RyR1 or FKBP12, was capable of forming functional Ca^{2+}-release channels, predominantly exhibiting sub-conductance states or partial openings to different levels. Upon co-expression of FKBP12, a substantial increase in stable channels with full conductances was observed, indicating for the first time that FKBP12 may stabilize Ca^{2+}-release channel behavior [5]. Single channel analyses of RyR1 incorporated into planar lipid bilayers after removal of FKBP12 with either FK506 or rapamycin further sustained the hypothesis that FKBP12 enhances cooperation among the four subunits of RyR and allows the channel to open to the full conductance state and to close tightly, thereby preventing a leak of Ca^{2+} from the SR [1, 2, 16, 17].

FKBP12.6 was first isolated and characterized by Sewell *et al.* during a screening study for the presence and abundance of FKBP and CaN isoforms in brain tissues [26]. Biochemical analysis revealed that FKBP12.6, rather than FKBP12, is associated with the canine cardiac RyR although FKBP12 is also present in heart tissue and even more abundant than FKBP12.6 [14, 29, 31]. The interaction appears to be highly specific; whereas FKBP12 can bind to and exchange with both RyR1 and RyR2, FKBP12.6 selectively binds to cardiac RyR2 [31]. In a recent study, selective binding of FKBP12.6 to RyR2 was found to be conferred by 3 out of 18 amino acid residues which differ between FKBP12.6 and FKBP12 [38].

Are there functional differences between FKBP12 and FKBP12.6 with respect to regulation of skeletal and cardiac muscle RyR1/RyR2, respectively? The results described so far are conflicting. In *in vitro* studies using the dissociation/reconstitution approach with RyRs incorporated into planar lipid bilayers, or ryanodine binding and Ca^{2+} loading assays of isolated SR vesicles, addition of FKBP12 or FKBP12.6 to "stripped" RyR1 preparations modulated the channel by restoring its quiescent behavior. In contrast, neither removal nor addition of FKBP12.6 to RyR2 had any effect on channel activity using the same methodological approach [4, 31]. In other studies, however, removal of FKBP12.6 by rapamycin or FK506 from RyR2 incorporated into planar lipid bilayers resulted in an increased open probability of the channel and the appearance of subconductance states, effects that are similar to those found with RyR1 [13, 37]. Moreover, McCall *et al.* observed a significant increase in steady-state twitch Ca^{2+} transients and contraction amplitudes in isolated rat ventricular myocytes after treatment with FK506, most likely due to an increased open probability of the RyR2 during E-C coupling and rest [18]. These studies support the hypothesis that FKBP12.6 modulates RyR2 activity in a similar manner as FKBP12 modulates RyR1 activity. The discrepancy between the individual studies underscores the complex nature of the SR Ca^{2+}-release process, a situation that may be difficult to reconstitute *in vitro*.

The facts became even more puzzling by the study of Shou *et al.*, who showed that FKBP12-knockout mice do have normal skeletal muscles but exhibit severe dilated cardiomyopathy. The majority of the FKBP12-deficient mice died between embryonic day 14.5 and birth because of cardiac defects that resembled the morphological features of heart failure in humans [28]. Unexpectedly, both skeletal and cardiac muscle RyRs from FKBP12-deficient mice showed similar alterations in single-channel behavior as compared to RyRs from wild-type mice, i.e. increased open probability of the channels and substrate activity. Since FKBP12.6 expression was apparently unchanged in FKBP12-knockout mice, but could not functionally substitute for FKBP12, this study indicates that FKBP12 modulates both the skeletal and the cardiac muscle RyR. The absence of skeletal muscle dysfunction was attributed to differences in E-C coupling mechanisms between skeletal and cardiac muscles. Thus, the precise role of FKBP12.6 in cardiac E-C coupling is still unclear.

Adenovirus-mediated gene transfer of FKBP12.6 in rabbit ventricular myocytes

Our present view of FKBP12/FKBP12.6 function is mainly based on experiments using an excess of immunosuppressive drugs (FK506 or rapamycin) in order to remove FKBP from the RyR. With the use of intact muscle preparations or isolated myocytes, however, high concentrations of the drug (≥10 μM) are necessary, because most of the drug is buffered by cytosolic FKBP12. Targets other than RyRs may thus as well be considered to underly the FK506/rapamycin-induced alterations in E-C coupling. In fact, duBell *et al.* provided evidence that FK506 increases Ca^{2+} transient amplitude in rat ventricular myocytes via SR-independent mechanisms through prolongation of the action potential due to inhibition of outward K^{+} currents [9].

In order to investigate the role of FKBP12.6 in cardiac E-C coupling, we used adenovirus-mediated gene transfer to overexpress FKBP12.6 in isolated rabbit ventricular myocytes [23]. Contractile behavior of FKBP12.6-transfected myocytes was analyzed by a video edge-detection system and compared to control-transfected myocytes.

Adenoviral vectors have become the method of choice for gene transfer into adult cardiac myocytes in primary culture. Importantly, adenovirus infection per se has no impact on contractile function of cardiomyocytes [25]. We generated a recombinant first generation adenovirus that carries the human FKBP12.6 gene under control of the CMV promoter together with the green fluorescent protein (GFP) as an independently expressed reporter gene (Ad-FKBP12.6-GFP). An adenovirus carrying only the GFP gene (Ad-GFP) served as a negative control in all experiments. After infection of cells with recombinant adenovirus, expression of the transgene increases over time, usually reaching a plateau at about 48 h after transfection. Accordingly, as shown by RT-PCR analysis, mRNA levels of FKBP12.6 in transfected cardiomyocytes were higher after a 48 h culture time, compared with a 24 h culture time following adenoviral infection (Fig. 3). Specific overexpression of FKBP12.6 was confirmed by simultaneous amplification of the endogenous FKBP12 gene. Constant amounts of detected FKBP12 transcripts demonstrated unchanged expression upon gene transfer of FKBP12.6. Interestingly, when PCR conditions were chosen such that amplification of FKBP12.6 was in the linear range, no endogenous FKBP12.6 expression was detected in the uninfected, or GFP-control virus-infected cells, whereas FKBP12 mRNA was readily detected (Fig. 3A). Only when more PCR cycles were conducted using the same samples was low level expression of endogenous FKBP12.6 evident, as shown in Fig. 3B. These results indicate that the FKBP12 expression level in rabbit cardiomyocytes is much higher than the expression level of FKBP12.6.

Myocyte shortening was measured at 24 h and at 48 h after virus infection by a video edge-detection system. Representative tracings of a single twitch of an Ad-GFP control, and an Ad-FKBP12.6-GFP- transfected myocyte are shown in Fig. 4. At 24 h after transfection (low level overexpression of FKBP12.6, see Fig. 3A), cell shortening was increased by 19% in Ad-FKBP12.6-GFP-infected cells compared to Ad-GFP-infected cells ($P=0.069$, $n=30$ each). A statistically significant increase in cell shortening by 22% ($P<0.05$, $n=42$ each) was established at 48 h post-transfection (high level overexpression of FKBP12.6). Thus, FKBP12.6 overexpression exerts a positive inotropic effect in rabbit ventricular myocytes.

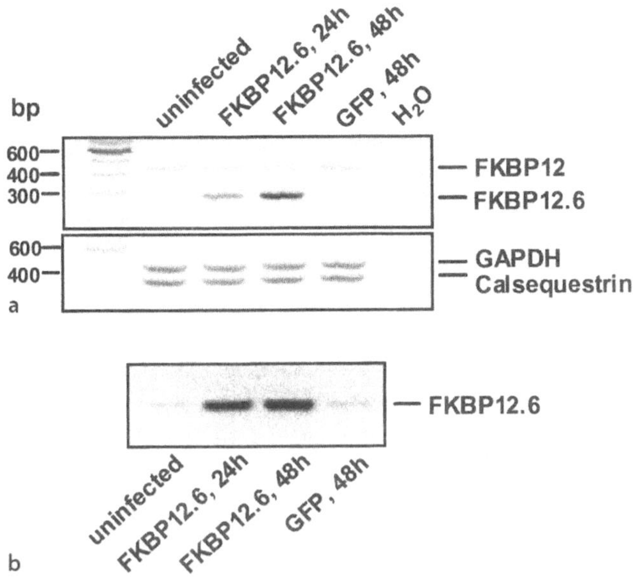

Fig. 3. RT-PCR analysis of Ad-FKBP12.6-GFP-transfected cardiomyocytes. **a** Rabbit ventricular myocytes were enzymatically isolated and plated onto 60 mm laminin-coated petri dishes at a density of 0.5×10^5 rod-shaped cells/cm^2. Myocytes were infected with Ad-FKBP12.6-GFP or Ad-GFP at a multiplicity of infection of 10 pfu/cell (MOI 10) for 2 h at 37 °C and cultured for 24 h/48 h in supplemented M199 medium. Thereafter, cells were harvested, total RNA was isolated and duplex RT-PCR analysis was performed with FKBP12 and FKBP12.6 specific primers. Duplex RT-PCR with glyceraldehyde-3-phosphate dehydrogenase (GAPDH) and calsequestrin-specific primers was performed separately to confirm equal cDNA load in each amplification reaction. FKBP12.6 mRNA was detectable after 24 h culture time following adenoviral infection and was considerably increased after 48 h culture time. Endogenous FKBP12 expression was similar in both Ad-FKBP12.6-GFP and Ad-GFP control-transfected cells, as well as in uninfected cells. Using PCR conditions ensuring amplification of FKBP12 and FKBP12.6 in the linear range, no FKBP12.6 mRNA expression could be detected in the uninfected nor Ad-GFP control-transfected myocytes. Only when additional PCR cycles were run could low level endogenous expression of FKBP12.6 be detected (**b**). Thus, adenovirus-mediated overexpression of FKBP12.6 does not affect endogenous FKBP12 expression level in rabbit ventricular myocytes.

Conclusions

There is compelling evidence that FKBPs play an essential role in E-C coupling in cardiac as well as in skeletal myocytes by modulating RyR activity. Yet, it is still unclear which FKBP isoform controls which RyR subtype and whether both FKBP isoforms are exchangeable with respect to their function in E-C coupling. Fleischer and coworkers convincingly showed that the skeletal muscle RyR1 of all five classes of vertebrates is associated with FKBP12 but can also exchange with FKBP12.6, whereas the cardiac muscle RyR2 selectively binds FKBP12.6 [24]. However, the latter has only been demonstrated for the canine RyR2 and it remains to be elucidated whether this holds true for other species. The data from the FKBP12-knockout mice

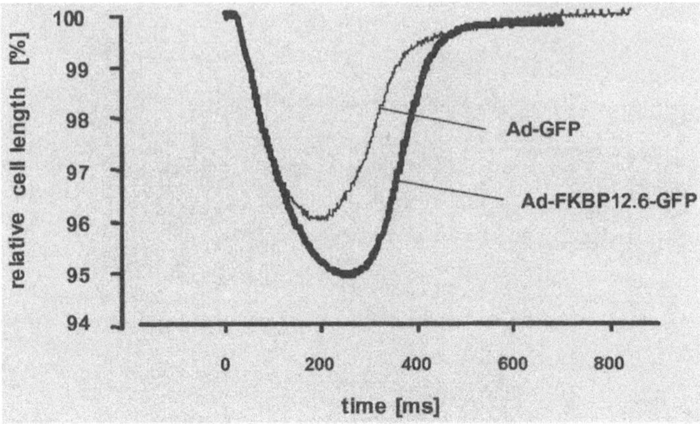

Fig. 4. Representative tracings of myocyte shortening experiments. Rabbit ventricular myocytes, plated onto laminin-coated 35 mm petri dishes, were infected with Ad-FKBP12.6-GFP or Ad-GFP at a MOI of 10 pfu/cell. Culture plates were placed in a heat-thermostated (37 °C) chamber on a microscope stage and myocytes were superfused with O_2-saturated M199 medium (1.8 mM external $CaCl_2$). Cells were electrically stimulated at 1 Hz via platinum electrodes. The image of the myocytes was recorded by a CCD camera and cell shortening was measured by an edge-detection system at a sampling rate of 240 Hz. At 48 h post-adenovirus infection, we observed a statistically significant increase in cell shortening by 22% in FKBP12.6 vs. GFP cells.

give rise to the assumption that FKBP12 may interact with both the skeletal muscle and the cardiac muscle RyR.

FKBP12 and FKBP12.6 are both expressed in heart tissue. By means of adenoviral gene transfer in isolated cardiomyocytes, we showed that overexpression of FKBP12.6 increases contractility of the myocytes through a yet undefined mechanism. At first glance, it seems to be contradictory that both overexpression of FKBP12.6 and removal of FKBP12.6 (or possibly FKBP12) from the RyR2 by FK506 treatment exert a positive inotropic effect. The latter can be explained by an increase in $[Ca^{2+}]_i$ transient amplitude due to an increased open time of the RyR and/or a prolongation of the action potential [9, 18]. However, the positive inotropic effect is at the cost of a 'leaky' SR, as indicated by the accelerated rest decay of SR Ca^{2+} content and the increase in Ca^{2+} spark frequency during rest [18]. From a physiological standpoint, FK506 treatment as a positive inotropic intervention would thus be disastrous, because of a high risk of arrhythmias. On the other hand, it is reasonable to speculate that overexpression of FKBP12.6 results in a more coordinated function of the RyR2 in a way that all channels may simultaneously open to the full conductance level upon activation and close tightly after inactivation.

The stoichiometry of FKBP12.6-binding sites per RyR tetramer was calculated to be one molecule FKBP12.6 per RyR subunit. Thus, the question of how the overexpression of FKBP12.6 may influence RyR2 activity, assuming that all FKBP12.6-binding sites are already occupied under normal conditions, arises. Yet, this does not seem to be the case. In binding studies of soluble ^{35}S-labeled FKBP12.6 to cardiac SR preparations, Timerman *et al.* estimated that about 17% of total FKBP12.6-binding sites in dog cardiac SR vesicles appear to be unoccupied [31].

In summary, we demonstrated that overexpression of FKBP12.6 increases basal contractility of cardiac myocytes. The SR Ca^{2+}-release channel and associated proteins may therefore represent promising molecular targets to improve SR function and thus cardiac performance.

References

1. Ahern GP, Junankar PR, Dulhunty AF (1997) Subconductance states in single-channel activity of skeletal muscle ryanodine receptors after removal of FKBP12. Biophys J 72:146–162
2. Ahern GP, Junankar PR, Dulhunty AF (1994) Single channel activity of the ryanodine receptor calcium release channel is modulated by FK-506. FEBS Letters 352:369–374
3. Arakawa H, Nagase H, Hayashi N, Fujiwara T, Ogawa M, Shin S, Nakamura Y (1994) Molecular cloning and expression of a novel human gene that is highly homologous to human FK506-binding protein 12 kDa (hFKBP-12) and characterization of two alternatively spliced transcripts. Biochem Biophys Res Commun 200:836–843
4. Barg S, Copello JA, Fleischer S (1997) Different interactions of cardiac and skeletal muscle ryanodine receptors with FK-506 binding protein isoform. Am J Physiol 272:C1726–C1733
5. Brillantes A-MB, Ondrias K, Scott A, Kobrinsky E, Ondriasová E, Moschella MC, Jayaraman T, Landers M, Ehrlich BE, Marks AR (1994) Stabilization of calcium release channel (ryanodine receptor) function by FK506-binding protein. Cell 77:513–523
6. Cameron AM, Nucifora FC, Fung ET, Livingston DJ, Aldape RA, Ross CA, Snyder SH (1997) FKBP12 binds the inositol 1,4,5-triphosphate receptor at leucine-proline (1400-1401) and anchors calcineurin to this FK506-like domain. J Biol Chem 272:27582–27588
7. Cameron AM, Steiner JP, Sabatini DM, Kaplin AI, Walensky LD, Snyder SH (1995) Immunophilin FK506 binding protein associates with inositol 1,4,5-triphosphate receptor modulates calcium flux. Proc Natl Acad Sci USA 92:1784–1788
8. Collins JH (1991) Sequence analysis of the ryanodine receptor: possible association with a 12 kDa, FK506-binding immunophilin/protein kinase C inhibitor. Biochem Biophys Res Commun 178:1288–1290
9. duBell WH, Wright PA, Lederer WJ, Rogers TB (1997) Effect of the immunosuppressant FK506 on excitation-contraction coupling and outward K^+ currents in rat ventricular myocytes. J Physiol 501.3:509–516
10. Fabiato A (1985) Time and calcium dependence of activation and inactivation of calcium-induced release of calcium from the sarcoplasmic reticulum of a skinned canine Purkinje cell. J Gen Physiol 85:247–289
11. Guo W, Campbell KP (1995) Association of triadin with the ryanodine receptor and calsequestrin in the lumen of the sarcoplasmic reticulum. J Biol Chem 270:9027–9030

12. Jayaraman T, Brillantes A-M, Timerman AP, Fleischer S, Erdjument-Bromage H, Tempst P, Marks AR (1992) FK506 binding protein associated with the calcium release channel (ryanodine receptor). J Biol Chem 267:9474–9477
13. Kaftan E, Marks AR, Ehrlich BE (1996) Effects of rapamycin on ryanodine receptor/Ca^{2+}-release channels from cardiac muscle. Circ Res 78:990–997
14. Lam E, Martin MM, Timerman AP, Sabers C, Fleischer S, Lukas T, Abraham RT, O'Keefe SJ, O'Neill EA, Wiederrecht GJ (1995) A novel FK506 binding protein can mediate the immunosuppressive effects of FK506 and is associated with the cardiac ryanodine receptor. J Biol Chem 270:26511–26522
15. Lokuta AJ, Meyers MB, Sander PR, Fishman GI, Valdivia HH (1997) Modulation of cardiac ryanodine receptors by sorcin. J Biol Chem 272:25333–25338
16. Marks AR (1997) Intracellular calcium-release channels: regulators of life and death. Am J Physiol 272:H597–H605
17. Mayrleitner M, Timerman AP, Wiederrecht G, Fleischer S (1994) The calcium release channel of sarcoplasmic reticulum is modulated by FK-506 binding protein: effect of FKBP-12 on single channel activity of the skeletal muscle ryanodine receptor. Cell Calcium 15:99–108
18. McCall E, Li L, Satoh H, Shannon TR, Blatter LA, Bers DM (1996) Effects of FK-506 on contraction and Ca^{2+} transients in rat cardiac myocytes. Circ Res 79:1110–1121
19. Meyers MB, Pickel VM, Sheu S-S, Sharma VK, Scotto KW, Fishman GI (1995) Association of sorcin with the cardiac ryanodine receptor. J Biol Chem 270:26411–26418
20. Michnick SW, Rosen MK, Wandless TJ, Karplus M, Schreiber SL (1991) Solution structure of FKBP, a rotamase enzyme and receptor for FK506 and rapamycin. Science 252:836–839
21. Moore JM, Peattie DA, Fitzgibbon MJ, Thomson JA (1991) Solution structure of the major binding protein for the immunosuppressant FK506. Nature 351:248–250
22. Noguchi N, Takasawa S, Nata K, Tohgo A, Kato I, Ikehata F, Yonekura H, Okamoto H (1997) Cyclic ADP-ribose binds to FK506-binding protein 12.6 to release Ca^{2+} from islet microsomes. J Biol Chem 272:3133–3136
23. Prestle J, Janssen A, Lehnart SE, Zeitz O, Janssen PML, Hasenfuss G (1999) Role of FKBP12.6 in excitation-contraction coupling in rabbit ventricular myocytes. Eur Heart J 20:44 (Suppl)
24. Qi Y, Ogunbunmi EM, Freund EA, Timerman AP, Fleischer S (1998) FK-binding protein is associated with the ryanodine receptor of skeletal muscle in vertebrate animals. J Biol Chem 273:34813–34819
25. Rust EM, Westfall MV, Metzger JM (1998) Stability of the contractile assembly and Ca^{2+}-activated tension in adenovirus infected adult cardiac myocytes. Mol Cell Biochem 181:143–155
26. Sewell TJ, Lam E, Martin MM, Leszyk J, Weidner J, Calaycay J, Griffin P, Williams H, Hung S, Cryan J, Sigal NH, Wiederrecht GJ (1994) Inhibition of calcineurin by a novel FK-506-binding protein. J Biol Chem 269:21094–21102
27. Shinkura N, Ikai I, Yamauchi A, Hirose T, Kawai Y, Inamoto T, Ozaki S, Iwai M, Bona B, Yamaoka Y (1999) Autoantibodies to FK506 binding protein 12 (FKBP12) in autoimmune diseases. Autoimmunity 29:159–170
28. Shou W, Aghdasi B, Armstrong DL, Guo Q, Bao S, Charng M-J, Mathews LM, Schneider MD, Hamilton SL, Matzuk MM (1998) Cardiac defects and altered ryanodine receptor function in mice lacking FKBP12. Nature 391:489–492
29. Timerman AP, Jayaraman T, Wiederrecht G, Onoue H, Marks A, Fleischer S (1994) The ryanodine receptor from canine heart sarcoplasmic reticulum is associated with a novel FK-506 binding protein. Biochem Biophys Res Commun 198:701–706

30. Timerman AP, Ogunbunmi E, Freund E, Wiederrecht G, Marks A, Fleischer S (1993) The calcium release channel of sarcoplasmic reticulum is modulated by FK-506 binding protein. J Biol Chem 270:22992–22999
31. Timerman AP, Onoue H, Xin H-B, Barg S, Copello J, Wiederrecht G, Fleischer S (1996) Selective binding of FKBP12.6 by the cardiac ryanodine receptor. J Biol Chem 271:20385–20391
32. Tripathy A, Xu L, Mann G, Meissner G (1995) Calmodulin activation and inhibition of skeletal muscle Ca^{2+}-release channel (ryanodine receptor). Biophys J 69:106–119
33. Thomson AW, Bonham CA, Zeevi A (1995) Mode of action of Tacrolimus (FK506): molecular and cellular mechanisms. Ther Drug Monit 17:584–591
34. Van Duyne GD, Standaert RF, Karplus PA, Schreiber SL, Clardy J (1993) Atomic structures of the human immunophilin FKBP-12 complexes with FK506 and rapamycin. J Mol Biol 229:105–124
35. Wagenknecht T, Radermacher M (1997) Ryanodine receptors: structure and macromolecular interactions. Curr Opin Struct Biol 7:258–265
36. Wang T, Li B-Y, Danielson PD, Shah PC, Rockwell S, Lechleider RJ, Martin J, Manganaro T, Donahoe PK (1996) The immunophilin FKBP12 functions as a common inhibitor of the TGF family type I receptors. Cell 86:435–444
37. Xiao R-P, Valdivia HH, Bogdanov K, Valdivia C, Lakatta EG, Cheng H (1997) The immunophilin FK506-binding protein modulates Ca^{2+} release channel closure in rat heart. J Physiol 500:343–354
38. Xin H-B, Rogers K, Qi Y, Kanematsu T, Fleischer S (1999) Three amino acid residues determine selective binding of FK506-binding protein 12.6 to the cardiac ryanodine receptor. J Biol Chem 274:15315–15319
39. Yamazawa T, Takeshima H, Sakurai T, Endo M, Iino M (1996) Subtype specificity of the ryanodine receptor for Ca^{2+} signal amplification in excitation-contraction coupling. EMBO J 15:6172–6177

Chapter 8

Adenovirus-mediated myocardial gene therapy

J. K. Donahue

Institute of Molecular Cardiobiology, Department of Medicine, Johns Hopkins University School of Medicine, Baltimore, MD, USA

Introduction

The introduction of genetic material to the heart showed promise when adenovirus vectors were demonstrated to easily and efficiently transfer reporter genes to isolated cardiac myocytes *in vitro* [17, 18]. Numerous possibilities for the new technology were readily apparent. The most obvious was the replacement of genetic defects in inherited disorders, such as the long QT syndrome and several types of hypertrophic and dilated cardiomyopathies. Even more exciting, however, was the prospect of using this technology to modify more common, acquired diseases including ischemic diseases, acquired cardiomyopathies and arrhythmias. Most of these diseases affect every cell in the heart, so therapeutic applications would require delivery of the gene of interest to a majority of the myocytes in a homogeneous pattern throughout the heart.

Enthusiasm for this new technology was quelled when several problems arose. Chief among these was the inability to translate the success of isolated myocyte gene transfer to the development of a successful *in vivo* model. Other problems included the lack of adequate control to manipulate the site, timing and amount of gene expression, and the inability to suppress the immune response to both the delivery vectors and the transgenes.

The majority of work in myocardial gene transfer has been performed using adenoviruses. This review will focus on the problems of gene delivery to the myocardium by examining the basic principles of adenovirus virology and virus-cell interactions before looking at the behavior of the virus in *ex vivo* models. In that way, a foundation can be laid that could potentially lead to the development of a successful *in vivo* delivery system.

Basic virology

The adenovirus was first identified in 1953 when Rowe et al. reported spontaneous degeneration of primary cell cultures of human adenoidal tissue [29], and pathogenicity in humans was confirmed in 1954 with linkage to an epidemic of upper respiratory tract infections among army recruits [16]. Interest in adenovirus research was originally sparked by the documentation of adenovirus-mediated oncogenesis [31]. The early history of the field was dominated by isolation and identification of multiple serotypes (currently there are 47 serotypes of human adenoviruses that are categorized in 7 subgroups [30]) and investigation of the interactions between viruses and cultured cell lines [5, 27, 28]. In the 1970s and 1980s, the physical structure of the virus was investigated, the genome was sequenced, and structural and functional proteins were identified and mapped to the genome [17, 19, 25, 32, 33]. In the late 1980s and 1990s the primary and secondary cellular receptors were discovered [2, 34]. Current interest in adenoviruses comes from their utility as agents of gene transfer for cell culture transformation and for human vaccines and gene therapy.

The adenovirus is a double-stranded DNA virus with a 35 kb genome. The genome is organized into early and late genes. The early genes are predominately those required for replication and transcription of the viral genome, and the late genes mainly encode virus structural proteins. Of primary interest to the gene therapist, the virus is capable of packaging DNA with a size ±5% of the wildtype [11]. To render the viruses replication-incompetent for gene therapy, the E1, E3 and sometimes E4 genes have been deleted. The removal of these sections of the genome provides up to 10.7 kb for insertion of the transgene, while preventing the adenovirus from replicating. Production of these replication-incompetent viruses requires use of a cell line with complementary DNA sequences to complete the virus genome, such as HEK 293 or 911 cells.(see Graham et al. for a review of adenovirus production and amplification [13]). Removal of the entire adenovirus-genome has been reported. The advantages of that approach are that the entire 35 kb becomes available for the transgene and the removal of the virus structural proteins from the genome may reduce the immune response during gene therapy [6]. The disadvantage is that the virus can no longer be manufactured in complementary cell lines, requiring co-infection with helper viruses for replication.

Structurally, the adenovirus is composed of an icosahedral protein shell, known as the capsid, and a series of appendages called fibers. The icosahedron is composed of hexagonal and pentagonal proteins called hexons and pentons, respectively. The hexons form the walls of the structure and the pentons are the vertices. Extending from each penton is a fiber protein consisting of a penton-attachment moiety, a stalk, and a globular head. The diameter of the adenovirus capsid in a five-fold symmetry orientation is 736 Å and the fiber length is 240–310 Å [25].

Virus-cell interactions

Together the fiber and penton proteins form the virus attachment unit. The so far its function is unknown. After attachment of the fiber to CAR, the body of the adenovirus is brought into close proximity to the cell allowing arginine-glycine-aspartate sequences on the penton protein to bind to cellular $\alpha_V\beta_3$ and $\alpha_V\beta_5$ integrins [34]. The integrins are cellular receptors for extracellular matrix proteins. Following multiple fiber and penton attachment events, the virus is internalized via receptor-mediated endocytosis [27].

To date, most adenovirus research has focused on attachment from the point of view of the virus.

In order to enhance the efficiency of adenovirus-mediated gene transfer, we took the opposite point of view and evaluated the virus-cell interaction from the perspective of the cell [9]. Infection was evaluated by using a recombinant adenovirus encoding the E. coli β-galactosidase gene and by staining cells with X-gal solution to identify infected cells. In this model, we evaluated the effect of changing virus and cell concentrations, temperature, exposure time, and culture media on success of infection (Fig. 1); we found that the virus attachment to the cell typifies a receptor-ligand interaction. The final percentage of infected cells (and thus gene transfer) is dependent on the amounts of both virions and cells as well as on the temperature, reaction time, and culture medium. The reaction has two components: virus diffusion to the cell surface and attachment of the virus to the receptor. When sufficient time is given for diffusion to occur, the final percentage of infected cells is related to the starting virus amount in a sigmoidal fashion (Fig. 2a). At 37 °C in culture dishes containing 1×10^5 cardiac myocytes, half-maximal infection occurs with 1×10^5 pfu of adenovirus and infection saturates at 100% when the total adenovirus amount is greater than 1×10^6 pfu. The dependence on the total amount of cellular receptors has not yet been demonstrated in this system, but we did find an inverse association between the percentage of infected cells and the total number of cells (Fig. 2b). For a constant 1×10^5 pfu of adenovirus, the final percentage of infected cells decreased with increasing cell number.

Dependence of virus attachment on temperature was also demonstrated using the same system (Fig. 3). Infection of 1×10^5 myocytes with 1×10^5 pfu of adenovirus at 37 °C resulted in half-maximal infection after

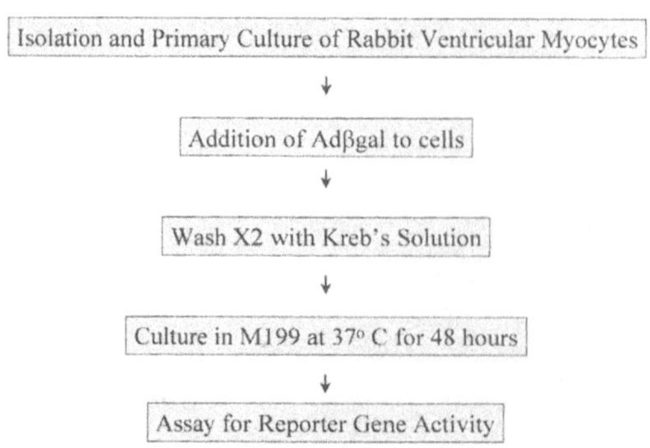

Fig. 1. Schematic of protocol for experiments in isolated ventricular myocytes.

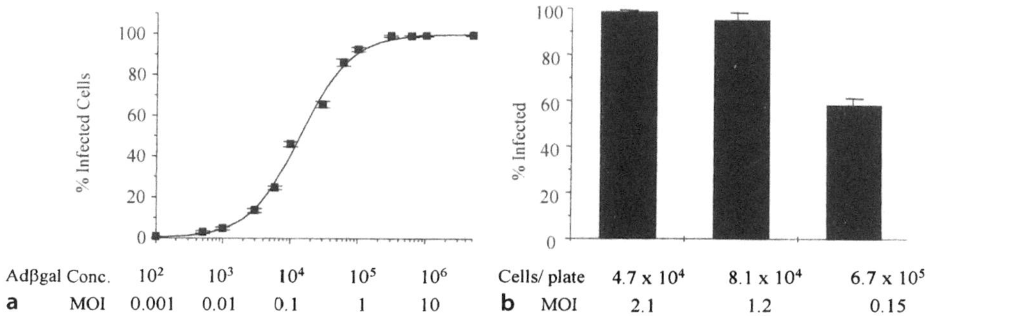

Fig. 2. Influence of virus and cell concentration on recombinant adenovirus infection in primary cultures of adult rabbit ventricular myocytes at 37°C. **a** Percentage of cells positive for β-galactosidase after 48 hr exposure to varying concentrations of Adβgal (1.0×10^5 cells/culture dish). **b** Percentage of cells positive for β-galactosidase with varying cell number after 48 h exposure to Adβgal (1.0×10^5 pfu in 1 ml of M199). MOI is the ratio of infectious particles to cells. n=3 for each data point.

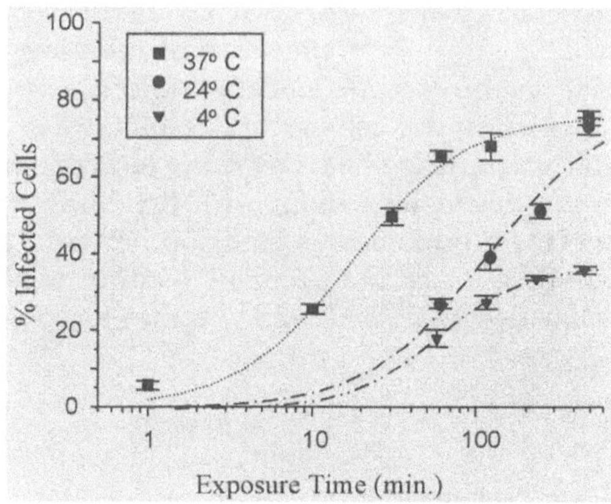

Fig. 3. Temperature effects on virus infection in isolated rabbit ventricular myocytes. Percentage of cells positive for β-galactosidase after 1 min to 8 h exposure to 1.0×10^5 pfu of Adβgal in 1.0 ml Kreb's solution at three different temperatures (8.9×10^4 cells/culture dish). Solid lines are logistical regression curves drawn through data. n=3 for each data point.

19.0±2.3 min. At 24 °C, the time to half-maximal infection was longer, requiring 216±42 min, but the final infection percentage of 76.3±3.7% was similar to that at 37 °C. At 4 °C, both the rate and final percentage were reduced. Half-maximal infection occurred in 60.2±1.4 min, and peak infection was only 37.9±0.3%. The time to half-maximal infection at 4 °C occurred sooner than at 24 °C, but the percentage of infected cells was much less, so the actual infection rate at 4 °C was also less. These results demonstrate a temperature dependence of both the infection rate and final percentage of infected cells. The effect on infection rate is likely secondary to changes in the diffusion rate and the energy of molecular collisions at different temperatures. The change in the total number of infected cells agrees with previous observations in HeLa cells [26]. Below 6 °C, virus binding to HeLa cells exhibited negative cooperativity and the binding of one virion inhibited subsequent virus binding to a given cell. Above 6 °C, positive cooperativity was noted, and the binding of an initial virion enhanced further virus binding. The degree of positive cooperativity in HeLa cells increased between 6 and 20 °C and was stable above 20 °C.

The behavior of the myocyte culture infection system with different culture media seems to be related to the presence or absence of inhibitors of infection (Fig. 4). In crystalloid media, such as culture media 199 (M199) or Kreb's solution, the percentage of Adβgal-infected cells is similar, 41.6±0.8% and 40.7±1.8%, respectively (p = NS). The presence of red blood cells inhibits infection (15.6±3.1% infection with hematocrit = 33%, $p<0.001$ relative to M199), and plasma has a smaller inhibitory effect (35.1±2.4% infection, $p<0.01$ relative to M199). Red blood cells bind the adenovirus fiber particle, so addition of red cells in effect adds a non-competitive inhibitor to the system. Likewise, addition of blood containing antibody has an inhibitory effect on the infection of cultured myocytes (0.07±0.03% infection, $p<0.001$ relative to M199). Iohexol, a non-ionic contrast agent used in coronary angiography, also has an inhibitory effect on infection (29.6±1.4%, $p<0.001$ compared to M199). We speculate that this effect may be from chelation of the virus by the negatively-charged organic acids in the structure of the molecule.

Based on the cell culture results, we suggest that the adenovirus-myocyte interaction resembles any other enzyme-substrate or receptor-ligand interaction and can be treated with the same types of analyses. Each presumably involves a bimolecular collision between a freely mobile particle and a relatively fixed cellular receptor leading to a cascade of intracellular events of which the end result may be measured. The reaction rate in these systems

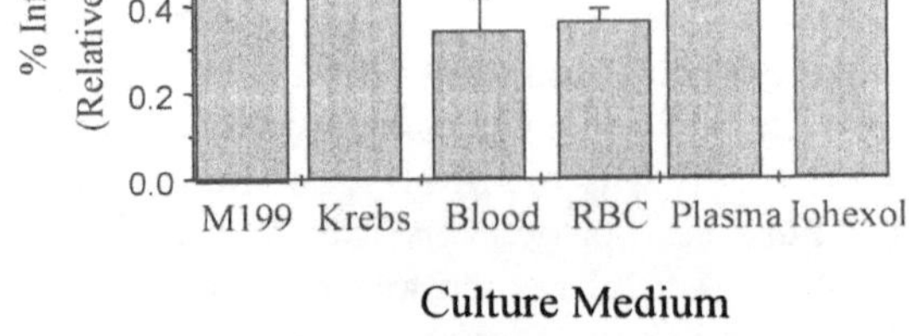

Fig. 4. Effects of culture media on virus infection in isolated rabbit ventricular myocytes. Percentage of cells positive for β-galactosidase after exposure to 1.0×10^5 pfu of Adβgal in different media for 2.0 h at 37 °C (4.4×10^4 cells/culture dish). Whole rabbit blood had a hematocrit of 33%, and isolated red blood cells (RBC) were diluted in Kreb's solution to a hematocrit of 33%. Iohexol was diluted in M199 to 20% by volume. n = 3 for each data point.

is determined by the probability of any particle colliding with a receptor at an energy greater than the reaction activation energy; thus the rate would be dependent on temperature and virus concentration. Since the reaction is ultimately irreversible and it occurs in a stoichiometric fashion, the final concentration of the product will be a function of the ratio of starting reactants at the completion of the reaction. Utilization of this model allows us to identify and optimize several parameters important to the adenoviral infection of ventricular myocytes and transfer these results to the *ex vivo* system.

Virus infection in an *ex vivo* System

Having evaluated the dependence of gene transfer on several basic parameters in the cell culture system, we sought an environment with the increased complexity of tissue interactions but with more control than could be achieved in the *in vivo* environment. Using a Langendorff perfusion model, we were able to evaluate the effects of the vasculature and of cell-cell interactions on adenovirus-mediated gene transfer. The basic model (Fig. 5) included cannulation of the ascending aorta of the explanted heart of a New Zealand white rabbit, followed by perfusion of the coronary vasculature by retrograde flow from the cannula, through the ascending aorta, and down the coronary arteries. During infection, coronary flow was controlled with a masterflex pump and the right ventricular outflow drained freely into a beaker. All experiments were performed at 37 °C and the total Langendorff perfusion time for all experiments was 180 min for uniformity. After infection and sufficient perfusion to allow time for virus internalization, the hearts were enzymatically digested and the resulting isolated myocytes were cultured for 48 hours to allow time for transgene expression. Like the cell culture model, the hearts were infected with a recombinant adenovirus encoding the gene for E. coli *β*-galactosidase, and the percentage of infected cells was quantified by counting blue cells after exposure to X-gal solution. Using this system, we evaluated the effects of coronary flow, virus exposure time, virus concentration, calcium concentration and exposure to agents known to modify vascular permeability.

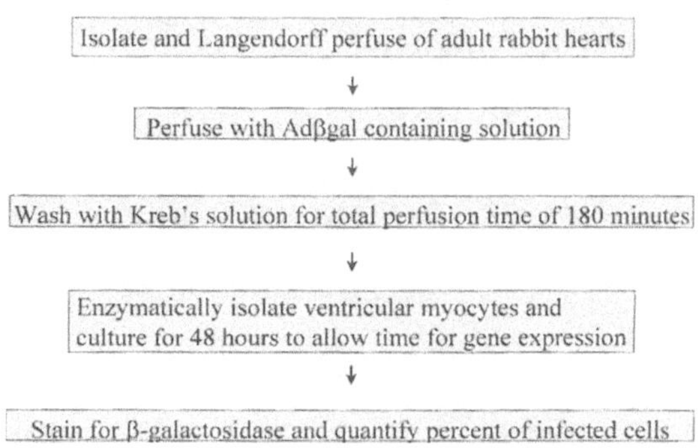

Fig. 5. Schematic of protocol for experiments in *ex vivo* perfused hearts.

Variation in coronary flow from 10–40 ml/min resulted in an increase in infection from 10.6±2.5% at a flow rate of 10 ml/min to 40.3±3.2% for flow rates of 30 ml/min or greater (Fig. 6). Although the decreased efficiency of gene transfer at 10 ml/min may have been related to reduced perfusion pressure, the improvement at higher flow rates was independent of perfusion pressure, which did not vary significantly for coronary flow rates between 20–40 ml/min. A more likely cause of the flow dependence is the presence of precapillary sphincters that open in response to increasing flow rates [22]. We surmise that flow above a critical rate opens all of the myocardial capillaries, maximizing the surface area for virus delivery and shortening diffusion distances to myocytes.

As observed in the cell culture system, virus concentration and exposure time in the Langendorff system were complementary variables (Fig. 7). Changes in virus concentration affected both the infection rate and the final percentage of infected cells, and therefore increasing concentration could compensate for decreasing exposure time. With a virus concentration of 1×10^8 pfu/ml, half-maximal infection occurred at 30 min and infection peaked at 40% after 60 min of virus exposure. Increasing the virus concentration to 1.6×10^9 pfu/ml reduced the time to half-maximal infection to 18 min and 96% of cells were infected after 30 min.

These data demonstrated the feasibility of reaching nearly all of the cells in an intact heart for adenovirus-mediated gene transfer, but the requirement of 30 minutes of isolated coronary perfusion would be difficult to attain in an intact animal. Consequently, we sought conditions that would produce gene transfer to more than 90% of myocytes after a brief exposure to virus

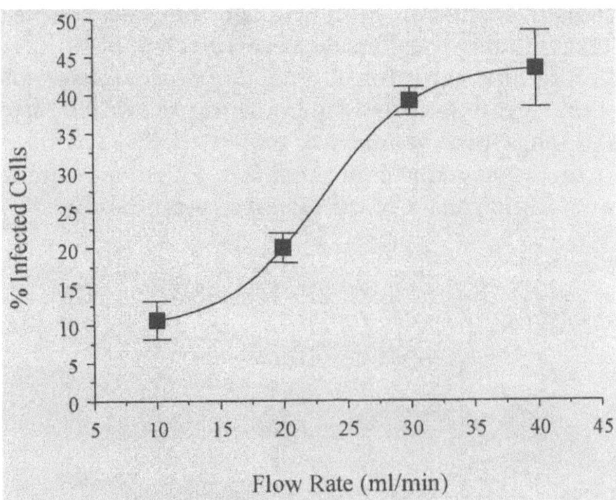

Fig. 6. Adβgal delivery to intact, Langendorff-perfused rabbit hearts at 37 °C. Percentage of myocytes positive for β-galactosidase following 2.0 h infections with 1.0×10^8 pfu/ml Adβgal at coronary flow rates ranging from 10 to 40 ml/min. n=3 for each data point.

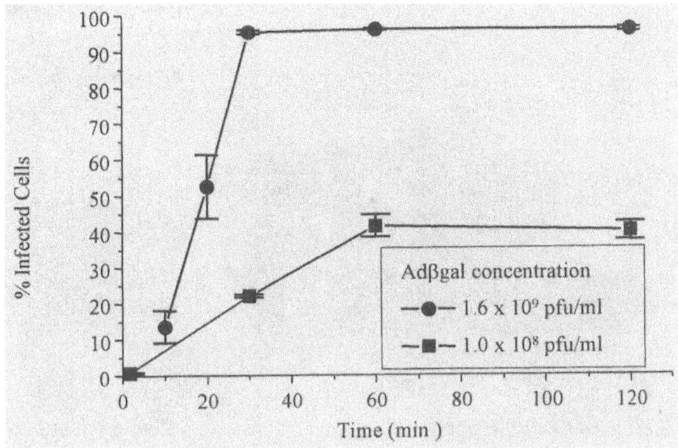

Fig. 7. Comparison of the time course of adenovirus infection at two virus concentrations. Explanted adult rabbit hearts were perfused with Ad*β*gal for up to 60 min. Baseline conditions included infection in Kreb's solution at 30 ml/min and 37 °C, followed by a virus-free perfusion with Kreb's solution. The total perfusion time was 180 min, independent of the infection time. n = 3 for each data point.

(Fig. 8a). A potential solution to this problem was to breakdown the vascular and extravascular barriers to virus diffusion. In a proof of principle experiment, we disrupted these barriers with a 30 second exposure to Kreb's solution containing 1 mg/ml trypsin immediately prior to infusion with the Ad*β*gal-containing solution. Compared to controls, treatment with trypsin followed by 30 min exposure to 1×10^8 pfu/ml Ad*β*gal resulted in a 3-fold increase in infection. The problem with this approach was the frequent deterioration in myocardial function after brief digestion. To overcome this difficulty, we used serotonin and bradykinin. Each of these agents has been shown in a variety of models to increase permeability of the vasculature at the post-capillary venular level [23, 24]. Treatment with 1×10^{-5} mol/L of serotonin or bradykinin for 15 min prior to infection with 1×10^8 pfu/ml Ad*β*bgal in the presence of 1×10^{-5} mol/L of serotonin or bradykinin led to an increase in infection to a similar degree as that seen with trypsinization. Unlike trypsin exposure, however, there was no functional detriment noted from these manipulations.

Following a similar line of reasoning, we postulated that brief exposure to solutions with low calcium concentration would increase capillary permeability by transiently disrupting endothelial tight junctions and possibly extracellular matrix attachment. Reduction in the extracellular calcium concentration by chelation with EDTA was previously shown to increase adenoviral gene transfer to hepatocytes [8]. Cardiac cells, however, do not tolerate similar treatment, since the elimination of calcium from the extracellular environment is toxic when calcium is re-introduced to myocytes [4]. A calcium concentration of 50 µmol/L is sufficient, however, to avoid this so-called "calcium paradox". Indeed, a 2 min wash-down of the calcium concentration to 50 µmol/L followed by 30 min exposure to 1×10^8

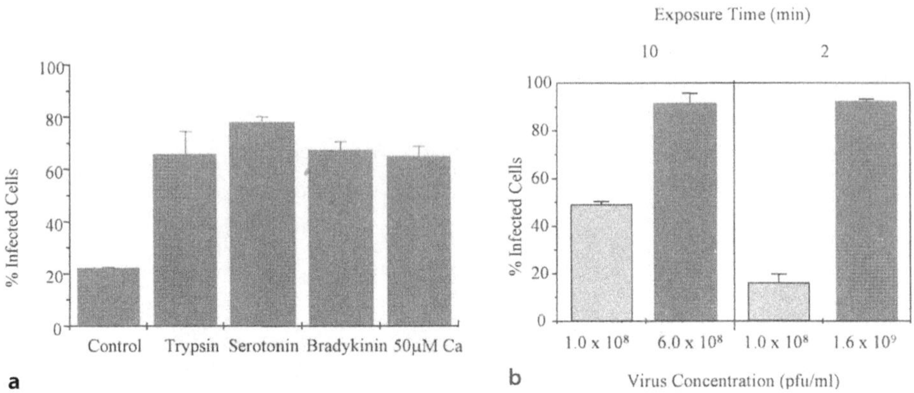

Fig. 8. Summary of the effects on adenovirus infection after pretreatment with moderators of microvascular permeability. **a** Langendorf perfused rabbit hearts were exposed to 1 mg/ml trypsin, 10^{-5} mol/L serotonin or bradykinin, or 50 μmol/L calcium-Kreb's prior to 30 min infection with 1.0×10^{8} pfu/ml of Ad*β*gal. **b** Pretreatment with 10^{-5} mol/L serotonin and 50 μmol/L calcium-Kreb's solution reduced the necessary adenovirus exposure time. Adult rabbit hearts were perfused with 10^{-5} mol/L serotonin in normal Kreb's solution for 15 min, followed by 10^{-5} mol/L serotonin in 50 μmol/L calcium-Kreb's for 3 min and infection in Kreb's with 50 μmol/L calcium, 10^{-5} mol/L serotonin, and Ad-*β*gal at the stated concentration for the stated time. n=3 for each data point.

pfu/ml Ad*β*gal in low calcium Kreb's solution caused an increase in infection similar to that seen with serotonin, bradykinin and trypsin (Fig. 8a).

Since the low calcium and serotonin manipulations had different effector sites, we speculated that a combination of the two protocols would be synergistic, allowing even greater levels of gene transfer over shorter periods of time. Pretreatment with 1×10^{-5} mol/L of serotonin in normal Kreb's solution for 13 min followed by 1×10^{-5} mol/L of serotonin in 50 μmol/L calcium-Kreb's for 2 min resulted in a significant improvement in infection. Using a virus concentration of 1.0×10^{8} pfu/ml, infection occurred in 49.4±1.0% of cells after 10 min virus exposure and 16.3±3.4% of cells after 2 min. To achieve our target of 90% infection at each time point, the virus concentration was increased. 10 min exposure to an Ad*β*gal concentration of 6.0×10^{8} pfu/ml produced 91.5±4.4% infection, and 2 min of virus exposure with 1.6×10^{9} pfu/ml resulted in 92.3±1.0% reporter gene delivery into cardiac myocytes (Fig. 8b).

Transfer of Findings to in vivo models

These data demonstrate that adenovirus-mediated gene transfer is essentially a diffusion-limited process, so optimization of parameters relevant to diffusion, such as virus and receptor concentration, particle size, and temperature, will increase the efficiency of gene transfer. Likewise, breaking down structural barriers by serotonin and low calcium exposure should improve results. The poor efficiency of adenovirus-mediated gene transfer in previously published *in vivo* models can be readily explained by these data. For the previously reported transplant models [12, 21], low temperature and slow flow rate would limit infection rate. In the coronary catheterization models [1, 23], the presence of blood and contrast dye would have inhibited myocyte infection, and poor flow rate, short exposure time and low virus concentration would have decreased infection efficiency. Pericardial delivery [20] and direct myocardial injection [14] would have the advantages of maintaining local virus concentration, but both would be limited from achieving generalized delivery by diffusional barriers. More recently, an *in vivo* delivery system used the above data to successfully deliver the phospholamban gene to rats after aortic and pulmonary artery cross-clamping [15].

In theory, success in in vivo models can be formulated using these findings. The most direct application would be to the transplant setting. With adequate safeguards to insure continued myocardial oxygenation and substrate delivery, adenovirus delivery through the coronary arteries could be achieved at 37 °C using the same system developed for Langendorff perfusion. With minor adjustments, the system could be modified for *in vivo* delivery in a cardiac surgery model. During peripheral bypass, the coronary circulation would be isolated and available for perfusion using the parameters identified in the above models. An additional advantage of these delivery systems is that the unattached virus would not be exposed to the entire body. Delivery during coronary catheterization does not have that safeguard, but it does have the advantage of delivery in a minimally invasive system. During catheterization, localized delivery is theoretically attainable using the same variables, but the permeability agents and virus would be delivered to the entire body.

In summary, the investigation of several basic variables in isolated cells and then in intact tissue has allowed us to identify parameters important for successful adenovirus-mediated gene transfer. The current challenge is to transfer this information to usable *in vivo* models and eventually into human subjects for gene therapy of a variety of congenital and acquired cardiac diseases.

References

1. Barr E, Carroll J, Kalynych AM, Tripathy SK, Kozarsky K, Wilson JM, Leiden JM (1994) Efficient catheter-mediated gene transfer into the heart using replication-defective adenovirus. Gene Therapy 1:51–58
2. Bergelson JM, Cunningham JA, Droguett G, Kurtjones EA, Krithivas A, Hong JS, Horwitz MS, Crowell RL, Finberg RW (1997) Isolation of a common receptor for coxsackie B viruses and adenoviruses 2 and 5. Science 275:1320–1323
3. Breil I, Koch T, Belz M, Vanackern K, Neuhof H (1997) Effects of bradykinin, histamine, and serotonin on pulmonary vascular resistance and permeability. Acta Physiologica Scandinavica 159:189–198

4. Chapman RA (1987) Calcium channels, the sodium-calcium exchange and intracellular sodium in the predisposition of the heart to the calcium paradox. Biomed Biochem Acta 46:S512–S516
5. Chardonnet Y, Dales S (1970) Early events in the interaction of adenoviruses with HeLa cells: I. penetration of type 5 and intracellular release of the DNA genome. Virology 40:462–477
6. Chen HH, Mack LM, Kelly R, Ontell M, Kochanek S, Clemens PR (1997) Persistence in muscle of an adenoviral vector that lacks all viral genes. Proc Natl Acad Sci USA 94:1645–1650
7. Chroboczek J, Bieber F, Jacrot B (1992) The sequence of the genome of adenovirus type 5 and its comparison with the genome of adenovirus type 2. Virology 186:280–285
8. de Roos WK, Fallaux FJ, Marinelli AW, Lazaris-Karatzas A, von Geusau AB, van der Eb MM, Cramer SJ, Terpstra OT, Hoeben RC (1997) Isolated-organ perfusion for local gene delivery: efficient adenovirus-mediated gene transfer into the liver. Gene Ther 4:55–62
9. Donahue JK, Kikkawa K, Johns DC, Marban E, Lawrence JH (1997) Ultrarapid, highly efficient viral gene transfer to the heart. Proc Natl Acad Sci USA 94:4664–4668
10. Fechner H, Haack A, Wang H, Wang X, Eizema K, Pauschinger M, Schoemaker R, Veghel R, Houtsmuller A, Schultheiss HP, Lamers J, Poller W (1999) Expression of Coxsackie adenovirus receptor and alpha-integrin does not correlate with adenovector targeting in vivo indicating anatomical vector barriers. Gene Therapy 6:1520–1535
11. Ghosh-Choudhury G, Haj-Ahmad Y, Graham FL (1987) Protein IX, a minor component of the human adenovirus capsid, is essential for the packaging of full length genomes. EMBO J 6:1733–1739
12. Gojo S, Kitamura S, Niwaya K, Yoshida Y, Sakaguchi H, Kawachi K (1996) *Ex vivo* gene transfer to transplanted heart grafts using adenoviral vector. Transplantation Proceedings 28:1818–1819
13. Graham FL, Prevec L (1995) Methods for construction of adenovirus vectors. Mol Biotechnol 3:207–220
14. Guzman RJ, Lemarchand P, Crystal RG, Epstein SE, Finkel T (1993) Efficient gene transfer into myocardium by direct injection of adenovirus vectors. Circ Res 73:1202–1207
15. Hajjar RJ, Schmidt U, Matsui T, Guerrero L, Lee K, Gwathmey JK, Dec G, Semigran M, Rosenzweig A (1998) Modulation of ventricular function through gene transfer in vivo. Proc Natl Acad Sci USA 95:5251–5256
16. Hilleman MR, Werner JH (1954) Recovery of new agents from patients with acute respiratory illness. Proc Soc Exp Biol Med 85:183–188
17. Kass-Eisler A, Falck-Pedersen E, Alvira M, Rivera J, Buttrick PM, Wittenberg BA, Cipriani L, Leinwand LA (1993) Quantitative determination of adenovirus-mediated gene delivery to rat cardiac myocytes *in vitro* and *in vivo*. Proc Natl Acad Sci USA 90:11498–11502
18. Kirshenbaum LA, MacLellan WR, Mazur W, French BA, Schneider MD (1993) Highly efficient gene transfer into adult ventricular myocytes by recombinant adenovirus. J Clin Invest 92:381–387
19. Kruijer W, van Schaik FM, Sussenbach JS (1980) Nucleotide sequence analysis of a region of adenovirus 5 DNA encoding a hitherto unidentified gene. Nucleic Acids Res 8:6033–6042
20. Lamping KG, Rios CD, Chun JA, Ooboshi H, Davidson BL, Heistad DD (1997) Intrapericardial administration of adenovirus for gene transfer. Am J Physiol 272:H310–H317

21. Lee J, Laks H, Drinkwater DC, Blitz A, Lam L, Shiraishi Y, Chang P, Drake TA, Ardehali A (1996) Cardiac and pulmonary replacement: cardiac gene transfer by intracoronary infusion of adenovirus vector-mediated reporter gene in the transplanted mouse heart. J Thorac Cardiovasc Surg 111:246–252
22. Marcus ML (1983) The coronary circulation in health and disease. McGraw-Hill, New York
23. Muhlhauser J, Jones M, Yamada I, Cirielli C, Lemarchand P, Gloe TR, Bewig B, Signoretti S, Crystal RG, Capogrossi MC (1996) Safety and efficacy of *in vivo* gene transfer into the porcine heart with replication-deficient, recombinant adenovirus vectors. Gene Therapy 3:145–153
24. Mullins RJ, Malias MA, Hudgens RW (1989) Isoproterenol inhibits the increase in microvascular membrane permeability produced by bradykinin. J Trauma 29:1053–1063
25. Nermut MV (1975) Fine structure of adenovirus Type 5: I. Virus capsid. Virology 65:480–495
26. Persson R, Svensson U, Everitt E (1983) Virus receptor interaction in the adenovirus system: II. Capping and cooperative binding of virions on HeLa cells. J Virol 46:956–963
27. Philipson L (1967) Attachment and eclipse of adenovirus. J Virol 1:868–875
28. Philipson L, Lonberg-Holm K, Pettersson U (1968) Virus-receptor interaction in an adenovirus system. J Virol 2:1064–1075
29. Rowe WP, Huebner RJ, Gilmore LK, Parrott RH, Ward TG (1953) Isolation of a cytopathogenic agent from human adenoids undergoing spontaneous degeneration in tissue culture. Proc Soc Exp Biol Med 84:570–573
30. Shenk T (1996) Adenoviridae: the viruses and their replication. In: Fields BN, Knipe DM, Howley PM (eds) Fields virology. Lippincott-Raven, Philadelphia, pp 2111–2148
31. Trentin JJ, Yabe Y, Taylor G (1962) The quest for human cancer viruses. Science 137:835–849
32. van Ormondt H, Maat J, van Beveren CP (1980) The nucleotide sequence of the transforming early region E1 of adenovirus type 5 DNA. Gene 11:299–309
33. Weeks DL, Jones NC (1983) E1A control of gene expression is mediated by sequences 5′ to the transcriptional starts of the early viral genes. Mol Cell Biol 3:1222–1234
34. Wickham TJ, Mathias P, Cheresh DA, Nemerow GR (1993) Integrins $\alpha_v\beta_3$ and $\alpha_v\beta_5$ promote adenovirus internalization but not virus attachment. Cell 73:309–319

CHAPTER 9

Adenovirus-mediated transfection of multicellular cardiac preparations

P. M. L. JANSSEN, S. E. LEHNART, J. K. DONAHUE, J. PRESTLE, E. MARBÁN, G. HASENFUSS

Department of Cardiology and Pneumology, University of Göttingen, Göttingen, Germany

Summary

The study of altered protein expression patterns in diseased myocardium has greatly contributed to our understanding of cardiac dysfunction. Adenovirus-mediated changes in this protein expression pattern in order to correct deregulated protein synthesis is currently undergoing widespread interest and is emerging as a possible future therapy. In an *in vitro* setting, most experiments to date have used primary adult myocyte cultures to study the impact of adenovirus-mediated gene transfer on the function of the myocardium. Several studies have already indicated that the isotonic shortening behavior of isolated myocytes can be successfully changed through adenoviral-mediated gene transfer. However, under cell culture conditions active loaded contractions do not occur as they do *in situ*, thereby hampering interpretation to this *in vivo* situation. Although multicellular cardiac preparations may not represent every single aspect of the beating heart, loading conditions can be influenced and these preparations have a multicellular architecture contracting under loaded conditions as occur in heart. The latter implies that impact of secretory factors and interaction between different cell types is possible. Moreover, cell-to-cell connections allow for passing-on of intracellular signals and physical loading conditions, between myocytes specifically, in these multicellular preparations.

We have used a Langendorff-based adenoviral gene-transfer protocol to the rabbit heart and cultured multicellular preparations from these hearts for several days. Basic contractility parameters did not change over time when such preparations were cultured, and physiological and pharmacological responses were well preserved. Although after 48 hours efficient and high levels of the transfected reporter-gene LacZ were observed in the individual myocytes of the preparation, contractile parameters and physiological/pharmacological responses were unaltered.

Introduction

In many pathophysiological conditions of the heart, the myocardial protein expression pattern deviates from the normal physiological situation. These changes can be causal, but can also be a consequencial adaptation to myocardial dysfunction that occurs to compensate loss of function. The study of altered protein expression patterns in diseased myocardium has greatly contributed to our knowledge of cardiac dysfunction. Changes of the myocardial expression pattern can be induced by neuro-humoral, mechanical, and pharmacological interventions. Also, in the last few decades a variety of gene-transfer techniques have been developed that can be employed to alter the protein expression pattern under *in vitro* and *in vivo* settings [2, 12, 13, 20]. When any of these interventions are employed *in vivo*, the functional consequences of the altered protein expression pattern can be assessed with conventional methods of organ physiology. However, *in vitro* evaluation of the functional effects of gene transfer has so far been limited to the study of isolated myocytes [1, 14, 17, 39, 40]. Although this is a valuable tool that has led and will continue to lead to many important findings [38], the lack of cell-to-cell connections, lack of the presence of and interaction between different cell types, and absence of loading conditions may severely hamper interpretation of the impact on contractile function.

Several techniques are currently available to assess contractile function *in vitro* in mammalian myocardium. Closely interpretable to the *in vivo* situation are whole heart experiments, both *in situ* (such as the open chest canine model) and *ex vivo* (Langendorff heart, working heart). Although these methods can be employed to study acute contractile responses, they cannot be employed for the study of gene transfer because they do not allow sufficient time (>24 hours) to pass between an event that triggers altered protein expression and the actual functional consequence of this altered protein pattern. Contractile function can also be studied in isolated myocardial multicellular preparations like papillary muscles or endocardial ventricular trabeculae. These preparations have been shown to be closely interpretable to the *in vivo* situation, since they display many, if not all, of the basic contractile regulatory mechanisms of the heart, including the Frank-Starling mechanism and ejection properties [4, 8, 41]. Isolated myocardial preparations are longitudinal running muscles in the heart and consist of myocytes, fibroblasts, and both endocardial and vascular endothelium. Recently, we developed an experimental chamber in which contractile function of rabbit and human muscles can be studied over several days [23, 24]. This approach now bridges the time between a trigger that changes the protein expression pattern and its functional alteration. Providing we can induce a widespread adenoviral gene transfer in the vast majority (~95%) of the individual cells in these preparations [9, 10], we would be able to link altered protein expression with its functional relevance. In this chapter we describe the combination of two techniques, multicellular preparation culture and efficient adenoviral-mediated gene transfer, which allow us to study the link between protein expression and myocardial contraction.

The myocardial culture system

We aimed to develop a system in which small myocardial trabeculae and/or papillary muscles could be kept contracting for several days. Several adaptations from more classical *in vitro* muscle experiments were a prerequisite in creating an *in vitro* environment that allows for successful culture of myocardial trabeculae for several days [23, 24]. The most important adaptation of a classical set-up (using crystalline perfusion solutions) is that protein synthesis must continue to take place in order to replace proteins that are lost because of natural turnover and also to be able to allow alterations in the protein expression pattern *per se*. Preserved protein synthesis implies that preparations have to be kept under conditions similar to a cell culture environment. We achieved this through development of a chamber (see Fig. 1) where temperature, pH, and bathing solutions are kept constant, while allowing for continuous measurement of contractile function. Furthermore, the use of a modified cell culture medium ensures that all essential nutritional compounds are available. Changing this solution every 6–12 hours ensures that all nutrients are readily available and break-down products are removed

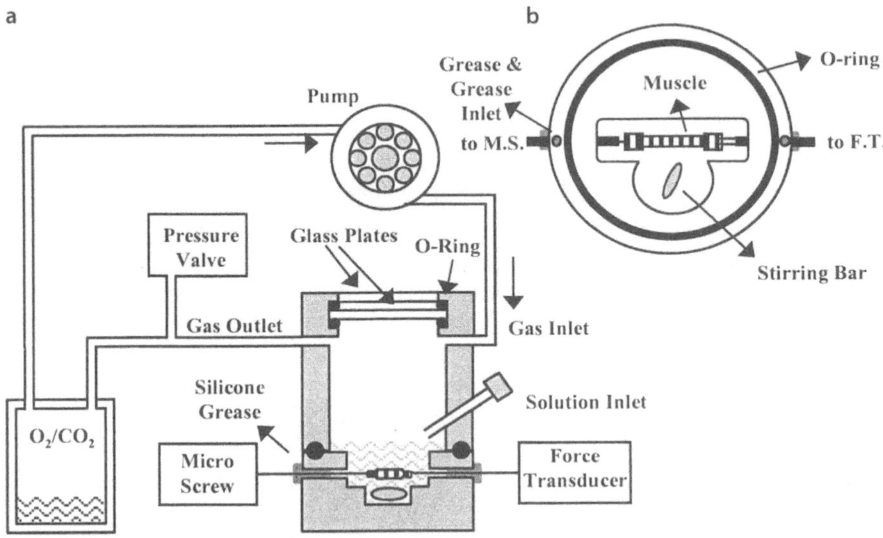

Fig. 1. Illustration depicting the trabecula culture system, modified after Janssen et al. [23]. **a** Suitable preparations (ave. diameter <350 μm, length 2–5 mm) are dissected from rabbit or human hearts and mounted in the system between a force transducer and micro-screw to adjust preload. The system is sealed off from the external environment to prevent evaporation of water and also to prevent bacterial contamination. A gas mixture of 95% O_2/5% CO_2 is pumped through the chamber to supply oxygen and to keep pH of the bicarbonate buffer constant. The top of the chamber has double walled glass to prevent condensation of water. **b** Top view and detail of the teflon muscle chamber. A small stirbar situated next to the muscle continuously stirs the solution. Muscles are mounted with the "basket and hook" method [8, 23, 41] to minimize damage to the preparation.

from the incubation solution. In this system, protein synthesis as indicated by measurement of incorporation of ^{3}H-leucine in 12-hour intervals remained stable over at least 72 hours [23]; in the first 12 hours protein synthesis amounted to 652±65 decays per minute per μg protein (n = 3), which was similar in preparations after 72 hours of culture (750±129 dpm/μg prot., n = 3).

Another important modification from a more classical muscle chamber is that the system is completely sealed off from the environment, thereby minimizing risk of bacterial contamination. Also, it prevents evaporation and concentration of the culture media over time. We have used this system to culture trabeculae from both rabbit hearts [23] and from hearts explanted from patients who underwent cardiac transplantation surgery [24]. In Fig. 2, average values are given for developed force (F_{dev}), diastolic force (F_{dia}), and time from peak tension to 50% relaxation ($RT_{50\%}$). As can be seen, very little change in these contractile parameters are observed after 48 hours in the system, both in the rabbit and in the human preparations. Other contractile parameters like time to peak tension, minimal and maximal derivative of force development, and time to 90% relaxation were also unaltered over time. Although contractile parameters of the individual muscles can fluctuate over time, possibly due to the steep force-length relation under the current conditions [29, 41], average values of these parameters allow for comparison between the beginning and the end of a 48-hour culture period.

In addition to baseline contractility, we investigated whether regulatory mechanisms remain intact after 48 hours of culture. Therefore we measured the contractile response to an addition of either endothelin-1 or iso-

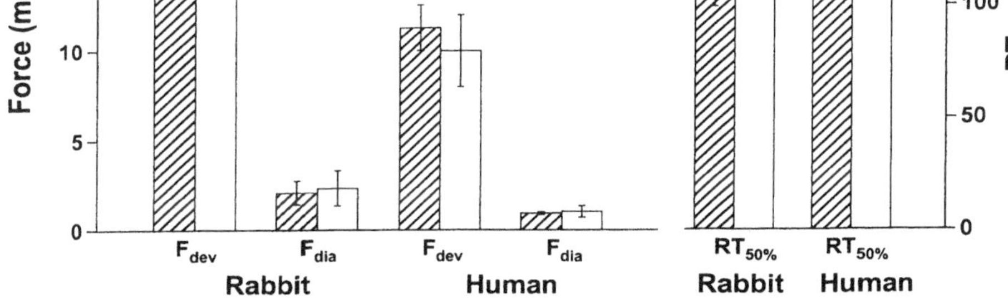

Fig. 2. Contractile parameters of rabbit and human trabeculae. Developed force (F_{dev}), diastolic force (F_{dia}), and time from peak tension to 50% relaxation ($RT_{50\%}$) of rabbit (n = 8) and human muscles (n = 10) at t = 0 (open bars) and after 48 hours (gray bars) of continuous contractions at 0.5 or 1 Hz in the trabeculae culture system (t = 48 h).

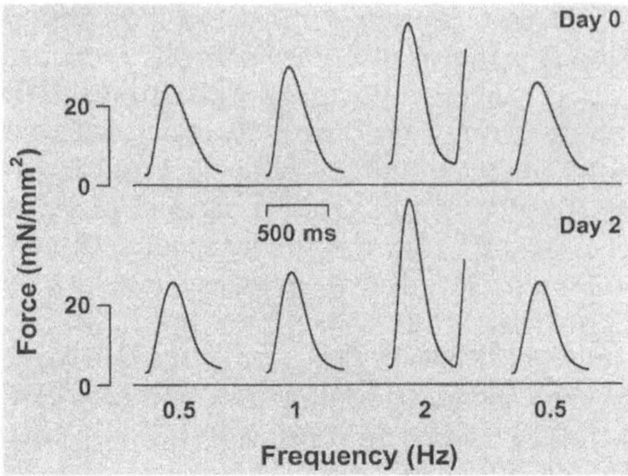

Fig. 3. Response to increase in stimulation frequency. Original recording of the force-frequency protocol in a human trabecula. The time between the two frequencies was about 5 min. No differences were observed between the start (day 0, top panel) and the end of the experiment (day 2, bottom panel).

proterenol (Fig. 3). After the addition of 1 μM isoproterenol, both rabbit and human trabeculae (left) responded with an increased force of contraction and an increased speed of relaxation (right). Addition of endothelin-1 (ET-1, 0.1 μM) increased force of contraction without altering speed of relaxation in rabbit trabeculae. The responses to these drugs indicate that the entire signal-transduction cascade through the receptor, second messenger, and effector is well preserved. However, although the observed response is very similar to those observed in freshly isolated trabeculae [19, 31], whether culture of these trabeculae changes the response over time to those agents has not yet been investigated.

An increase in the stimulation frequency under physiological conditions results in increased force of contraction in almost all mammals, including the rat [30], rabbit [11], and human [32, 37]. It has been established that during cardiac failure this behavior is altered: an increase in stimulation frequency results in a blunted- or even negative force-frequency relationship in patients with end-stage heart failure [32, 37]. To further characterize our system, we investigated the force-frequency behavior after multiday cultivation of the preparations and whether it had changed from its initial behavior. In 7 from the 11 human preparations studied we observed that frequency potentiation of force was preserved up to 2 Hz. In all these muscles, force-frequency behavior was unchanged after 48 hours (example in Fig. 4). Muscles that displayed a flat (n=1) or a negative (n=3) force-frequency behavior also remained unchanged.

In conclusion, in the trabeculae culture system, preparations can be kept contracting for several days without adversely impacting basic contractile behavior, and display preserved responses to pharmacological and physiological stimuli.

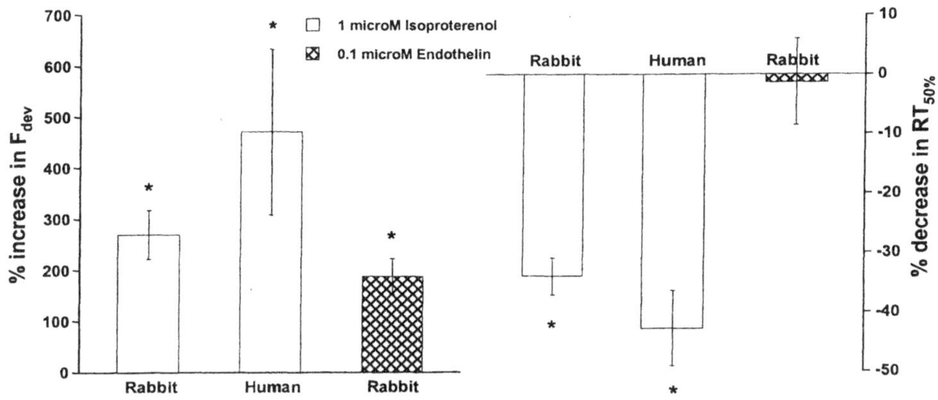

Fig. 4. Response to isoproterenol and endothelin. After 48 or 72 hours of contractions, the contractile response to isoproterenol (open bars) was preserved in rabbit and human trabeculae. Upon stimulation with 1 μM isoproterenol, both rabbit and human preparations responded with an increase in force development (left panel) and an abbreviation of duration of relaxation (right panel). Endothelin (ET-1, 0.1 μM, gray bars) also increased force development in preparations from the rabbit (left), but did not change twitch timing parameters (right). *denotes a significant ($p<0.05$) change from control.

Adenoviral gene transfer

In the recent past, several gene transfer techniques have been developed to replace missing cellular proteins or to express therapeutic gene products. Myocardial gene therapy may become a promising approach for the treatment of myocardial disorders [5, 20, 28, 29, 35]. Meanwhile, numerous studies have demonstrated the feasibility of recombinant adenoviruses as gene delivery systems to the heart [1, 9, 10, 13, 14, 18, 33]. *In vitro* studies have already demonstrated the feasibility of adenoviral gene transfer to possibly combat arrhythmias by overexpression of a potassium channel gene that resulted in increased K^+ currents and shortened action potential duration in failing cardiac myocytes [35]. Likewise, contractility of the cardiac myocyte has been shown to improve upon overexpression of the sarcoplasmic Ca^{2+}-ATPase (SERCA) in cardiac myocytes through enhanced SR Ca^{2+}-uptake and shortening of the prolonged intracellular Ca^{2+} transients [14].

Although the adenoviral-mediated gene transfer is a promising tool and may even become a future therapeutic approach for heart failure and/or arrhythmias, most of the studies are limited by a low efficiency of gene transfer. In sharp contrast to the isolated cardiomyocytes that can be easily and effectively transfected by low titers of adenoviral vectors, transfection of cardiomyocytes in a multicellular setting, as in the intact heart, has proven to be difficult. Only a few studies have been able to show effective expression of adenovirally introduced proteins in the working heart [18, 29]. Moreover, a strong immunogenicity and unknown intrinsic toxicity of the vector system against the host cell [12, 43] limit *in vivo* adenoviral infection of the heart.

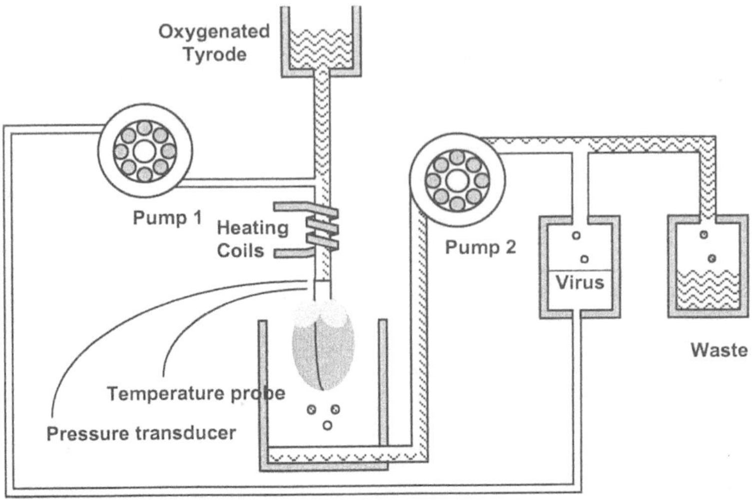

Fig. 5. Illustration depicting adenoviral transfection with the Langendorff set-up [9, 10]. The heart is mounted in the set-up and is gravity perfused (30–40 ml/min) retrogradely through the aorta with regular oxygenated Tyrode's solution (gray waves pathway). After washout of all the blood, the heart is subjected to 1 hour of controlled flow perfusion (30 ml/min) with a circulating buffer containing $1.6 \cdot 10^9$ pfu/ml adenovirus (clear pathway). During all protocols, temperature (controlled to 37 °C) and perfusion pressure are recorded. Following washout of the virus with oxygenated Tyrode's solution, the heart is dismounted and multicellular preparations are dissected, also under sterile conditions.

The tight endothelial cell layer surrounding the myocytes is the main hurdle that is limiting transfection efficiency in most previously mentioned studies. This barrier can be overcome by either physically enlarging the gap between the endothelial cells via increased perfusion pressure or with pharmaceutical interventions like serotonin application. Reducing this barrier now allows for high level efficiency of adenoviral transfection in nearly 100% of the myocytes in the heart [9, 10]. With this technique, retrograde flow-controlled perfusion of rabbit hearts in a Langendorff mode is used to transfect the myocytes (Fig. 5). After stabilization of the beating heart, the heart is perfused at an increased pressure with a physiological salt buffer containing a very high virus concentration (up to 1.6×10^9 pfu/ml). After adequate washout of the virus at normal perfusion pressures, 95% of the myocytes have been shown to be successfully transfected [9, 10]. Thus, by overcoming the endothelial barrier, it is possible to efficiently transfect cardiac myocytes by adenoviral vectors in their multicellular longitudinal setting.

After using this method to transfect the myocytes, we dissected multicellular preparations from these hearts and cultivated these preparations in the experimental chamber we developed. Possible alterations in contractile function can be directly studied in these preparations while significant levels of the protein of interest are synthesized and become functionally meaningful.

Contractile function and transgene expression of transfected trabeculae

The combination of the trabeculae culture system and the adenoviral-mediated gene transfer protocol allows for measurement of contractile function before, during, and after the protein expression pattern has been changed. This complicated approach was necessary since pilot experiments revealed that simply incubating the preparations with high titers of virus resulted in only a low transfection percentage of the myocytes (<10%), even though nearly 100% of endothelial cells were transfected. In Fig. 6, the contractile parameters F_{dev}, F_{dia}, and $RT_{50\%}$ are given at the beginning of the experiment and after 48 hours of continuous contractions. LacZ-transfected trabeculae and sham-transfected (same Langendorff perfusion protocol without virus) retained their function over time. Also, baseline contractile function of these preparations is very similar and not significantly different from those that were not subjected to the virus-perfusion protocol at all (e.g., Fig. 2). In addition, the isoproterenol response after virus transfer was not different from the response observed in non-transfected preparations. Thus, these data clearly demonstrate that, under the conditions used, no adverse effect on contractile function of the virus-transfection protocol was observed.

To detect the alteration of the protein expression pattern after transfection of the LacZ gene, both control and LacZ-transfected trabeculae were stained with X-gal, the substrate for *β*-galactosidase (LacZ). The staining

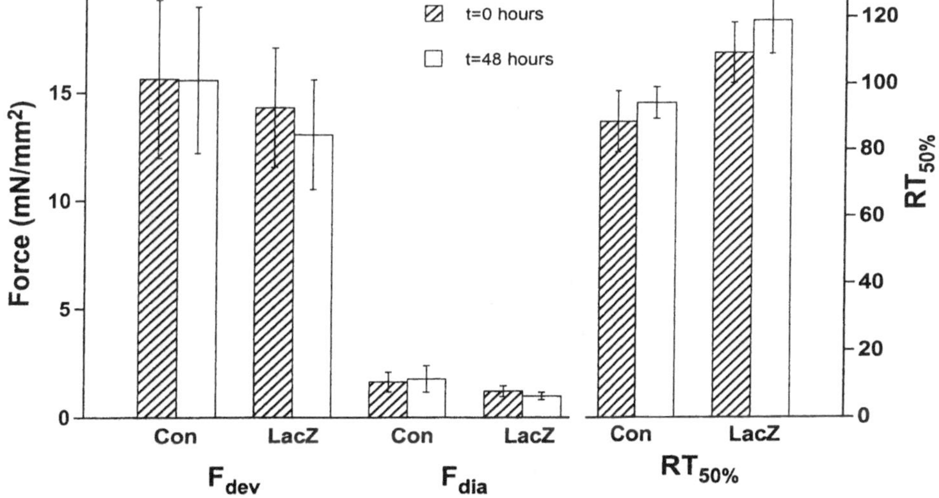

Fig. 6. Contractile parameters of transfected trabeculae. Rabbit trabeculae are dissected from hearts subjected to control perfusion (no virus) or to perfusion with adenovirus encoding for the LacZ gene. Developed force (F_{dev}), diastolic force (F_{dia}), and time from peak force to 50% relaxation ($RT_{50\%}$) of control (n=11) and LacZ-transfected preparations (n=12) at t=0 (open bars) and after 48 hours of continuous contractions (gray bars).

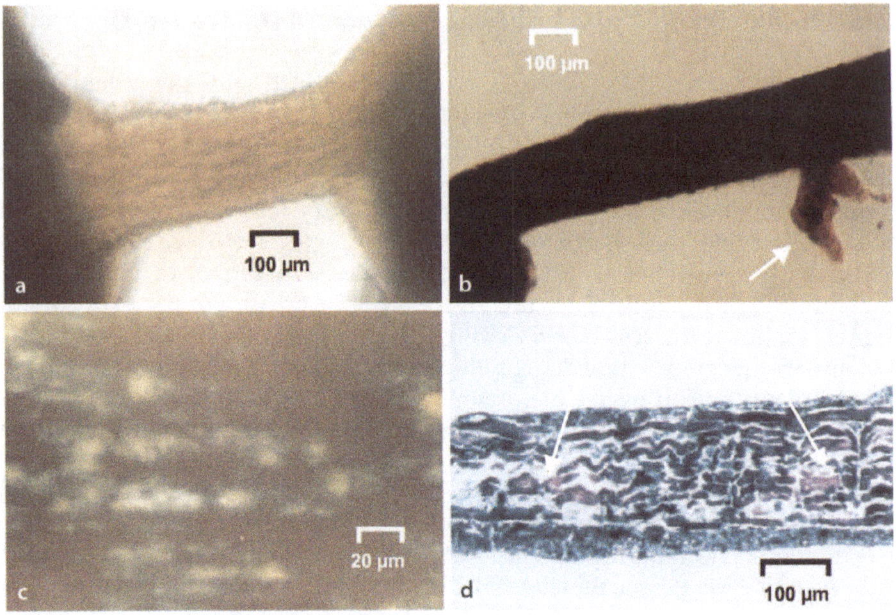

Fig. 7. Transgene expression in multicellular preparations. **a** Control muscle (non-transfected) stained for LacZ expression with X-Gal; no blue staining is observed. **b** LacZ-transfected muscle after 2 days of continuous contractions in the set-up; widespread blue staining can easily be observed in this preparation. Interestingly, it can be seen that within the small side-branch (indicated by the arrow), only staining in the center can be observed. The outer cell layers died in the first few hours of the experiment due to calcium overload after this side-branch was severed and these cells did not survive long enough to allow for the expression of the β-galactosidase transgene. **c** Section of a LacZ-transfected muscle; also in the core of the muscle, widespread β-galactosidase expression is detected. **d** Histological section of a LacZ-transfected muscle; nearly all myocytes are transfected, indicated by the intense blue staining. This preparation was counterstained with HE (pink) to visualize non-transfected myocytes (see arrows).

protocol was performed at an alkaline pH of 8.5 to avoid false-positive staining. In Fig. 7b, a macroscopic picture of a LacZ-transfected trabecula is shown. As can be easily seen, almost the entire trabecula is stained blue, indicating widespread and high levels of LacZ expression. This is in sharp contrast to control trabeculae (Fig. 7a) that were entirely devoid of any blue staining. Figure 7c shows that in the core of larger preparations myocytes are also transfected. In Fig. 7d a HE-counterstained histological section is shown where it is evident that the vast majority of myocytes express the transfected gene. Only a few myocytes show poor transgene expression (examples indicated by the arrows).

Thus, the combination of the trabeculae culture and efficient adenoviral gene transfer allows for the expression of transgenes, while simultaneously allowing the impact on contractile function to be assessed in an *in vitro* setting.

Discussion

By use of the adenoviral perfusion protocol in intact hearts [9, 10], it is possible to program high levels of transgene expression into myocardial preparations that can be subsequently followed [23, 24] to correlate changes in protein expression with changes in contractility. Also, demonstration of a lack of adverse effects on myocardial function despite robust overexpression of adenoviral transgenes in these preparations is important in the light of upcoming gene therapy protocols in the future.

Currently, different methods are employed to deliver transgenes to the myocardium. In an *in vivo* setting, direct injection techniques have been shown to induce infection of the myocardium [12, 15]; transgene expression only occurs in myocytes situated in or very close to the needle tract. Other techniques including intrapericardial injection [13], combined aortic and pulmonary artery clamping (18); and catheter-based delivery [2] were developed over the years and transfection efficiencies have improved, although consistent results of >50% myocyte throughout the entire heart transfection have not yet been achieved. Surely, the transfection efficiency is important but we should keep in mind that the protein of interest mainly dictates whether a near 100% efficiency is a prerequisite for alteration of function (e.g., when blocking a pharmacological response) or if a small population of transfected cells suffices (e.g., when the recombinant protein is secreted into the global circulation). However, for proof-of-principle studies, unambiguous results can only be obtained when transfection efficiency is sufficiently high. Currently, *in vivo* transfection techniques are still hampered by a robust host immune response [12, 43], inducible promotors [6] could help reduce the immune response. Thus, combination of the above mentioned points necessitates interpretation of results from these *in vivo* studies to be done with due care.

In *in vitro* settings, the primary culture of adult cardiomyocytes is often used to study effects of adenovirus-mediated transfection of recombinant proteins on contractility [1, 14, 35, 39, 40] and has contributed to our understanding of myocardial (dys-)function. However, quantitative investigation of the primary heart function, contraction, is hampered by methodological problems that limit interpretation of these isolated myocyte data to the *in vivo* situation. First, incubation of myocytes with adenovirus does not reflect the more complex situation of gene delivery to the intact heart [2, 9, 12, 15, 42]. Second, electrically stimulated myocytes shorten against almost zero load, which does not reflect the loading conditions of the working heart [4, 8, 23]. Third, the amount of shortening diminishes over the first few days in primary culture when not continuously stimulated at a physiologically meaningful frequency [3] or when not attached [16], and over extended time periods morphological changes occur with concurrent deviation of function [7]. Fourth, and most importantly, isolated myocytes are devoid of connections to both neighboring cells of the same cell type and to different cell types within the heart (myocytes, endothelial cells, smooth muscle cells, fibroblasts). This cell-to-cell connection is of crucial importance in regulating contractility and passing on loading conditions and signals between cells [22]. Also, factors like NO [36] or angiotensin [26] are released by one cell type, thereby co-regulating function of other cell types in the heart.

The use of cultured multicellular preparations (trabeculae and papillary muscles), of which loading conditions can be varied and which consist of the different cell types of the heart, overcomes several of the aforementioned limitations [23, 24]. Furthermore, the use of the *ex vivo* Langendorff perfusion protocol overcomes low transfection efficiencies by widening the gaps between the endothelial cells, thus, allowing for the adenovirus to dock to its receptor on the myocytes [9, 10]. The combination of these two methods now allows for efficient and high level expression of transgenes while contractile function can be continuously assessed. The observed absence of reporter gene influence on contractile function is in close agreement with studies that also reported no effects of the LacZ transgene on cardiac myocytes [17, 28]. In addition to the absence of impact on contractile function, adenoviral transfer of the LacZ reporter gene did not affect β-adrenergic signaling as assessed by stimulation of myocardial preparations with isoproterenol after 48 hours. Therefore, in contrast to a report on neonatal myocytes [34], adenoviral infection of multicellular preparations of adult hearts does not seem to enhance β-adrenergic signaling. Although the current adenoviral vectors might have limitations in "long-term" expression (months/years), the fast and robust expression makes them especially useful in these "short-term" expression experiments (days/weeks). Also, using the trabecula culture method for the assessment of the expression of recombinant transgenes on myocardial function might offer specific advantages over transgenic animal models. Developmental adaptation in transgenic animals often results in a new phenotype that is difficult to differentiate for the specific effects of the transgene expression on myocardial function from secondary effects. For instance, transgenic mice overexpressing calsequestrin [25] or serca2a also exhibit increased transcription of other physiologically important proteins like phospholamban and the Na^+-Ca^{2+} exchanger [21]. In conclusion, multi-day assessment of myocardial contractile function during the establishment of transgene expression can be used to investigate both the time course and functional effects of proteins introduced into intact myocardial tissue. Furthermore, the approach reported here may be important in investigating possible molecular approaches to the therapy of human heart failure on the level of the working myocardium.

References

1. Akhter SA, Skaer CA, Kypson AP, McDonald PH, Peppel KC, Glower DD, Lefkowitz RJ, Koch WJ (1997) Restoration of β-adrenergic signaling in failing cardiac ventricular myocytes via adenoviral-mediated gene transfer. Proc Natl Acad Sci USA 94:12100–12105
2. Barr E, Carroll J, Kalynych AM, Tripathy SK, Kozarsky K, Wilson JM, Leiden JM (1994) Efficient catheter-mediated gene transfer into the heart using replication-defective adenovirus. Gene Ther 1:51–58
3. Berger HJ, Prasad SK, Davidoff AJ, Pimental D, Ellingsen O, March JD, Smith TW, Kelly RA (1994) Continual electric field stimulation preserves contractile function of adult ventricular myocytes in primary culture. Am J Physiol 266 (Heart Circ Physiol 35):H341–H349
4. Bers DM (1997) Ca^{2+} sparks, jumping the gap from the cell to cardiac muscle. Circ Res 81:636–638
5. Brodde OE, Michel MC, Zerkowski HR (1995) Signal transduction mechanisms controlling cardiac contractility and their alterations in chronic heart failure. Cardiovasc Res 30:570–584
6. Burcin MM, Schneider G, Kochanek S, Tsai SY, O'Maley BW (1999) Adenovirus-mediated regulable target gene expression in vivo. Proc Natl Acad Sci USA 96:355–360
7. Claycomb WC, Palazzo MC (1980) Culture of the terminally differentiated adult cardiac muscle cell: a light and scanning microscope study. Dev Biol 80:466–482
8. de Tombe PP, Little WC (1994) Inotropic effects of ejection are myocardial properties. Am J Physiol 266 (Heart Circ Physiol 35):H1202–H1213
9. Donahue JK, Kikkawa K, Johns DC, Marbán E, Lawrence JH (1997) Ultrarapid, highly efficient viral gene transfer to the heart. Proc Natl Acad Sci USA 94:4664–4668
10. Donahue JK, Kikkawa K, Thomas AD, Marbán E, Lawrence JH (1998) Acceleration of widespread adenoviral gene transfer to intact rabbit hearts by coronary perfusion with low calcium and serotonin. Gene Ther 5:630–634
11. Edman KA, Johannsson M (1976) The contractile state of rabbit papillary muscle in relation to stimulation frequency. J Physiol (Lond) 254:565–581
12. French BA, Mazur W, Geske RS, Bolli R (1994) Direct *in vivo* gene transfer into porcine myocardium using replication-deficient adenoviral vectors. Circulation 90:2414–2424
13. Fromes Y, Salmon A, Wang Y, Collin H, Rouche A, Hagege A, Schwartz K, Fiszman MY (1999) Gene delivery to the myocardium by intrapericardial injection. Gene Ther 6:683–688
14. Giordano FJ, He H, McDonough P, Meyer M, Sayen R, Dillmann WH (1997) Adenovirus-mediated gene transfer reconstitutes depressed sarcoplasmic reticulum Ca^{2+}-ATPase levels and shortens prolonged cardiac myocyte Ca^{2+} transients. Circulation 96:400–403
15. Guzman RJ, Lemarchand P, Crystal RG, Epstein SE, Finkel T (1993) Efficient gene transfer into myocardium by direct injection of adenovirus vectors. Circ Res 73:1202–1207
16. Haddad J, Decker ML, Hsieh LC, Lesch M, Samarel AM, Decker DS (1988) Attachment and maintenance of adult rabbit cardiac myocytes in primary culture. Am J Physiol 255 (Cell Physiol 24):C19–C27
17. Hajjar RJ, Schmidt U, Kang JX, Matsui T, Rosenzweig A (1997) Adenoviral gene transfer of phospholamban in isolated rat cardiomyocytes. Rescue effects by concomitant gene transfer of sarcoplasmic reticulum Ca^{2+}-ATPase. Circ Res 81:145–153

18. Hajjar RJ, Schmidt U, Matsui T, Guerrero JL, Lee KH, Gwathmey JK, Dec JW, Semigran MJ, Rosenzweig A (1998) Modulation of ventricular function through gene transfer *in vivo*. Proc Natl Acad Sci USA 95:5251–5256
19. Hasenfuss G, Mulieri LA, Allen PD, Just H, Alpert N (1996) Influence of isoproterenol and ouabain on excitation-contraction coupling, cross-bridge function, and energetics in failing human myocardium. Circulation 94:3155–3160
20. Hasenfuss G (1998) Calcium pump overexpression and myocardial function. Implications for gene therapy of myocardial failure. Circ Res 83:966–968
21. He H, Giordano FJ, Hilal-Dandan R, Choi DJ, Rockman HA, McDonough PM, Bluhm WF, Meyer M, Sayen MR, Swanson E, Dillmann WH (1997) Overexpression of the rat sarcoplasmic reticulum Ca^{2+} ATPase gene in the heart of transgenic mice accelerates calcium transients and cardiac relaxation. J Clin Invest 100:380–389
22. Hynes RO (1992) Integrins: versatility, modulation, and signaling in cell adhesion. Cell 69:11–25
23. Janssen PML, Lehnart SE, Prestle J, Lynker JC, Salfeld P, Just H, Hasenfuss G (1998) The trabecula culture system: a novel technique to study contractile parameters over a multiday time period. Am J Physiol 274 (Heart Circ Physiol 43):H1481–H1488
24. Janssen PML, Lehnart SE, Prestle J, Hasenfuss G (1999) Preservation of contractile characteristics of human myocardium in multi-day cell culture. J Moll Cell Cardiol 31:1419–1427
25. Jones LR, Suzuki YJ, Wang W, Kabayashi YM, Ramesh V, Franzini-Armstrong C, Cleemann L, Morad M (1998) Regulation of Ca^{2+} signaling in transgenic mouse cardiac myocytes overexpressing calsequestrin. J Clin Invest 101:1385–1393
26. Katwa LC, Campbell SE, Tyagi SC, Lee SJ, Cicila GT, Weber KT (1997) Cultured myofibroblasts generate angiotensin peptides de novo. J Mol Cell Cardiol 29:1375–1386
27. Kentish JC, ter Keurs HEDJ, Ricciardi L, Bucx JJJ, Noble MIM (1986) Comparison between the sarcomere length-force relations of intact and skinned trabeculae from rat right ventricle. Circ Res 58:755–768
28. Kirshenbaum LA, Angelides KJ, Schneider MD (1994) Detection of exogenous gene expression in live adult ventricular myocytes after adenoviral gene delivery. Circulation 90:2124–2125
29. Kypson AP, Peppel K, Akhter SA, Lilly RE, Glower DD, Lefkowitz RJ, Koch WJ (1998) *Ex vivo* adenovirus-mediated gene transfer to the adult rat heart. J Thorac Cardiovasc Surg 115:623–630
30. Layland J, Kentish JC (1999) Positive force- and $[Ca^{2+}]_i$-frequency relationships in rat ventricular trabeculae at physiological frequencies. Am J Physiol 276 (Heart Circ Physiol 45):H9–H18
31. Li K, Steward DJ, Rouleau JL (1991) Myocardial contractile actions of endothelin-1 in rat and rabbit papillary muscles. Role of endocardial endothelium. Circ Res 69:301–312
32. Mulieri LA, Hasenfuss G, Leavitt B, Allen PD, Alpert NR (1992) Altered myocardial force-frequency relation in human heart failure. Circulation 85:1743–1750
33. Näbauer M, Kaab S (1998) Potassium channel down-regulation in heart failure. Cardiovasc Res 37:324–334
34. Novotny J, Gustafson B, Kvapil P, Ransnas LA (1994) Adenovirus infection of myocardial cells induces an enhanced sensitivity to β-adrenergic agonists by increasing the concentration of the stimulatory G-protein. Biochem Mol Biol Int. 34:993–1001
35. Nuss HB, Johns DC, Kaab S, Tomaselli GF, Kass D, Lawrence JH, Marbán E (1996) Reversal of potassium channel deficiency in cells from failing hearts by adenoviral gene transfer: a prototype for gene therapy for disorders of cardiac excitability and contractility. Gene Ther 3:900–912

36. Palmer RM, Ferrige AG, Moncada S (1987) Nitric oxide release accounts for the biological activity of endothelium-derived relaxing factor. Nature 327:524–526
37. Pieske B, Kretschmann B, Meyer M, Holubarsch C, Weirich J, Posival H, Minami K, Just H, Hasenfuss G (1995) Alterations in intracellular calcium handling associated with the inverse force-frequency relation in human dilated myocardium. Circulation 92:1169–1178
38. Piper HM, Isenberg G (1989) Isolated Adult Cardiomyocytes. CRC Press., Inc Boca Raton, Florida
39. Prestle J, Baudet S, Janssen AP, Weisser J, Pieske B, Janssen PML, Hasenfuss G (1999) Blunted positive inotropic response to endothelin-1 in rabbit ventricular myocytes upon adenovirus-mediated overexpression of protein kinase Cε. Circulation (abstract in press) 100:1–191
40. Prestle J, Janssen PML, Janssen AP, Lehnart SE, Zeitz O, Hasenfuss G (1999) Adenovirus-mediated overexpression of FKPB12.6 increases contractility in isolated rabbit ventricular myocytes. Circulation (abstract in press) 100:1–629
41. ter Keurs HEDJ, Rijnsburger WH, van Heuningen R, Nagelsmit MJ (1980) Tension development and sarcomere length in rat cardiac trabeculae: evidence of length-dependent activation. Circ Res 46:703–714
42. von Harsdorf R, Schott RJ, Shen YT, Vatner SF, Mahdavi V, Nadal-Ginard B (1993) Gene injection into canine myocardium as a useful model for studying gene expression in the heart of large mammals. Circ Res 72:688–695
43. Yang Y, Nunes FA, Berencsi K, Furth EE, Gonczol E, Wilson JM (1994) Cellular immunity to viral antigenes limits E1-deleted adenoviruses for gene therapy. Proc Natl Acad Sci USA 91:4407–4411

CHAPTER 10

Myocardial-specific gene delivery

W.-M. FRANZ [1], O. J. MÜLLER [1], H. A. KATUS [1], G. VON DEGENFELD [2], G. STEINBECK [2], P. BOEKSTEGERS [2]

[1] Medizinische Klinik II, Medizinische Universität zu Lübeck, Lübeck, Germany

[2] Medizinische Klinik I, Klinikum Großhadern der LMU, München, Germany

Introduction

Somatic gene therapy represents a promising approach for the treatment of inherited and acquired heart diseases. In contrast to final stadium cancer or rare inherited diseases, established pharmacological, catheter-based or surgical alternatives for treatment of cardiac disorders frequently exist. Therefore, the safety of the vector system and its application requires careful consideration in cardiac gene therapy approaches. An ideal vector system should be immunologically tolerated, allow gene expression specifically in the myocardium, and should be administered with high efficacy as specific as possible.

Besides correction of inherited cardiomyopathies by gene transfer of the intact gene, conditions such as heart failure, cardiac hypertrophy, arrhythmias, and ischemic heart disease are targets for new cardiac gene therapeutic approaches. Positive inotropy could be induced in rabbits by adenoviral transfer of components of the β-signaling pathway [37] or in transgenic rats overexpressing the SERCA2a gene in the myocardium [8] suggesting a potential role in future therapeutic approaches of heart failure. Table 1 provides an overview of genes revealing beneficial effects in animal models of congestive heart failure. Myocardial hypertrophy could be prevented in an animal model by inhibiting the stress-regulated MAP-kinase cascade [7]. Adenoviral transfer of the human K^+ channel HERG significantly reduced early afterdepolarizations in an in vitro model of cardiac arrhythmia [38]. Finally, preliminary clinical trials in ischemic heart disease with plasmid DNA or adenoviral transfer of the angiogenic factor VEGF revealed positive effects on subjective and objective parameters of myocardial ischemia [32, 47]. Although these clinical studies showed promising effects, one should be aware that there may be a potential inflammatory response: recently a patient enrolled in a study of hepatic gene transfer died from acute hepatic failure after adenoviral transfer [30]. Further side effects may be caused by expression of the therapeutic gene in other organs due to the use of strong, but unspecific promoters. Moreover, the route of application via a thoracotomy is associated with a considerable procedural risk and therefore not applicable to a broad range of patients. Therefore, routine clinical applications require a vector system with cardiac-specific expression of the

Table 1. Positive inotropy by gene transfer

Gene	Reference
β_2-adrenergic receptor	Maurice et al. 1999 [37]
β-adrenergic receptor kinase 1 inhibitor	Rockman et al. 1998 [46]
Sarcoplasmic reticulum Ca^{2+}-ATPase 2a	Baker et al. 1998 [1] Franz et al. 2000 [8]
Sarcoplasmic reticulum Ca^{2+}-ATPase 1a	Loukianov et al. 1998 [33]
Mutated phospholamban (dominant negative)	He et al. 1999 [18]

therapeutic gene. Additionally, new delivery systems need to be developed to decrease the risk of vector application by surgical approaches. This article emphasizes recent findings which may contribute to the development of a gene transfer system for cardiac-specific gene expression:

Characterization of cardiac-specific promoters for transcriptional control of gene expression.

Development of a new percutaneous transluminal delivery system for myocardial vector transfer.

Vectors for myocardial gene transfer

Plasmid DNA – also called "naked DNA" – was succesfully used for therapeutic gene transfer in the clinical study of Losordo and coworkers [32]. A disadvantage of this approach is the high amount of plasmid DNA due to a low transfer rate even in combination with local injections. A more efficient method is liposomal transfer. However, this method resulted in high extracardiac expression levels [53]. Furthermore, retroviral vectors also enable gene delivery into the myocardium [43]. As the retroviral DNA is integrated into the genome of the host cell, a mutagenic effect may be possible. Therefore, this system might not be the first choice for therapeutic gene transfer in patients. Recombinant adenoviral vectors have been shown to be a highly efficient vector system for gene delivery into the myocardium [2, 14, 17, 22]. Unlike retroviral vectors, adenoviruses infect non-dividing cardiomyocytes very efficiently and show 50- to 100-fold higher gene expression in rat myocardium after direct injection of viral particles compared with injection of plasmid DNA alone [22, 26]. In addition, adenoviral vectors can accommodate large inserts and can be easily prepared in high titers (10^{10}–10^{12} plaque forming units (pfu)/ml). In most models, however, gene expression is transient after adenoviral infection and inflammation is observed in tissue expressing the transgene [57]. Table 2 summarizes the properties of recombinant adenoviruses. Recently, a new generation of adenoviral vectors was developed lacking the complete viral backbone, providing an increase in packaging capacity to 28–34 kb. These

Table 2. Recombinant adenoviruses as vectors for myocardial gene transfer

Advantages	Disadvantages
Highly efficient gene transfer	Gene transfer and expression not restricted to target cells
Infection of postmitotic celles	Immune response
Large DNA-inserts	Incidence of hepatic failure in one patient
Broad host range	

vectors enable prolonged gene expression and reduced immune response, but their persistence in the heart has not yet been tested [27, 39]. Having the recent death of a patient in mind receiving a high dose of conventional adenoviral vectors, adenoviral gutless vectors are expected to prevent such incidents. Finally, progress has been made in the development of adeno-associated virus (AAV) vectors. AAV are considered as a promising vehicle for therapeutic gene transfer because they are naturally replication deficient and can only replicate in the presence of a helper virus such as adenovirus. Furthermore, AAV which have never been associated with any human disease like other viral vectors can infect several human cell types including cardiomyocytes [34]. To prevent a potential contamination by the helper virus, Xiao and coworkers [56] developed a method to cotransfect only a subset of adenoviral helper genes sufficient to enable AAV amplification. The limitation of AAV vectors is currently the lack of sufficient titers for *in vivo* studies. A clinical application would require the development of new approaches for large-scale production.

Identification of promoter sequences for cardiac-specific gene expression

Previous studies analyzed the efficiency of different routes of administration to infect heart muscle cells *in vivo* using adenoviral vectors [19, 23]. These experiments showed that even direct injection into the heart resulted in transgene expression in many other tissues including thymus, lung and liver, raising important safety concerns. For example, a strong expression of the *Drosophila Shaker* potassium channel was reported in liver after intracardiac injection of the recombinant adenovirus AdShK [20]. As noted by the authors, this may have phenotypic consequences since the hepatocyte membrane potential determines the rate of bile acid uptake. Therefore, the question of how to restrict gene expression to heart muscle cells needs to be addressed for potential gene therapy applications.

Targeted expression may be achieved by using a tissue-specific promoter sequence. Suitable promotors need to be characterized in transgenic animal models because only a correctly targeted expression into a defined tissue or cell type of a transgenic animal provides the confirmation that a

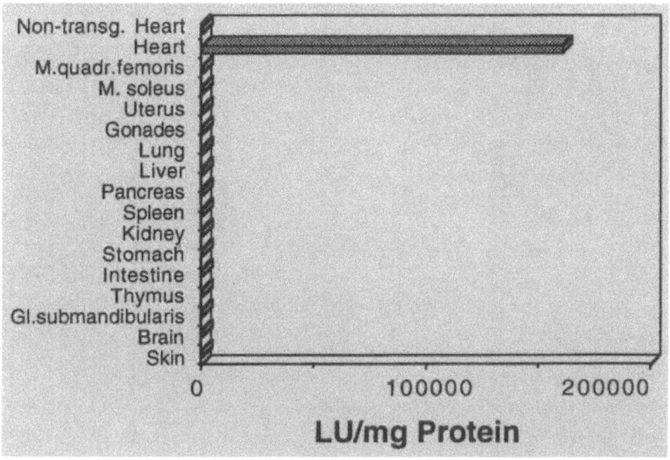

Fig. 1. Luciferase activities [in light units (LU) per mg protein] in representative organs of adult transgenic mice harboring a 2.1 kb mlc2v-Luc transgene. Except for ventricular myocardium only background activities were detected.

regulatory sequence fulfills the criteria for an appropriate promoter [11]. For identification of a cardiac-specific promoter, we analyzed the myosin light chain (MLC)-2v promoter since expression of protein and mRNA are confined to ventricular myocardium. Transgenic lines were established in which the luciferase reporter gene was controlled by a 2.1 kb MLC-2v promoter fragment [9, 10]. Luciferase activity was specifically detected in ventricular myocardium in four independent transgenic lines (Fig. 1). This study demonstrated that the 2.1 kb MLC-2v promoter sequence harbors the regulatory elements required for ventricle-specific gene expression. Table 3 lists further regulatory sequences with predominant activity in cardiac tissue. However, not all promoters listed there have been used routinely for specific gene expression. For targeted expression into ventricular myocardium the MLC-2v promoter is suitable as shown in several transgenic and adenoviral studies [8, 11, 48]. Another frequently used regulatory sequence is the α-myosin heavy chain (MHC) promoter which is active both in ventricular and atrial tissue in transgenic mice [51, 52]. The atrial natriuretic factor (ANF) promoter allows a targeted expression in atrial myocardium in adult mice under normal conditions [50]. As this promoter is upregulated in hypertrophic ventricular cardiomyocytes, the ANF regulatory sequence can be used to target gene expression in hypertrophy [55]. In an approach to target gene expression specifically to ischemic myocardium, Prentice et al. fused a hypoxia-responsive enhancer element with the α-MHC promoter [42]. This chimeric promoter enabled a strong induction by hypoxia in tissue culture and by ischemia *in vivo*.

Table 3. Promoters with cardiac activity in transgenic mice

Heart-specific promoters	Further activity in	Reference
Atrium		
Atrial natriuretic factor (ANF)	Hypothalamus	Seidman et al. 1991 [50]
A1 adenosine receptor (A1AR)	Brain	Rivkees et al. 1999 [45]
Ventricle		
Myosin light chain-2 (MLC-2v)	None	Lee et al. 1992 [29] Franz et al. 1993 10]
β-myosin heavy chain (β-MHC)	Skeletal muscle	Rindt et al. 1993 [44]
Dystrophin*	None	Kimura et al. 1997 [25]
Atrium and ventricle		
α-myosin heavy chain (α-MHC)	Lung	Subramaniam et al. 1991 [52]
α-skeletal actin	Skeletal muscle (high), stomach (low)	Petropoulos et al. 1989 [41] Brennan et al. 1993 [6]
M-creatine kinase (CK-M)	Skeletal muscle (high), lung, brain	Johnson et al. 1989 [21]
Myoglobin	Skeletal muscle	Parsons et al. 1993 [40]
Myosin light chain-3F (MLC-3F)	Skeletal muscle	Kelly et al. 1995 [24]
α-B-crystallin	Skeletal muscle, lens	Gopal-Srivastava et al. 1995 [13]
Cardiac actin	Skeletal muscle, blood vessels	Biben et al. 1996 [3]
Adenylosuccinate synthetase	Skeletal muscle	Lewis et al. 1996 [31]
Phospholamban	None	Haghighi et al. 1997 [16]
Conductive tissue (AV node)		
Troponin I (TnI)	Skeletal muscle, cartilage	Zhu et al. 1995 [58]

* no expression in left ventricle

Adenoviral vectors with targeted expression in the myocardium

In order to target genes and the corresponding proteins to defined regions within the heart such as atrium and/or ventricle, we compared the rat cardiac α-MHC promoter with the MLC-2v promoter with regard to their cardiac selectivity and their differences in atrial and ventricular gene expression [11, 48]. For these experiments several recombinant adenoviral vectors with luciferase and LacZ reporter genes were constructed by homologous recombination (Fig. 2). Following transthoracal puncture of the cardiac cavity in anesthesized newborn Sprague-Dawley rats, 2×10^9 pfu of the recombinant adenoviruses Ad-RSV-βgal, Ad-Luc, Ad-RSV-Luc, Ad-MHC-Luc or Ad-MLC-Luc were injected into the cardiac cavity in a 20 µl volume using a 27½ gauge tuberculin syringe.

The spatial distribution of transduced heart muscle cells after intracavitary injection of adenoviruses was assessed by injection of a recombinant adenovirus expressing the β-galactosidase reporter-gene under control of the rous sarcoma virus (RSV) promoter (Ad-RSV-βgal). After sectioning

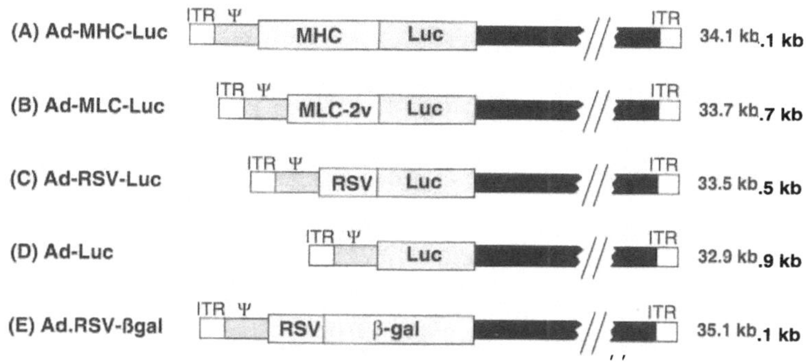

Fig. 2. Schematic drawing of the replication-defective adenoviruses Ad-mhcLuc, Ad-mlcLuc, Ad-rsvLuc, Ad-Luc, and Ad-RSV-βgal. Viruses (**A**)–(**D**) were harboring the luciferase reporter gene (replacing the E1-region) driven by (**A**) the α-mhc promoter, (**B**) the mlc-2v promoter, (**C**) the rsv promoter, and (**D**) no promoter (*ITR* Inverted Terminal Repeat, Ψ adenoviral packaging sequence, *rsv* Rous Sarcoma Virus promoter, *mlc-2v* myosin light chain-2 promoter, α-mhc α-myosin heavy chain promoter, *Luc* luciferase, *β-gal* β-galactosidase).

and transgene staining, we found by visual inspection that approximately half of the myocardial β-galactosidase activity resulted from direct myocardial injection along the needle track into the heart, whereas only a few cardiomyocytes stained blue in the remaining myocardium (Fig. 3).

Extracardiac vector distribution after intracardiac injections could be detected by PCR amplification of viral DNA in intercostal muscle, thymus, lung, diaphragm and liver, independent of the injected recombinant virus (Fig. 4B). Adenoviral DNA was detected in similar amounts both in ventricular and atrial tissue. Increasing sensitivity by Southern blot hybridization of PCR products identified adenoviral DNA in low amounts in all tissues investigated (Fig. 4C).

A further set of analyses addressed the specificity of reporter gene expression after intracardiac injection of the recombinant adenoviruses Ad-MHC-Luc and Ad-MLC-Luc. Luciferase activities were determined in atrial and ventricular myocardium, in intercostal muscle, thymus, lung, diaphragm, abdominal wall muscle, liver, stomach, spleen, and quadriceps femoris muscle. Reporter gene expression was compared with the positive control virus Ad-RSV-Luc and the negative control virus Ad-Luc. Adenovirus Ad-MHC-Luc and Ad-MLC-Luc harboring the heart muscle-specific promoters revealed the highest reporter gene expression in the heart. Ad-MHC-Luc-infected animals showed additional luciferase activity in lung and liver tissue (Fig. 5). In contrast, adenoviral Ad-MLC-Luc transfer resulted in cardiac-specific gene expression with background activities at or below the negative control. Ad-RSV-Luc led to the highest luciferase activity in heart and intercostal muscle and showed a substantial level of reporter gene expression in thymus, diaphragm, lung and a lower abundance in the abdominal wall muscle, liver and spleen. Reporter activity of Ad-MLC-Luc in the heart was 20-fold higher in comparison to Ad-Luc and

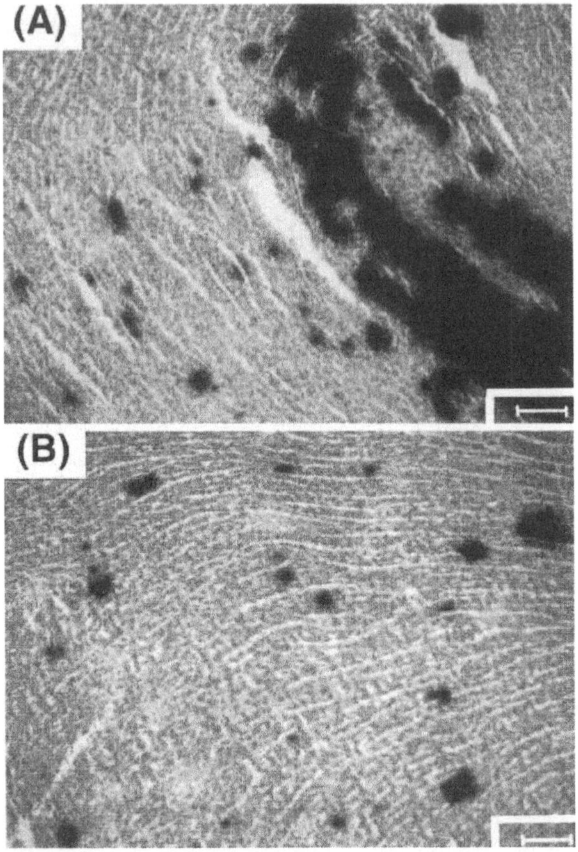

Fig. 3. Histological detection of β-galactosidase activity in the myocardium 5 days after intracavitary injection of Ad-RSV-βgal. **A** Photomicrograph of a histological section through the apical site of injection and **B** through the central part of the heart. In each panel blue staining shows β-galactosidase activity. Bar represents 100 µm [48].

reached 11% of the expression obtained by Ad-RSV-Luc. Ad-MHC-Luc gave a 6.5-fold higher luciferase activity in the heart compared to Ad-Luc, corresponding to 3% of the Ad-RSV-Luc activity. To study the regional differences of reporter gene expression in atrial and ventricular myocardium, the four recombinant adenoviruses containing the luciferase reporter gene were injected into the cardiac cavity accordingly. While Ad-MLC-Luc showed high luciferase activity in the ventricle, luciferase expression levels in the atrium were comparable to the negative control Ad-Luc. The ratio of light emission for ventricular to atrial tissue is shown for the four recombinant adenoviruses in Fig. 6. While Ad-RSV-Luc, Ad-MHC-Luc and Ad-Luc injection led to an approximately 2-fold higher luciferase activity in the ventricle, Ad-MLC-Luc injection gave a 35-fold higher luciferase activity in the ventricular compared to the atrial tissue. These data demonstrate that in contrast to the 1.0 kb α-MHC promoter Ad-MLC-Luc is specifically active in the ventricle of neonatal rats. Therefore, the MLC-2v regulatory sequence appears to be suitable for targeting gene expression specifically into ventricular myocardium.

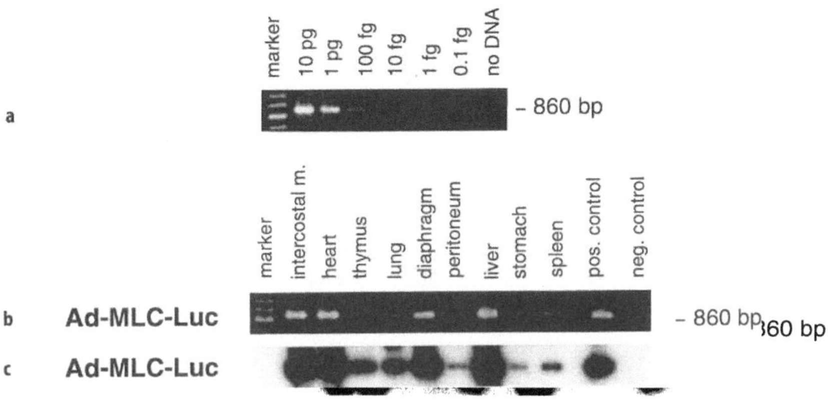

Fig. 4. Detection of adenoviral DNA in nine tissues after intracavitary injection of the representative adenovirus Ad-mlcLuc. **a** Agarose gel (2.4%) showing specific 860 bp PCR-product amplified from decreasing amounts of Ad del324 DNA. For templates, 100 ng of rat genomic DNA were mixed together with the following amounts of viral DNA: 10 pg (lane 1); 1 pg (lane 2); 100 fg (lane 3); 10 fg (lane 4); 1 fg (lane 5); 0.1 fg (lane 6); no viral DNA (lane 7). A 100 bp ladder served as the molecular weight standard (lane M). **b** Agarose gel (2.4%) showing 860 bp PCR-product amplified from 100 ng genomic DNA isolated from the indicated organs after intracavitary injection of Ad-mlcLuc. PCR reactions containing 100 ng of rat genomic DNA mixed with 1 pg Ad del324 DNA or without addition of viral DNA served as positive and negative controls, respectively. **c** Southern blot analysis of the same Ad-mlcLuc-infected animal using the specific, ^{32}P-radiolabeled 860 bp amplification product as a probe.

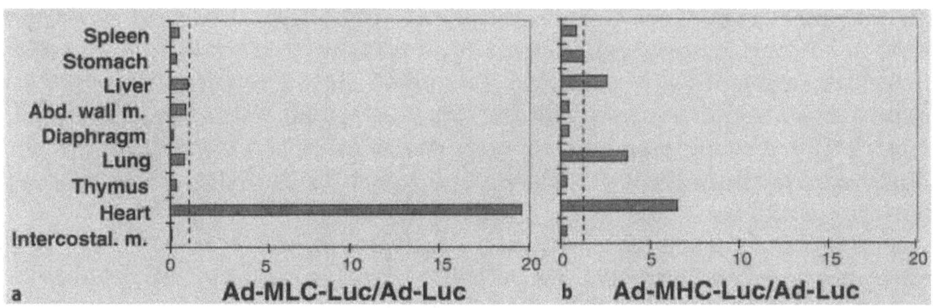

Fig. 5. Ratio of luciferase activity for recombinant adenovirus Ad-mlcLuc **a** and Ad-mhcLuc **b** related to the promoterless virus Ad-Luc in 9 different tissues expressed in two bar diagrams. All bars left of the dashed line, representing a ratio of 1, express background luciferase activities.

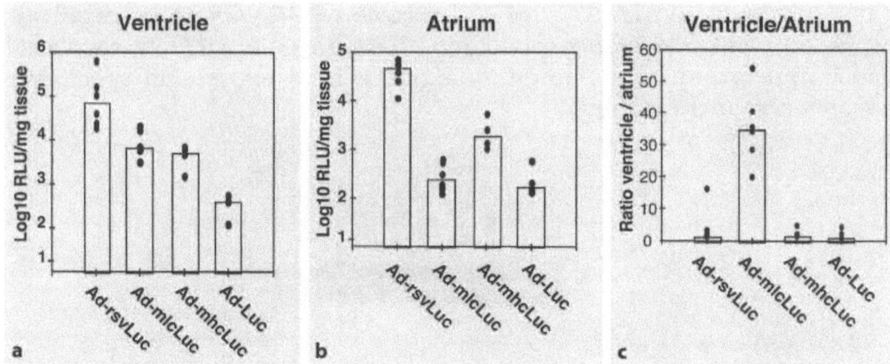

Fig. 6. Luciferase activity in **a** ventricular and **b** atrial myocardium after intracavitary injection of recombinant adenoviruses Ad-rsvLuc, Ad-mlcLuc, Ad-mhcLuc or Ad-Luc. Panel **c** shows the ratio of luciferase activity in ventricle to atrium for each adenoviral construct. A dot represents the value of an individual animal; the bar represents the median. Ad-rsvLuc and Ad-mlcLuc (n=6); Ad-mhcLuc and Ad-Luc (n=4).

Percutaneous transluminal retrograde gene delivery (PTRGD) – a new approach for vector delivery

In animal models, vectors are usually applied by direct injection into the myocardium or the cardiac cavity. These techniques are limited by either patchy or low vector transfer. Direct delivery of an adenoviral vector into coronary arteries by a percutaneous transluminal approach resulted in rather low efficiency [35]. Also pericardial delivery did not provide transmural gene expression [28, 36]. Table 4 summarizes the properties of various delivery approaches with regard to potential clinical application. Homogeneous myocardial gene transfer in a defined target area might be preferable for future clinical approaches. One of the major limitations of cardiac gene transfer via the coronary circulation is the short adhesion time of the vector with endothelium and cardiomyocytes resulting in a systemic distribution of the vector. In a rat model, transfer efficiency could be increased by simultaneously clamping the aorta and pulmonary artery for a brief period of time enabling repeated passage of the vector through the coronary circulation [17]. For future clinical use in patients, a less invasive system for efficient delivery of adenoviral vectors is required. Previous studies have shown that selective retroinfusion of the coronary veins enhance myocardial concentrations of β-blockers or calcium antagonists in ischemic myocardium [15, 49]. Moreover, pressure-regulated retroinfusion allowed targeting of dobutamine specifically to ischemic myocardium without systemic effects [54]. Selective suction and pressure-regulated retroinfusion of oxygenized blood into the coronary vein revealed a high efficacy in preserving regional myocardial function during balloon angioplasty in high-risk patients [5]. Under the assumption of a prolonged vector attach-

Table 4. Modes of application

	Advantages	Disadvantages
Intravenous	Fast, easy to perform	Low titers in target tissue; broad viral spread
Percutaneous transluminal		
▪ arterial	Selective application	Low titers in target tissue
▪ venous (retroinfusion)	Expression in the region of a certain coronary artery	Block of coronary artery required
Surgical		
▪ intramuscular (after CABG)	Distinct area of expression	Expression limited to needle track
– (minimal invasive)	Distinct area of expression	Additionally: risk of anesthesia
▪ pericardial	Homogeneous distribution in pericardial cavity	Predominantly epicardial expression, anesthesia required

ment the potential of retroinfusion for adenoviral gene transfer was analyzed.

The principle of selective pressure-regulated retroinfusion for regional myocardial gene delivery was reported in detail in Boekstegers et al. [5] (Fig. 7). Figure 8 demonstrates the catheterization procedure in a patient undergoing PTCA of the proximal left anterior descending artery (LAD) under protection of retroinfusion. The adenoviral experiments were carried out in German farm pigs (24 kg ± 4 kg). After anesthesia and endotracheal intubation, catheter introducer sheaths were placed in the right carotid artery (8F Cordis, Miami, USA) and right external jugular vein (8.5 F, Arrows, Reading, USA). For insertion of a 3.0 mm PTCA balloon into the LAD, a 7 F guiding catheter (Cordis) was placed in the left coronary artery. The orifice of the coronary sinus was catheterized with a 7 F left Amplatz II coronary diagnostic catheter (Cordis). After retrograde injection of contrast agent into the coronary sinus for confirming correct placement, a high support coronary guide wire (0.018 in., Cook) was advanced through the coronary sinus into the anterior cardiac vein accompanying the LAD. A 6 F four lumen retroinfusion catheter was inserted through the coronary sinus and advanced until its tip was located in the anterior interventricular vein. After removing the guide wire, the balloon of the retroinfusion catheter was inflated via the first channel, which is connected to the pressure-controlled balloon pump. The second and third channels are connected to a high pressure reservoir channel. The fourth was used for continuous monitoring of the coronary venous pressure. The virus solution was added to the retroinfusion line through a stopcock valve. The retroinfusion pressure was set 20 mmHg above the systolic plateau pressure in the coronary vein. For the start of continuous selective pressure-regulated retroinfusion, the balloon tip of the retroinfusion catheter was inflated to a constant pressure of 150 mmHg. A valve opened and provided retrograde delivery of the

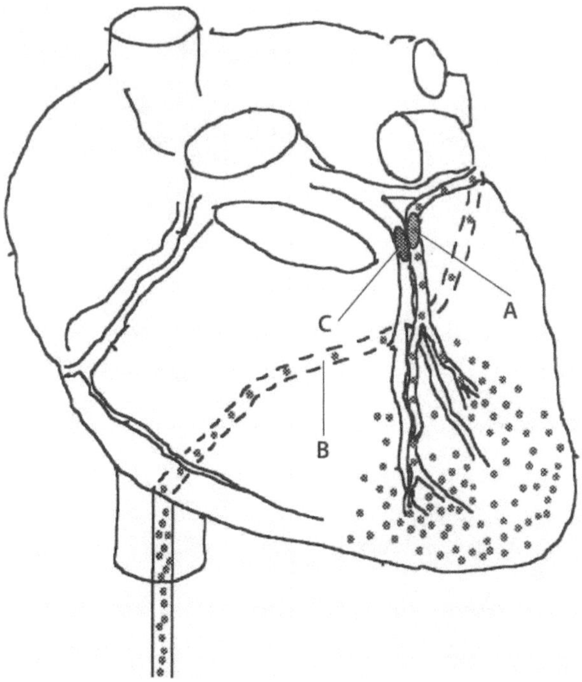

Fig. 7. Principle of retroinfusion: **A** position of the retroinfusion catheter tip during selective synchronized suction and retroinfusion in the anterior interventricular vein. **B** retroinfusion catheter placed through the femoral vein. **C** occlusion site of the LAD.

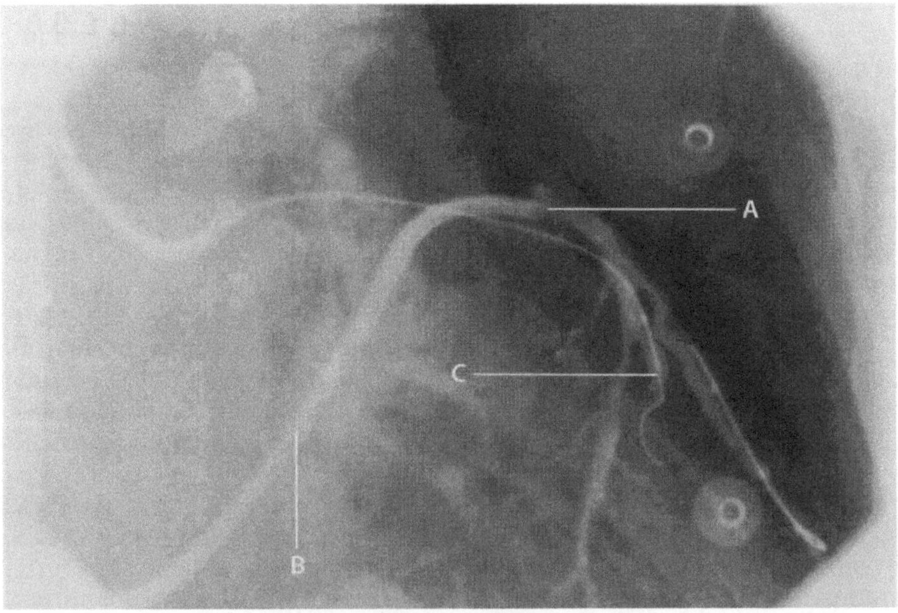

Fig. 8. Angiographic sequence of catheterization procedure in a patient with selective suction and pressure-regulated retroinfusion undergoing PTCA of a proximal stenosis of the LAD. **A**, **B**, and **C** are corresponding to Fig. 7. (Reprinted from [5]).

vector solution driven by the high pressure in the reservoir until the preset retroinfusion pressure was reached (Fig. 9). Now 25 ml of the vector solution were infused over 10 min via the retroinfusion line while retrograde blood flow was regulated by the valve within milliseconds to adjust coronary venous pressure to the preset value.

Determination of luciferase activity showed high levels of reporter gene expression throughout the targeted LAD region seven days after retrograde adenoviral gene transfer by selective retroinfusion (Fig. 10). Furthermore, transmural transfection and – even more important – gene expression were present in significant amounts. For analysis of spatial distribution in the retroinfusion experiments, histological assessment of *β*-galactosidase was performed seven days after delivery of an adenoviral vector expressing *β*-galactosidase. Semiquantiative evaluation revealed 15–25% of *β*-galactosidase-positive cells. The pattern of distribution itself appeared inhomogeneous. Extra-cardiac adenoviral transfection was analyzed by PCR and luciferase activities were determined [5]. None of the tissues tested showed any evidence for extra-cardiac infection. Selectivity of gene transfer to the LAD region was confirmed by the observation that both PCR for adenoviral sequences and reporter gene activities were negative for all probes of the control region (circumflex artery) in contrast to the LAD probe.

The use of percutaneous transluminal retrograde gene delivery (PTRGD) through the coronary vein enabled a highly efficient adenoviral gene trans-

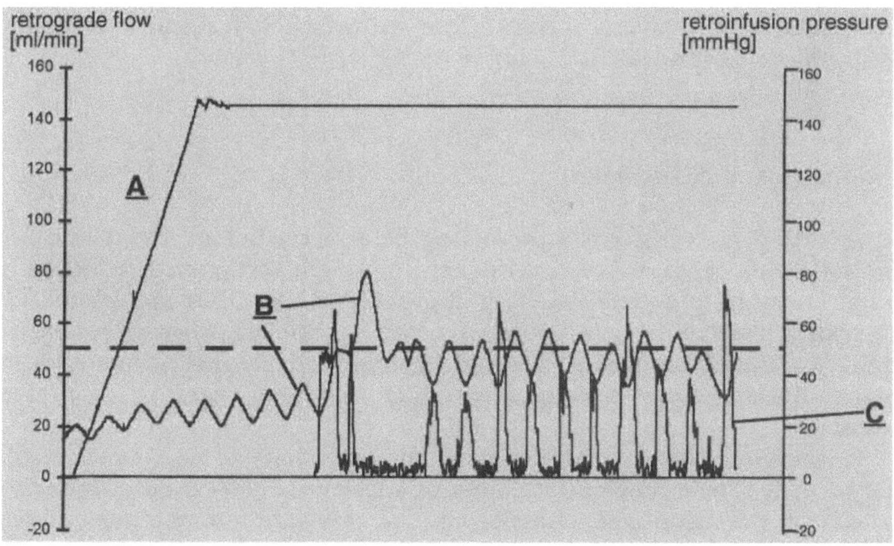

Fig. 9. Modified retroinfusion technique for gene transfer: original registration of continuous selective pressure-regulated retroinfusion: **A** balloon pressure [mmHg]; **B** retroinfusion pressure in the coronary vein [mmHg]; **C** retrograde transcatheter saline flow [ml/min]; *dashed line* = preset retroinfusion pressure (50 mmHg). (Reprinted from [4]).

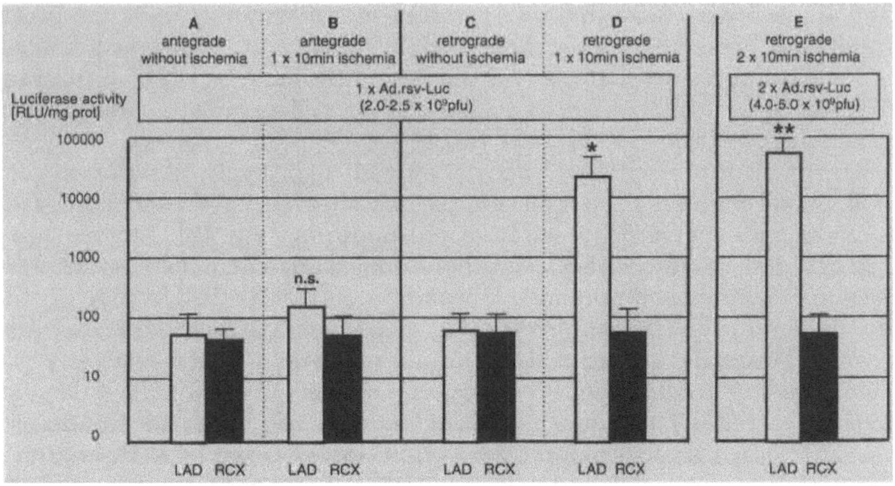

Fig. 10. Comparison of antegrade and retrograde delivery of adenoviral vectors with and without ischemia: mean luciferase activity in myocardial probes of the targeted LAD and nontargeted CX region. Group A = antegrade delivery without ischemia (10 min) (2.0–2.5×109 pfu Ad.rsv-Luc), group B = antegrade delivery during 10 min of ischemia (2.0–2.5×109 pfu Ad.rsv-Luc), group C = retrograde delivery without ischemia (10 min) (2.0–2.5×109 pfu Ad.rsv-Luc), group D = retrograde delivery during 1×10 min of ischemia (2.0–2.5×109 pfu Ad.rsv-Luc), group E = retrograde delivery during 2×10 min of ischemia (4.0–5.0×109 pfu. Ad.rsv-Luc). n.s. = non significant, * = $p<0.001$ vs. group B, ** = $p<0.01$ vs. group D. (Reprinted from [4]).

fer targeted to the ischemic myocardium with limited systemic contamination in a porcine model [4].

Summary and conclusion

Therapeutic gene transfer is a promising field in cardiology. However, clinical application requires the development of a safe vector system. Recently, a tragic incident in a gene targeting approach into the liver underlined the danger of a possible immunogenic effect of the current delivery systems in certain patients. The use of so-called "gutless" adenoviral vectors lacking the viral backbone are expected to provide the safety required for clinical studies.

A further important consideration is the specificity of expression of the targeted gene. Since previous attempts of adenoviral gene transfer have not allowed for precise gene expression in the myocardium, the goal of our studies was the development of an approach for safe gene delivery into the myocardium. We presented evidence that the heart muscle-specific myosin-light-chain 2 promoter retains its *in vivo* specificity of gene expression in the myocardium after incorporation into an adenoviral vector. Therefore, this promoter should be suitable for cardiac-specific expression of potentially therapeutic genes.

Local application of the vector is also a limitation for gene therapeutic approaches. Intracavitary injections are limited by the confined area of vector distribution around the needle track, whereas in the remaining myocardium only 1–2% of the cardiomyocytes were transfected. For an efficient gene therapy approach, however, a more homogeneous distribution is required. Therefore, we established a new percutaneous transluminal retrograde gene delivery system (PTRGD). Based on experiences with efficient myocardial application of different drugs by sective pressure-regulated retroinfusion of coronary veins, this delivery system was modified and successfully used for transfer of reporter genes into the targeted LAD region. Interestingly, no reporter activities were detected in different layers of the circumflex region. Additionally, PCR for the adenoviral vector was positive in the LAD specimen but not in the circumflex territory or extracardiac tissue, indicating at least only very small systemic contamination by the vector. Further studies analyzing the transfer of potential therapeutic genes will validate future clinical use of PTRGD.

Combination of the tissue specificity of the MLC-2v promoter with the efficient local transfer via PTRGD and improved adenoviral vectors might enable the use of recombinant adenoviruses to treat heart muscle diseases.

References

1. Baker DL, Hashimoto K, Grupp IL, Ji Y, Reed T, Loukianov E, Grupp G, Bhagwhat A, Hoit B, Walsh R, Marban E, Periasamy M (1998) Targeted overexpression of the sarcoplasmic reticulum Ca^{2+}-ATPase increases cardiac contractility in transgenic mouse hearts. Circ Res 83:1205–1214
2. Barr E, Carroll J, Kalynych AM, Tripathy SK, Kozarsky K, Wilson JM et al (1994) Efficient catheter-mediated gene transfer into the heart using replication defective adenovirus. Gene Ther 1:51–58
3. Biben C, Hadchouel J, Tajbakhsh S, Buckingham M (1996) Developmental and tissue-specific regulation of the murine cardiac actin gene *in vivo* depends on distinct skeletal and cardiac muscle-specific enhancer elements in addition to the proximal promoter. Dev Biol 173:200–212
4. Boekstegers P, von Degenfeld G, Giehrl W, Heinrich D, Hullin R, Kupatt C, Steinbeck G, Baretton G, Middeler G, Katus HA, Franz WM (2000) Myocardial gene transfer by selective pressure-regulated retroinfusion of coronary veins. Gene Therapy 7:232–240
5. Boekstegers P, Giehrl W, von Degenfeld G, Steinbeck G (1998) Selective suction and pressure-regulated retroinfusion: an effective and safe approach to retrograde protection against myocardial ischemia in patients undergoing normal and high risk percutaneous transluminal coronary angioplasty. J Am Coll Cardiol 31:1525–1533
6. Brennan KJ, Hardeman EC (1993) Quantitative analysis of the human α-skeletal actin gene in transgenic mice. J Biol Chem 268:719–725
7. Choukroun G, Hajjar R, Fry S, del Monte F, Haq S, Guerrero JL, Picard M, Rosenzweig A, Force T (1999) Regulation of cardiac hypertrophy in vivo by the stress-activated protein kinases/c-Jun NH(2)-terminal kinases. J Clin Invest 104:391–398

8. Franz WM, Degenhardt M, Mueller O, Lorenzen HP, Wagner K, Lange M, Hanssen E, Katus HA (2000) Overexpression of sarcoplasmic reticulum Ca^{2+} ATPase in the hearts of transgenic rats is associated with markedly enhanced myocardial contractility and elevated blood pressure. Circ Res (submitted)
9. Franz WM, Brem G, Katus HA, Klingel K, Hofschneider PH, Kandolf R (1994) Characterization of a cardiac-selective and developmentally upregulated promoter in transgenic mice. Cardioscience 5:235–243
10. Franz WM, Breves D, Klingel K, Brem G, Hofschneider PH, Kandolf R (1993) Heart-specific targeting of firefly luciferase by the myosin light chain-2 promoter and developmental regulation in transgenic mice. Circ Res 73:629–638
11. Franz WM, Mueller OJ, Hartong R, Frey N, Katus HA (1997) Transgenic animal models: new avenues in cardiovascular physiology. J Mol Med 75:115–129
12. Franz WM, Rothmann T, Frey N, Katus HA (1997) Analysis of tissue-specific gene delivery by recombinant adenoviruses containing cardiac-specific promoters. Cardiovasc Res 35:560–566
13. Gopal-Srivastava R, Haynes JII, Piatigorsky J (1995) Regulation of the murine αB-crystallin/small heat shock protein gene in cardiac muscle. Mol Cell Biol 15:7081–7090
14. Guzman RJ, Lemarchand P, Crystal RG, Epstein SE, Finkel T (1993) Efficient gene transfer into myocardium by direct injection of adenovirus vectors. Circ Res 73:1202–1207
15. Haga Y, Uriuda Y, Bjorkman JA, Hatori N, Johansson L, Nordlander R, Sjoquist PO, Ryden L (1994) Ischemic and nonischemic tissue concentrations of felodipine after coronary venous retroinfusion during myocardial ischemia and reperfusion: an experimental study in pigs. J Cardiovasc Pharmacol 24:298–302
16. Haghighi K, Kadambi VJ, Koss KL, Luo W, Harrer JM, Ponniah S, Zhou Z, Kranias EG (1997) In vitro and in vivo promoter analyses of the mouse phospholamban gene. Gene 203:199–207
17. Hajjar RJ, Schmidt U, Matsui T, Guerrero JL, Lee KH, Gwathmey JK, Dec GW, Semigran MJ, Rosenzweig A (1998) Modulation of ventricular function through gene transfer in vivo. Proc Natl Acad Sci (USA) 95:5251–5256
18. He H, Meyer M, Martin JL, McDonough PM, Ho P, Lou X, Lew WY, Hilal-Dandan R, Dillmann WH (1999) Effects of mutant and antisense RNA of phospholamban on SR $Ca(^{2+})$-ATPase activity and cardiac myocyte contractility. Circulation 100:974–980
19. Huard J, Lochmüller H, Acsadi G, Jani A, Massie B, Karpati G (1995) The route of administration is a major determinant of the transduction efficiency of rat tissues by adenoviral recombinants. Gene Ther 2:107–115
20. Johns DC, Nuss HB, Chiamvimonvat N, Ramza BM, Marban E, Lawrence JH (1995) Adenovirus-mediated expression of a voltage-gated potassium channel in vitro (rat cardiac myocytes) and in vivo (rat liver). J Clin Invest 96:1152–1158
21. Johnson JE, Wold BJ, Hauschka SD (1989) Muscle creatine kinase sequence elements regulating skeletal and cardiac muscle expression in transgenic mice. Mol Cell Biol 9:3393–3399
22. Kass Eisler A, Falck Pedersen E, Alvira M, Rivera J, Buttrick PM, Wittenberg BA et al (1993) Quantitative determination of adenovirus-mediated gene delivery to rat cardiac myocytes *in vitro* and *in vivo*. Proc Natl Acad Sci (USA) 90:11498–11502
23. Kass Eisler A, Falck Pedersen E, Elfenbein DH, Alvira M, Buttrick PM, Leinwand LA (1994) The impact of developmental stage, route of administration and the immune system on adenovirus mediated gene transfer. Gene Ther 1:395–402
24. Kelly R, Alonso S, Tajbakhsh S, Cossu G, Buckingham M (1995) Myosin light chain 3F regulatory sequences confer regionalized cardiac and skeletal muscle expression in transgenic mice. J Cell Biol 129:383–396

25. Kimura S, Abe K, Suzuki M, Ogawa M, Yoshioka K, Kaname T, Miike T, Yamamura K (1997) A 900 bp genomic region from the mouse dystrophin promoter directs lacZ reporter expression only to the right heart of transgenic mice. Dev Growth Diff 3:257–265
26. Kirshenbaum LA, MacLellan WR, Mazur W, French BA, Schneider MD (1993) Highly efficient gene transfer into adult ventricular myocytes by recombinant adenovirus. J Clin Invest 92:381–387
27. Kochanek S, Clemens PR, Mitani K, Chen HH, Chan S, Caskey T (1996) A new adenoviral vector: replacement of all viral coding sequences with 28 kb of DNA independently expressing both full-length dystrophin and β-galactosidase. Proc Natl Acad Sci USA 93:5731–5736
28. Lamping KG, Rios CD, Chun JA, Ooboshi H, Davidson BL, Heistad DD (1997) Intrapericardial administration of adenovirus for gene transfer. Am J Physiol 272:H310–317
29. Lee KJ, Ross RS, Rockman HA, Harris AN, O'Brien TX, van Bilsen M, Shubeita HE, Kandolf R, Brem G, Price J, Evans SM, Zhu H, Franz WM, Chien KR (1992) Myosin light chain-2 luciferase transgenic mice reveal distinct regulatory programs for cardiac and skeletal muscle-specific expression of a single contractile protein gene. J Biol Chem 267:15875–15885
30. Lehrman S (1999) Virus treatment questioned after gene therapy death. Nature 401:517–518
31. Lewis AL, Guicherit OM, Datta SK, Hanten GR, Kellems RE (1996) Structure and expression of the murine muscle adenylosuccinate synthetase gene. J Biol Chem 271:22647–22656
32. Losordo DW, Vale PR, Symes JF, Dunnington CH, Esakof DD, Maysky M, Ashare AB, Lathi K, Isner JM (1998) Gene therapy for myocardial angiogenesis: initial clinical results with direct myocardial injection of phVEGF165 as sole therapy for myocardial ischemia. Circulation 98:2800–2804
33. Loukianov E, Ji Y, Grupp IL, Kirkpatrick DL, Baker DL, Loukianova T, Grupp G, Lytton J, Walsh RA, Periasamy M (1998) Enhanced myocardial contractility and increased Ca^{2+} transport function in transgenic hearts expressing the fast-twitch skeletal muscle sarcoplasmic reticulum Ca^{2+}-ATPase. Circ Res 83:889–897
34. Maeda Y, Ikeda U, Shimpo M, Ueno S, Ogasawara Y, Urabe M, Kume A, Takizawa T, Saito T, Colosi P, Kurtzman G, Shimada K, Ozawa K (1998) Efficient gene transfer into cardiac myocytes using adeno-associated virus (AAV) vectors. J Mol Cell Cardiol 30:1341–1348
35. Macgovern CJ, Mack CA, Zhang J, Hahn RT, Ko W, Isom OW, Crystal RG, Rosengart TK (1996) Direct in vivo gene transfer to canine myocardium using a replication-deficient adenovirus vector. Ann Thorac Surg 62:425–433
36. March KL, Woody M, Mehdi K, Zipes DP, Brantly M, Trapnell BC (1999) Efficient in vivo catheter-based pericardial gene transfer mediated by adenoviral vectors. Clin Cardiol 22:I23–29
37. Maurice JP, Hata JA, Shah AS, White DC, McDonald PH, Dolber PC, Wilson KH, Lefkowitz RJ, Glower DD, Koch WJ (1999) Enhancement of cardiac function after adenoviral-mediated in vivo intracoronary beta2-adrenergic receptor gene delivery. J Clin Invest 104:21–29
38. Nuss HB, Marban E, Johns DC (1999) Overexpression of a human potassium channel suppresses cardiac hyperexcitability in rabbit ventricular myocytes. J Clin Invest 103:889–896
39. Parks RJ, Chen L, Anton M, Sankar U, Rudnicki MA, Graham FL (1996) A helper-dependent adenovirus vector system: removal of helper virus by Cre-mediated excision of the viral packaging signal. Proc Natl Acad Sci USA 93:13565–13570

40. Parsons WJ, Richardson JA, Graves KH, Williams RS, Moreadith RW (1993) Gradients of transgene expression directed by the human myoglobin promoter in the developing mouse heart. Proc Natl Acad Sci USA 90:1726–1730
41. Petropoulos CJ, Rosenberg MP, Jenkins NA, Copeland NG, Hughes SH (1989) The chicken skeletal muscle α-actin promoter is tissue specific in transgenic mice. Mol Cell Biol 9:3785–3792
42. Prentice H, Bishopric NH, Hicks MN, Discher DJ, Wu X, Wylie AA, Webster KA (1997) Regulated expression of a foreign gene targeted to the ischemic myocardium. Cardiovasc Res 35:567–574
43. Qin L, Chavin KD, Ding Y, Tahara H, Favaro JP, Woodward JE, Suzuki T, Robbins PD, Lotze MT, Bromberg JS (1996) Retrovirus-mediated transfer of viral IL-10 gene prolongs murine cardiac allograft survival. J Immunol 156:2316–2323
44. Rindt H, Gulick J, Knotts S, Neumann J, Robbins J (1993) *In vivo* analysis of the murine β-myosin heavy chain gene promoter. J Biol Chem 268:5332–5338
45. Rivkees SA, Chen M, Kulkarni J, Browne J, Zhao Z (1999) Characterization of the murine A1 adenosine receptor promoter, potent regulation by GATA-4 and Nkx2.5. J Biol Chem 274:14204–14209
46. Rockman HA, Chien KR, Choi DJ, Iaccarino G, Hunter JJ, Ross J Jr, Lefkowitz RJ, Koch WJ (1998) Expression of a beta-adrenergic receptor kinase 1 inhibitor prevents the development of myocardial failure in gene-targeted mice. Proc Natl Acad Sci USA 95:7000–7005
47. Rosengart TK, Lee LY, Patel SR, Sanborn TA, Parikh M, Bergman GW, Hachamovitch R, Szulc M, Kligfield PD, Okin PM, Hahn RT, Devereux RB, Post MR, Hackett NR, Foster T, Grasso TM, Lesser ML, Isom OW, Crystal RG (1999) Angiogenesis gene therapy: phase I assessment of direct intramyocardial administration of an adenovirus vector expressing VEGF121 cDNA to individuals with clinically significant severe coronary artery disease. Circulation 100:468–474
48. Rothmann T, Katus HA, Hartong R, Perricaudet M, Franz WM (1996) Heart muscle-specific gene expression using replication defective recombinant adenovirus. Gene Ther 3:919–926
49. Ryden L, Tadokoro H, Sjoquist PO, Regardh C, Kobayashi S, Corday E, Drury JK (1991) Pharmacokinetic analysis of coronary venous retroinfusion: a comparison with anterograde coronary artery drug administration using metoprolol as a tracer. J Am Coll Cardiol 18:603–612
50. Seidman CE, Schmidt EV, Seidman JG (1991) cis-dominance of rat atrial natriuretic factor gene regulatory sequences in transgenic mice. Can J Physiol Pharmacol 69:1486–1492
51. Subramaniam A, Gulick J, Neumann J, Knotts S, Robbins J (1993) Transgenic analysis of the thyroid elements in the alpha-cardiac myosin heavy chain gene promoter. J Biol Chem 268:4331–4336
52. Subramaniam A, Jones WK, Gulick J, Wert S, Neumann J, Robbins J (1991) Tissue-specific regulation of the α-myosin heavy chain gene promoter in transgenic mice. J Biol Chem 266:24613–24620
53. Thierry AR, Lunardi-Iskandar Y, Bryant JL, Rabinovich P, Gallo RC, Mahan LC (1995) Systemic gene therapy: biodistribution and long-term expression of a transgene in mice. Proc Natl Acad Sci USA 92:9742–9746
54. von Degenfeld G, Giehrl W, Boekstegers P (1997) Targeting of dobutamine to ischemic myocardium without systemic effects by selective suction and pressure-regulated retroinfusion. Cardiovasc Res 35:233–240
55. von Harsdorf R, Edwards JG, Shen YT, Kudej RK, Dietz R, Leinwand LA, Nadal-Ginard B, Vatner SF (1997) Identification of a cis-acting regulatory element conferring inducibility of the atrial natriuretic factor gene in acute pressure overload. J Clin Invest 100:1294–1304

56. Xiao X, Li J, Samulski RJ (1998) Production of high-titer recombinant adeno-associated virus vectors in the absence of helper adenovirus. J Virol 72:2224–2232
57. Yang Y, Nunes FA, Berencsi K, Furth EE, Gonczol E, Wilson JM (1994) Cellular immunity to viral antigens limits E1-deleted adenovirus for gene therapy. Proc Natl Acad Sci USA 91:4407–4411
58. Zhu L, Lyons GE, Juhasz O, Joya JE, Hardeman EC, Wade R (1995) Developmental regulation of troponin I isoform genes in striated muscles of transgenic mice. Dev Biol 169:487–503

CHAPTER 11

Transfection studies using a new cardiac 3D gel system

T. ESCHENHAGEN, C. FINK [1], T. RAU, U. REMMERS [1], J. WEIL [1], W.H. ZIMMERMANN, S. AIGNER [2], H.M. EPPENBERGER [2], T. WAKATSUKI [3], E.L. ELSON [3]

Department of Clinical Pharmacology and Toxicology, Institute of Experimental and Clinical Pharmacology and Toxicology, University of Erlangen-Nuremberg, [1] Institute of Experimental and Clinical Pharmacology, University Hospital Eppendorf, University of Hamburg, Germany, [2] ETH Zürich, Switzerland, [3] Department of Biophysics and Molecular Biochemistry, Washington University, School of Medicine, St. Louis, MO, USA

Summary

This paper summarizes recent progress in reconstituting embryonic chick or neonatal rat cardiac myocytes to a 3-dimensional heart tissue-like structure ("engineered heart tissue", EHT). The EHT is anchored to Velcro-coated silicone tubes, by which it can be attached to an isometric force transducer to measure steady (diastolic) and twitch (systolic) forces generated by the myocytes. EHTs exhibit a highly organized network of elongated, mostly longitudinally aligned cardiac myocytes with well-developed myofilaments, cross-striation, and cell-to-cell contacts, which cause EHT to beat coherently. This allows for simple measurement of the isometric force of contraction (0.1–0.5 mN) in standard organ baths. We show that cardiac myocytes within EHTs are easily and effectively transduced with adenovirus coding for β-galactosidase or green fluorescence protein. Adenovirus-mediated gene transfer does not affect basal, calcium, nor isoprenaline-stimulated force of contraction. Thus, EHTs are a suitable model to study the impact of short-term genetic manipulation on force of contraction.

Introduction

Cardiac myocytes are terminally differentiated postmitotic cells that cannot be cultured as permanent cell lines. Thus, primary cultures of neonatal rat or embryonic chick cardiac myocytes, introduced into cardiovascular research more than 40 years ago, serve as a standard *in vitro* model and are now indispensable tools to study mechanisms of cardiac hypertrophy and gene expression under defined *in vitro* conditions [19]. Although myocytes cultured in a 2-dimensional (2D) monolayer retain many characteristics of the cardiac phenotype such as spontaneous beating, are stable for up to 90 days [16], and are easily manipulated by pharmacological, mechanical or genetic means, they also exhibit significant shortcomings.

- 2D myocyte cultures lack the defined 3D architecture of the intact heart which is a complex, muscular organ made up of multiple cell types.
- Relatively pure cultures of myocytes can be only maintained by serum deprivation and the addition of cytostatics that prevent overgrowth by non-myocytes. The influence of these factors on the biological outcome is largely unknown.
- Measurement of contractile force, the main function of cardiac myocytes, is severely limited in 2D cultures.

The present paper summarizes attempts to overcome some of these limitations by establishing a new 3D cell culture model ("engineered heart tissue", EHT) that allows the impact of genetic manipulation of cardiac myocytes to be studied under defined conditions.

Materials and methods

Casting Velcro-anchored EHTs

EHTs were prepared either from embryonic chick or neonatal rat hearts. Details of the technique have been described previously [6, 23]. Here, only the principle is presented. Cardiomyocytes were isolated from 9–11 day chick embryos or from 0–3 day old neonatal rat hearts by a combined trypsin/collagenase (chick) or serial trypsin digestion (rat). In the standard protocol, a cell/collagen master mix was prepared for 8 EHTs (1 culture dish) and kept on ice until casting. 1.33 ml collagen type I (rat tail; 3.6 mg/ml 0.1% acetic acid, Upstate Biotechnology, Lake Placid, NY) was mixed with 1.33 ml 2× concentrated culture medium (2× DMEM, 20% horse serum, 4% chick embryo extract, 200 µg/ml streptomycin, 200 U/ml penicillin G; all from Gibco BRL), neutralized with 182 µl 0.1 M NaOH, and finally mixed with 1.48 ml cell suspension. Rat EHTs required addition of 0.48 ml extracellular matrix basement membrane from Engelbreth-Holm-Swarm tumor (Harbor Bio-Products, Tebu, Frankfurt, FRG; in the following referred to as Matrigel), this volume was substituted by culture medium in chick EHTs. Cell density was $15 \times 10^6/8$ EHTs in rat and $5.6 \times 10^6/8$ EHTs in chick. For each EHT 0.6 ml of the ice cold cell/collagen mix was poured into a well (17×10×4 mm; length×width×thickness) of the culture dish (10 cm diameter) that contained a layer of silicone rubber with 8 rectangular wells each holding one set of Velcro-coated silicone tubes (7–8 mm length, 3 mm outer, 2 mm inner diameter) kept at a fixed distance with a metal wire spacer (15×8×8 mm, length×width×height). The mixture was allowed to gel at 37 °C for 60 min before culture medium (20 ml) was added to the dish. Medium was changed after overnight incubation and then every other day.

Phallodin actin stain

Chick EHTs (day 10) were fixed overnight in 4% formaldehyde in PBS, 4 °C, and shock-frozen in isopentane at −80 °C. Flat cryo sections (10 μm) were thaw-mounted (30 min at room temperature) on poly-L-lysine-coated slides, postfixed in 3% paraformaldehyde in PBS for 20 min, 2× rinsed with PBS, treated with 0.2% Triton X-100 in PBS for 15 min, rinsed 2× with PBS, and incubated with FITC-phalloidin (0.2 units/μl PBS) for 1 h. After 2× washing with PBS, the preparation was viewed and photographed on a Leica TCS NT Confocal Scanner.

Adenovirus-mediated gene transfer

The feasibility of EHTs as a model for transfection studies was tested by infection with recombinant replication-deficient adenovirus type 5 encoding *β*-galactosidase (Ad5LacZ) or the green fluorescence protein (Ad5GFP) under the control of a CMV promoter. Ad5LacZ was a kind gift from Dr. Harold Prentice, Glasgow, UK, Ad5GFP was constructed using the protocol and the vectors provided by Dr. B. Vogelstein [11]. The virus was propagated in human embryonic kidney 293 cells (HEK 293) using a modified Hirt protocol and purified by discontinuous CsCl gradient centrifugation. Virus titer was determined by DNA-quantification after deproteination of the virus (21 μg = 1 pmole = 6.23×10^{11} virus particles). The titer of biologically active virus (bav) was determined by infection of cardiac myocytes in monolayer cultures with serial dilutions and amounted to about 1/30 of the virus count. Rat EHTs were infected on day 6 with a multiplicity of infection (MOI) of 50 and incubated for an additional 48–72 h with complete culture medium. *β*-Galactosidase staining and histology was performed as described previously [6]. GFP fluorescence was viewed and photographed on a Zeiss Axioplan microscope.

Isometric force measurement

Seventy two hours after infection with Ad5LacZ or vehicle (Ctr), i.e., on day 9 of culturing, EHTs were removed from the culture dish and individually suspended in thermostated organ bathes in modified Tyrode's solution (NaCl 119.8, KCl 5.4, $CaCl_2$ 0.4, $MgCl_2$ 1.05, NaH_2PO_4 0.42, $NaHCO_3$ 22.6, Na_2EDTA 0.05, ascorbic acid 0.28, glucose 5.0 mM). After stabilization without pacing to record the spontaneous beating rate, EHTs were electrically stimulated with rectangular pulses (5 ms, 20% above threshold) via 2 platinum wire electrodes (150 μm diameter, 1 cm; placed on both sides of the immersed EHT) at a standard frequency of 1.0 Hz and equilibrated. Preload was stepwise adjusted from the original (spacer) length (L_0) to L_{max}, i.e., the length at which EHTs developed maximal force. Contractile activity was evaluated with a PC assisted system (BMON2, Ingenieurbüro Jäckel, Hanau, FRG). Twitch parameters were amplitude, i.e., the difference between diastolic (resting) and maximal systolic tension, twitch duration, i.e., time between start of twitch and 80% relaxation, and resting tension, i.e., diastolic tension. EHTs were exposed to increasing concentrations of calcium (0.4–2.4 mM) and, after washing 3×, to isoprenaline (0.1–1000 nM).

Statistics

All values presented are arithmetic means±SEM. "n" indicates the number of samples (i.e., EHTs). Student's t-test for paired observations was used in all cases to compare force of contraction before and after interventions. Student's t-test for unpaired observations was used for all other experiments. A p-value of less than 0.05 was considered significant.

Results

Requirements for the reconstitution of chick and rat cardiac myocytes to EHTs

Embryonic chick cardiac myocytes spontaneously formed EHTs when mixed with neutralized collagen I and cultured in the presence of standard culture medium (DMEM, 10% horse serum, 2% chick embryo extract). The cells rapidly spread into the matrix; they formed cell-to-cell contacts; and they compressed and contracted the cell/collagen gel into a flat, biconcave sheet spanning the gap between the Velcro-coated tubes (Fig. 1). Two to four days after seeding, EHTs started to beat coherently and rhythmically at a frequency of about 1 Hz. In contrast, neonatal rat cardiac myocytes remained rounded and isolated from each other in the matrix without beating, which is in accord with a former study [20]. By varying the culture conditions, we found that formation of spontaneously and coherently beating rat EHTs depended on supplementation of the reconstitution mix with Matrigel in a concentration-dependent manner. Contractile force, as determined in the organ bath, increased from 0 (no Matrigel) to 0.12±0.005 (5% Matrigel; n=17/24), 0.22±0.02 (10% Matrigel; n=9/12), and 0.27±0.05 mN (15% Matrigel; n=11/16). Rat EHTs also needed a higher initial cell density (1.9×10^6 cells/EHT=2.5-fold chick). Interestingly, a cell density $>2.3\times10^6$ cells/EHT reproducibly failed to produce beating EHTs. Both rat and chick EHT performed better when cultured in the presence of chick embryo extract, but did not absolutely depend on it. We routinely obtained approximately 1.1 EHTs (2.1×10^6 cells)/neonatal rat heart and 1.4–2.9 EHTs ($1-2\times10^6$ cells/embryonic chick heart).

Morphological aspects

Cardiac myocytes changed the gel dimension from an original size (length×width×thickness) of approximately 11×10×5.5 mm (the 0.6 ml drop

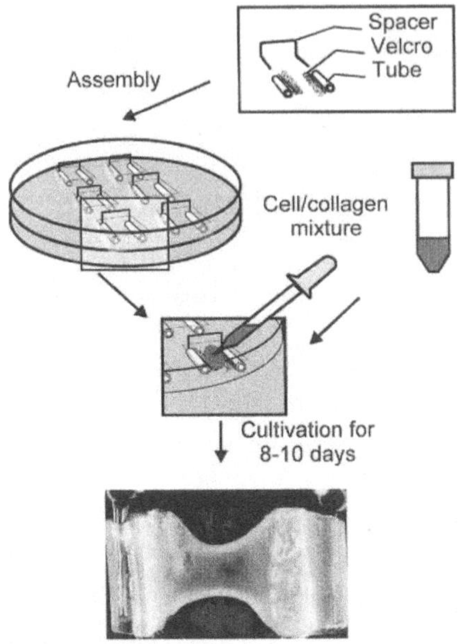

Fig. 1. Experimental setup to cast EHTs. Strips of Velcro (thick side) are glued to silicone tubes. 6–8 pairs of Velcro-coated tubes are assembled by stainless steel wire spacers and put in rectangular wells (17×10×4 mm) cut into a layer of silicone rubber in a 100 mm glass culture dish. The assembly is autoclaved before use. The cell/collagen/Matrigel mix is poured into each well between the two tubes and put in the 37 °C incubator for about 60 min before addition of 20 ml complete culture medium. After 6–10 days of cultivation, the typical biconcaval EHTs form and span the gap between the two tubes.

evenly distributed between the two Velcro-coated tubes) to EHTs with an average size of approximately 11×6×0.4 mm (rat) or 11×6×0.2 mm (chick). The tissue-like structure spanning the gap between the two tubes had a biconcave shape with an increased density of cells at the free lateral edges and sparse cell population of the central part (Fig. 1). Microscopically, cardiac myocytes at the free lateral edges of the gel (width approximately 200–500 μm) were mostly longitudinally oriented (parallel to the edge), while cells in the central parts formed a multidirectional network (Fig. 2). Actin staining with FITC-labeled phalloidin revealed highly organized myofibrils and clear cross-striation. The confocal image nicely revealed the network-like character with end-to-end and side-to-side contacts between cardiac myocytes (Fig. 2). Generally, chick EHTs had a more compact architecture than rat EHTs in which cells rather formed a loose network (see Fig. 3). In rat EHTs, cell remnants without nuclei laid intermingled between the differentiated myocytes. As judged by immunohistochemical means, the proportion of cardiac myocytes in chick EHTs was >80% [6].

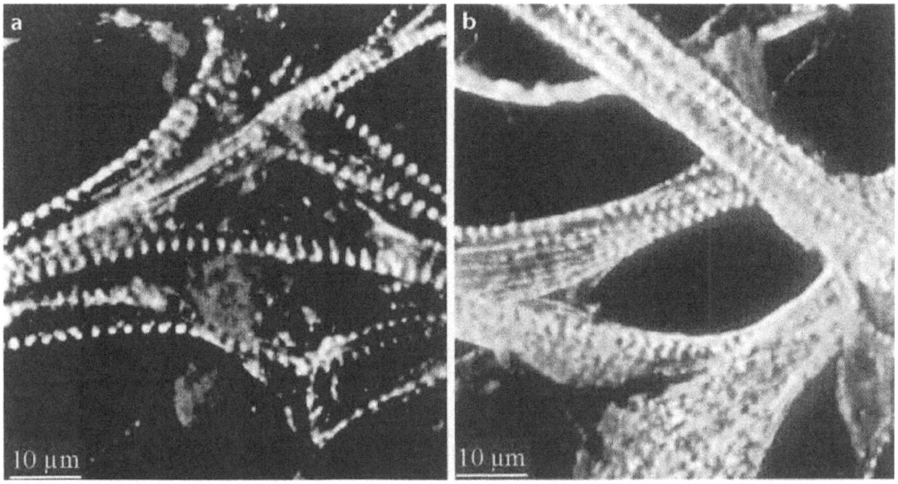

Fig. 2. Confocal images of chick EHTs. Cryo-sections (10 µm) from formaldehyde-fixed chick EHTs (day 10) were incubated with FITC-labeled phalloidin (specific actin stain) and viewed by confocal laser scanning microscopy. **a** shows a normal image; **b** an image in shadow technique. Both images were taken from the central region of chick EHTs and show well-developed myofibrils, cross-striation, and end-to-end and side-to-side contacts between myocytes.

Genetic manipulation

To test their applicability as an *in vitro* transgenic model, rat EHTs were infected with recombinant adenovirus type 5 carrying the cDNA for the two most commonly used marker genes, bacterial β-galactosidase (Ad5LacZ) and green fluorescence protein (Ad5GFP), respectively. Infection with both virus at a MOI of 50 yielded high gene transduction rates that reached 100% throughout the EHT without apparent morphological signs of cell toxicity (Fig. 3). Whereas Ad5LacZ-infected EHTs had to be fixed and stained for analysis, GFP transduction could be easily monitored in living cells with a standard fluorescence microscope. This enabled us to observe transducted cardiac myocytes contracting as a green luminous network spanning the entire EHT (Fig. 3).

Adenovirus-mediated gene transfer does not affect contractile behavior

Ad5LacZ-infected and mock-infected rat EHTs were subjected to isometric force measurements in the organ bath to study whether Ad5-mediated overexpression of marker genes *per se* affects contractile force of EHTs (Fig. 4). Neither basal force of contraction nor the positive inotropic effects of calcium or isoprenaline differed between control and Ad5LacZ-infected EHTs. Similarly, contraction kinetics were unchanged (time to 80% relaxation 145±6.4 in Ctr vs. 148±9.1 ms in Ad5LacZ, n=6 each).

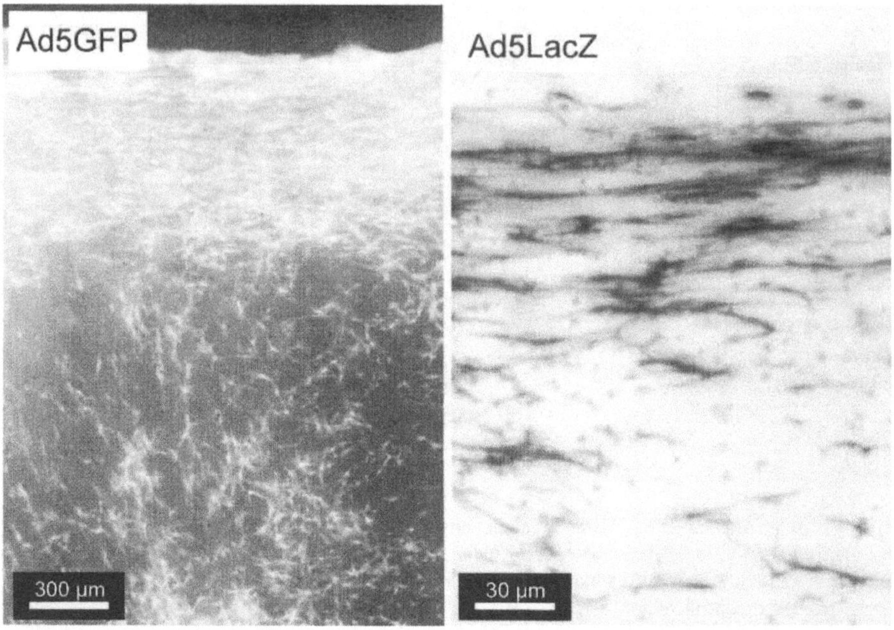

Fig. 3. Adenovirus-mediated gene transfer into EHTs. **a** Low power fluorescence photomicrograph of approximately 2/3 of width of a rat EHT *in situ*, 3 days after infection with Ad5GFP (MOI 50). Note the dense network of longitudinally oriented green cells at the free edge (upper part) and the "bridge-like" concentration of cells toward the center that appear to connect the two edges (only the upper free edge is seen on the photograph). **b** High power photomicrograph of a paraffin section (10 µm) of a rat EHT, 3 days after infection with Ad5LacZ (MOI 50). The EHT had been shortly formaldehyde-fixed, stained with 0.5 mg/ml X-gal, postfixed, embedded in paraffin, and cut parallel to the plane of the tissue (flat). Sections were counterstained with hematoxylin and eosin. The photomicrograph shows one of the two free lateral edges (top of photograph) of an EHT. Note that all viable cells stain strongly blue and only the rounded cell remnants that lay intermingled between the longitudinally oriented myocytes show light hematoxylin-eosin staining.

Discussion

This paper summarizes our recent progress in developing a new technique suitable to culture embryonic chick or neonatal rat cardiac myocytes in a 3D matrix to form spontaneously and coherently beating engineered heart tissue (EHT). The principle and details have been published previously [6, 23]. The main advantages of this culture technique are

- the 3D structure that surpasses monolayers in resembling intact heart architecture,
- inherent inhibition of dedifferentiation and overgrowth by non-cardiomyocytes in the presence of serum and absence of cytostatics that is probably the consequence of the 3D structure,
- the possibility to determine contractile force in standard organ baths,

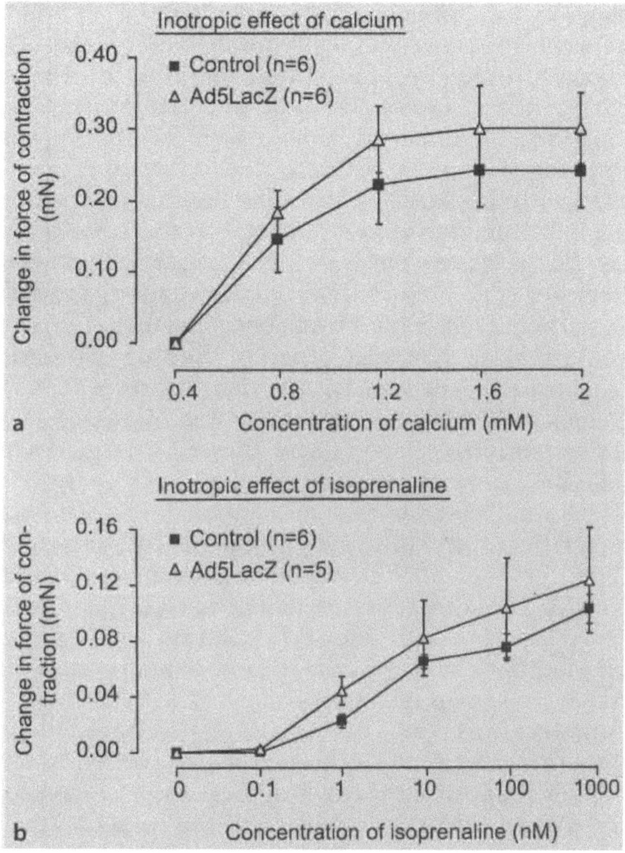

Fig. 4. Effect of adenovirus-mediated gene transfer on force of contraction. EHTs were infected with Ad5LacZ (MOI 50) or mock-infected (control) on day 6, cultured for an additional 3 days, suspended in individual organ baths, connected to an inductive force transducer, electrically paced at 1 Hz, stretched to the original (spacer) length, and equilibrated. **a** The positive inotropic effect of calcium was evaluated by cumulatively increasing the extracellular calcium concentration from 0.4 to 2.0 mM, 5 min each. **b** The positive inotropic effect of isoprenaline was tested after washing 3× with 0.4 mM Tyrode's solution. Isoprenaline concentrations were cumulatively increased from 0.1–1000 nM. Ordinates present the change in force of contraction in mN from predrug values, which did not differ between control and Ad5LacZ.

- the stability over long periods of cultivation (weeks) and the stability of force measurements, and
- the simplicity of genetic manipulation in comparison with intact heart tissues.

As demonstrated for immature chick and rat cardiac myocytes, the technique is applicable for different species but had to be modified to work with rat neonatal cardiac myocytes. The main prerequisite for rat cardiac myocytes to spread in the collagen matrix, to develop cell contacts, and to beat coordinately was the presence of Matrigel. Matrigel is a commercially available ascites fluid from mice with Engelbreth-Holm-Swarm tumors and, according to the manufacturer, contains high amounts of laminin (55%), collagen IV (30%), entactin (10%), heparin sulphate proteoglycan (5%), IGF-1 (11–24 ng/ml), and a number of other growth factors. At present, the identity of factor(s) that account for its permissive effect on rat EHT formation is unknown but we assume that IGF-1 or other soluble factors are important. This is because EHTs made without Matrigel in the reconstitution mix that were cultured in the same dish with EHTs made with Matrigel also started to beat coherently (not shown). IGF-1 has antiapoptotic activity [22] and one may speculate that IGF-1 (and probably a number of other factors) help to prevent execution of an apoptotic program that may be initiated by cell isolation. A second prerequisite was that cell density was 2.5-fold higher than in embryonic chick EHTs. When cell density was increased even further EHTs did not start synchronous beating and showed a large fraction of apparently dead cells. These observations suggest that an increase in cell density up to a certain degree facilitates cell-cell contact formation which is likely one of the most critical factors in establishing 3D collagen cultures. Above the critical cell density, metabolic problems may occur. It should be noted that cell death (or lack of adherence to the plastic surface) also occurs in standard 2D cultures in the first 24 h after cell isolation where such cells are removed with each medium change, while cell remnants remain in the 3D matrix.

We have shown previously that chick EHTs form a relatively dense heart muscle-like structure of longitudinally oriented cells at the lateral free edges. In contrast, the central regions are relatively sparsely populated by more star-shaped cells [6]. Confocal laser microscopy of phalloidin actin-stained chick EHTs also showed in the center of the matrix highly differentiated cardiac myocytes that were interconnected, albeit less regularly oriented than at the free edges. The reason for the nonhomogeneity of cell size, shape, and orientation is probably that cells at the free edges are exposed to higher longitudinal strain than those in the center. Strain or load is a growth stimulus [17] and cardiac myocytes align parallel to the direction of load [21]. Both reactions could lead cells at the edges to undergo hypertrophy and those in the center not or to a lesser extent. In support of this notion is the result of experiments in which chick and rat EHTs were exposed to a motorized cyclic stretch for 6 days. Stretch-induced hypertrophy of cardiac myocytes at the free lateral edges, an increase in RNA and protein yield, and a 3-5-fold increase in contractile force [7]. DNA content and [^{3}H]-thymidine incorporation were not significantly affected, indicating that hypertrophy and not hyperplasia accounted for the observed effects. Also [^{3}H]-thymidine incorporation rates are about 20–100 times lower in 3D EHT than in 2D cultures and decrease over time of cultivation [6]. This argues against the relevance of hyperplasia in this system.

The original objective of developing a 3D model for cardiac myocytes was to create a model that combines the advantages of 2D cardiac cell culture, namely easy genetic manipulation and defined *in vitro* conditions, with the possibility to directly measure the main function of cardiac cells, namely force of contraction. This is made possible by anchoring the 3D matrix to Velcro-coated tubes (surface enlargement), by allowing the cells to impose a contractile load that is resisted by the spacer that keeps the tubes at a defined distance (thereby preventing shrinkage of the 3D culture as seen in classical fibroblast/collagen gel e.g. [3], and by the simple method for attaching the EHTs in organ baths to force transducers. For EHTs to be a suitable test bed for genetic manipulations, two requirements had to be fulfilled: 1) high transfection rates and 2) lack of nonspecific effects of gene transfer vectors. We have chosen replication-deficient recombinant Ad5 because it is, at present, the most effective gene transfer vector for cardiac myocytes [12], is easy to prepare in high titers, and relatively easy to construct. Here we show that gene transfer with both Ad5LacZ and Ad5GFP was highly efficient and reached 100% of viable cells (Fig. 3). A higher MOI (50) was necessary for the transduction of 3D cultures than for the transduction of 2D cultures where we routinely obtain 100% efficiency at a MOI of 3–10. The lower efficiency of Ad5 in EHT is likely due to problems of access, because we have found previously that gene transfer efficiency decreased between day 6 and 10. In this period the thickness of EHTs decreases; thus, the density of the cells and matrix likely increases and this may decrease the accessibility of the cells to the virus. Infection with Ad5LacZ or Ad5GFP did not induce apparent signs of cell toxicity. That infection with Ad5LacZ also does not affect any of the parameters of contractile performance is shown in Fig. 4. Twitch amplitude, twitch duration as well as the response to increasing concentrations of calcium or isoprenaline were identical in the uninfected control and infected EHTs. This suggests that Ad5-mediated up-regulation of the stimulatory G protein Gsα that had been observed in an early study [18] does not occur in our system or occurs but does not affect contractile parameters. Thus, EHTs appear to be a suitable model to investigate the consequences of genetic manipulation, i.e., overexpression or antisense suppression of certain cardiac genes, on cardiac contractility, beating frequency, and morphology. Such experiments are relatively simple and quick and may provide important information prior or in addition to work with transgenic animals.

The model also has a number of shortcomings:

One is the nonhomogeneity of cell distribution/growth with the consequence that different parts of the structure contribute differently to contractile force as determined in the organ bath. We have recently reduced the width of tubes and thereby the fraction of loosely populated central parts. As expected, the smaller EHTs were more evenly populated and developed the same force. Further progress has resulted from chronic stretch and a different geometry [23].

EHTs are made from immature cells that, at least in 2D cell culture, exhibit signs of dedifferentiation. Morphological analysis suggests that the cardiac myocytes when cultured in 3D EHTs differentiate (Fig. 2 and [6]). Also, the force of contraction, when continuously recorded over >4 weeks, increase considerably with time [23]. Nevertheless, the degree of differentiation over time of cultivation in EHTs has yet to be thoroughly investigated. The tissue-like structure of EHTs does not fully resemble intact heart architecture, and it is evident that the system, even though closer to physiological conditions than the 2D cultures, is still an artificial system. Hence, it must compete with other recent methods that allow consequences of short-term genetic manipulation to be studied under relatively stable and physiological conditions.

Successful attempts have been made to inject adenoviruses into the coronary arteries *in vivo* and monitor alterations in heart function [10, 14], to perfuse whole hearts with adenovirus *in vitro* and either reimplant them heterotopically [13] or culture the infected cells or isolated heart muscle strips from those hearts *in vitro* [5] (and the paper from the Hasenfuss group, this issue, chapter 9), or to transduce freshly isolated adult cardiac myocytes and study alterations in shortening [9, 15]. At present it may be favorable to study the impact of genetic manipulations in different models to reduce the likelihood of model-specific artifacts and eventually to find the most favorable applications for each model.

The development of EHTs may be of interest also with regard to recent attempts to engineer heart tissue *in vitro*. One study used simulated microgravity to culture cardiac myocytes on microcarrier beads and detected some three-dimensional organization [1]. The same group found that neonatal rat cardiac cells (total population), when cultured in rotating bioreactors, spontaneously form a tissue-like structure even in the absence of exogenous matrix. This exciting finding suggests that formation of organotypic structures represents an intrinsic capacity to re-establish complex, 3-dimensional cardiac organization *in vitro* [2]. Another group used a biodegradable polymer scaffold to which cardiac myocytes attached and formed a contractile cell-polymer construct [4]. These new developments offer clinical promise, and it appears that specifically designed EHTs could be useful as tissue equivalents for *in vivo* tissue repair.

Acknowledgments. The study was supported by grants from the German Research Foundation (Deutsche Forschungsgemeinschaft) to T.E. (Es 88/6-1 and Es 88/8-19).

References

1. Akins RE, Schroedl NA, Gonda SR, Hartzell CR (1997) Neonatal rat heart cells cultured in simulated microgravity. In Vitro Cell Dev Biol Anim 33:337–343
2. Akins RE, Boyce RA, Madonna ML, Schroedl NA, Gonda SR, McLaughlin TA, Hartzell CR (1999) Cardiac organogenesis in vitro: reestablishment of three-dimensional tissue architecture by dissociated neonatal rat ventricular cells. Tissue Engineering 5:103–118

3. Burgess ML, Carver WE, Terracio L, Wilson SP, Wilson MA, Borg TK (1994) Integrin-mediated collagen gel contraction by cardiac fibroblasts. Effects of angiotensin II. Circ Res 74:291–298
4. Carrier RL, Papadaki M, Rupnick M, Schoen FJ, Bursac N, Langer R, Freed LE, Vunjak-Novakovic G (1999) Cardiac tissue engineering: cell seeding, cultivation parameters and tissue construct characterization. Biotechnol Bioengin 64:580–589
5. Donahue JK, Kikkawa K, Johns DC, Marban E, Lawrence JH (1997) Ultrarapid, highly efficient viral gene transfer to the heart. Proc Natl Acad Sci USA 94:4664–4668
6. Eschenhagen T, Fink C, Remmers U, Scholz H, Wattchow J, Weil J, Zimmermann WH, Dohmen HH, Schäfer H, Bishopric N, Wakatsuki T, Elson EL (1997) Three dimensional reconstitution of embryonic cardiomyocytes in a collagen matrix: a new heart muscle model system. FASEB J 11:683–694
7. Fink C, Remmers U, Weil J, Eschenhagen T (1998) Chronic stretch markedly improves contractile force of engineered heart tissue. Circulation 98 (Suppl 1):1–838
8. Giordano FJ, He H, McDonough P, Meyer M, Sayen MR, Dillmann WH (1997) Adenovirus-mediated gene transfer reconstitutes depressed sarcoplasmic reticulum Ca^{2+}-ATPase levels and shortens prolonged cardiac myocyte Ca^{2+} transients. Circulation 96:400–403
9. Hajjar RJ, Kang JX, Gwathmey JK, Rosenzweig A (1997) Physiological effects of adenoviral gene transfer of sarcoplasmic reticulum calcium ATPase in isolated rat myocytes. Circulation 95:423–429
10. Hajjar RJ, Schmidt U, Matsui T, Guerrero JL, Lee KH, Gwathmey JK, Dec GW, Semigran MJ, Rosenzweig A (1998) Modulation of ventricular function through gene transfer in vivo. Proc Natl Acad Sci USA 95:5251–5256
11. He TC, Zhou S, da Costa LT, Yu J, Kinzler KW, Vogelstein B (1998) A simplified system for generating recombinant adenoviruses. Proc Natl Acad Sci USA 95:2509–2514
12. Kass-Eisler A, Leinwand LA (1997) DNA- and adenovirus-mediated gene transfer into cardiac muscle. Methods Cell Biol 52:423–437
13. Kypson A, Hendrickson S, Akhter S, Wilson K, McDonald P, Lilly R, Dolber P, Glower D, Lefkowitz R, Koch W (1999) Adenovirus-mediated gene transfer of the beta2-adrenergic receptor to donor hearts enhances cardiac function. Gene Ther 6(7):1298–1304
14. Maurice JP, Hata JA, Shah AS, White DC, McDonald PH, Dolber PC, Wilson KH, Lefkowitz RJ, Glower DD, Koch WJ (1999) Enhancement of cardiac function after adenoviral-mediated in vivo intracoronary beta2-adrenergic receptor gene delivery. J Clin Invest 104:21–29
15. Meyer M, Bluhm WF, He H, Post SR, Giordano FJ, Lew WY, Dillmann WH (1999) Phospholamban-to-SERCA2 ratio controls the force-frequency relationship. Am J Physiol 276:H779–785
16. Mohamed SN, Holmes R, Hartzell CR (1983) A serum-free, chemically-defined medium for function and growth of primary neonatal rat heart cell cultures. In Vitro 19:471–478
17. Morgan HE, Baker KM (1991) Cardiac hypertrophy. Mechanical, neural, and endocrine dependence. Circulation 83:13–25
18. Novotny J, Gustafson B, Kvapil P, Ransnas LA (1994) Adenovirus infection of myocardial cells induces an enhanced sensitivity to beta-adrenergic agonists by increasing the concentration of the stimulatory G protein. Biochem Mol Biol Int 34:993–1001
19. Simpson PC (1990) Regulation of hypertrophy and gene transcription in cultured heart muscle cells. In: Molecular Biology of the Cardiovascular System. Alan R Liss, Inc, pp 125–133

20. Souren JEM, Schneijdenberg C, Verkeleij AJ, Van Wijk R(1992) Factors controlling the rhythmic contraction of collagen gels by neonatal heart cells. In Vitro Cell Dev. Biol 28A:199–204
21. Vandenburgh HH, Solerssi R, Shansky J, Adams JW, Henderson SA, Lemaire J (1995) Response of neonatal rat cardiomyocytes to repetitive mechanical stimulation in vitro. Ann NY Acad Sci 752:19–29
22. Wang L, Ma W, Markovich R, Chen JW, Wang PH (1998) Regulation of cardiomyocyte apoptotic signaling by insulin-like growth factor I. Circ Res 83:516–522
23. Zimmermann H, Fink C, Kralisch D, Remmers U, Weil J, Eschenhagen T: Three-dimensional Engineered Heart Tissue From Neonatal Rat Cardiac Myocytes. Biotech Bioengin (manuscript submitted)

CHAPTER 12

Cellular mechanisms of cardiac arrhythmias – do they play a role in heart failure?

D. J. BEUCKELMANN, L. PRIEBE, U. C. HOPPE
Department of Medicine III,
University of Cologne, Germany

Arrhythmias in heart failure

Patients with severe heart failure are at high risk to die suddenly. In the majority of these patients, sudden death is thought to be due to ventricular tachyarrhythmias. The mechanisms underlying these lethal arrhythmias are largely unknown. However, in animal models of heart failure and in humans, there is evidence that reentry as well as non-reentrant mechanisms may play a role (Table 1).

On a cellular level, three possible mechanisms may underlie arrhythmias (Fig. 1):

- early afterdepolarization
- delayed afterdepolarization
- abnormal impulse formation.

In animal models, calcium influx through voltage-gated calcium channels during the plateau phase of the action potential through reactivation of the inactivated channel has been shown to cause early afterdepolarizations (EAD). Cation influx through the non-specific calcium-activated cation channel ($I_{ns(Ca)}$) or sodium influx through the electrogenic Na/Ca exchanger (I_{NaCa}) was found to underlie delayed afterdepolarizations (DAD). It is characterized by a depolarization of the cell membrane after the preceding action potential has ended. In contrast to pacemaker cells of the sinus or AV node ventricular cells are quiescent under physiological conditions.

Table 1. Mechanisms of sudden cardiac death in heart failure

Tachyarrhythmias
■ Reentry mechanisms
macro-reentry
micro-reentry
■ Abnormal impulse formation
■ Triggered arrhythmias
early afterdepolarization
delayed afterdepolarization

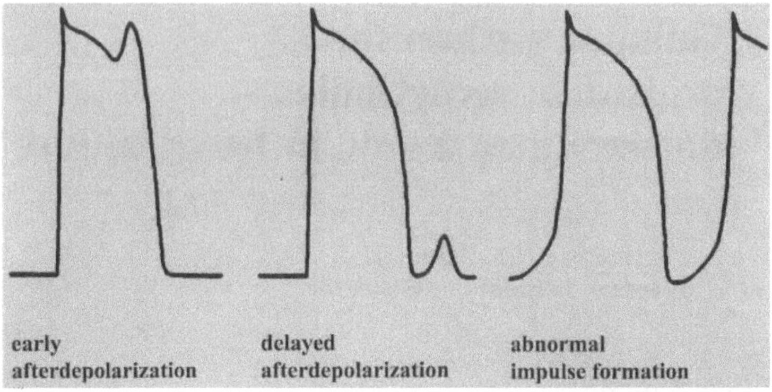

Fig. 1. Schematic diagram of possible cellular mechanisms of arrhythmias. Early afterdepolarizations are triggered by a preceding action potential during its plateau phase. Delayed afterdepolarizations are triggered by a preceding action potential after its complete repolarization. Abnormal impulse formation is caused by spontaneous depolarization of the working myocardium.

However, abnormal impulse formation may occur, when these cells start to depolarize spontaneously, possibly through activation of the pacemaker current I_f. However, it is unknown what influence these currents may have on triggered activity in human ventricular myocardium. In recent years, quantitative studies on ionic currents in human ventricular cells have greatly enlarged our knowledge about characteristics of the human action potential and its underlying ion movements in patients with heart failure. In this paper we summarize the data available on possible cellular mechanisms of arrhythmias in heart failure.

Action potential and repolarizing K^+ currents in heart failure

Heart failure is characterized by structural and functional changes within the heart which have a significant impact on cardiac electrical activity. At the cellular level, heart failure is accompanied by changes of calcium handling proteins and channel proteins governing cardiac repolarization. Prolongation of the action potential is a prominent feature of human ventricular myocardium from patients with severe heart failure [6]. In some of these studies, great variations in shape and duration of the action potentials have been found. Nevertheless, an unequivocal result was that the action potential is prolonged in human ventricular myocytes isolated from patients with heart failure compared to controls. Fig. 2 shows examples of human ventricular action potentials from failing and non-failing myocytes. Although their form and shape is variable, action potentials from failing myocytes are prolonged by approximately 50% at a frequency of 0.5 Hz. This has also been reported to occur in a variety of species and animal models of cardiac failure and hypertrophy. Prolongation of the action potential has been associated with an increased incidence of EADs.

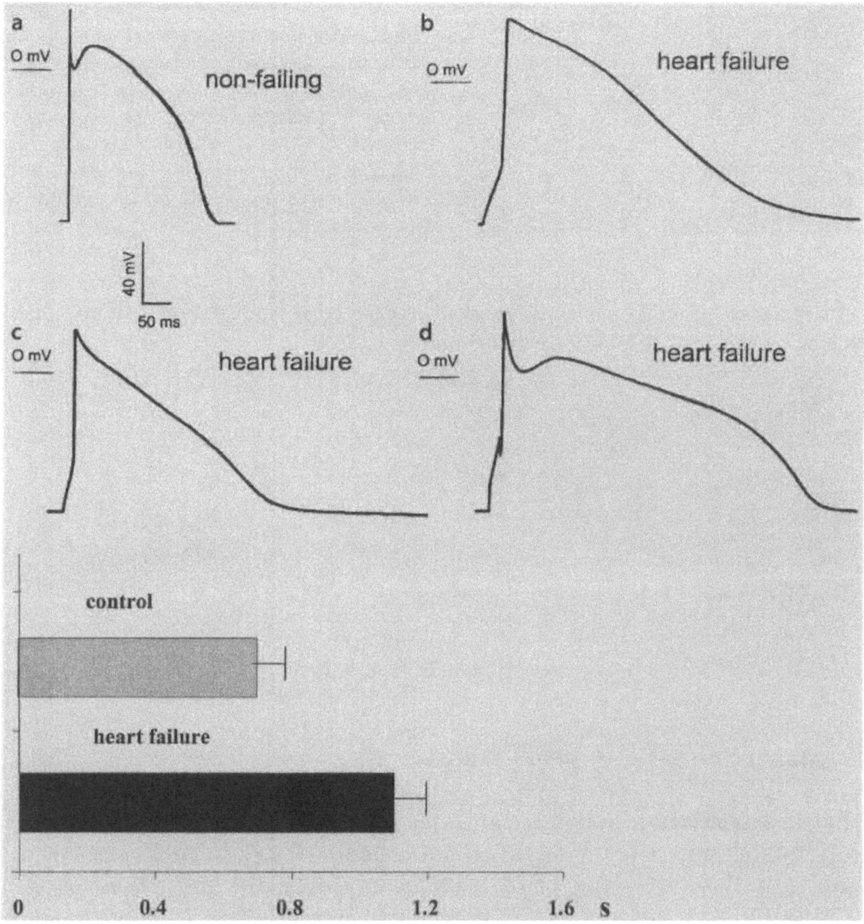

Fig. 2. Measured action potentials in non-failing (**a**) and failing myocytes (heart failure: **b–d**). Note the great variability in shape and duration of action potentials in failing myocytes.
Average action potential duration in human ventricular myocytes stimulated at 0.5 Hz under current clamp conditions.

The various currents underlying the human ventricular action potential are schematically depicted in Fig. 3. Various ionic currents have been shown to be altered in heart failure. The inward rectifier K^+ current (I_{K1}) [4, 32] and the transient outward K^+ current (I_{to}) [4, 41] have been found to be reduced by some groups, although this finding was not undisputed. Wettwer et al. [58] have found no significant alterations in current densities and kinetics of I_{to} in failing in comparison to non-failing myocytes. In Table 2 the alterations of various K^+ currents are summarized. Current densities and kinetics of the L-type Ca^{2+} current (I_{Ca}), however, have been shown to be unaltered by most groups [5, 37, 45].

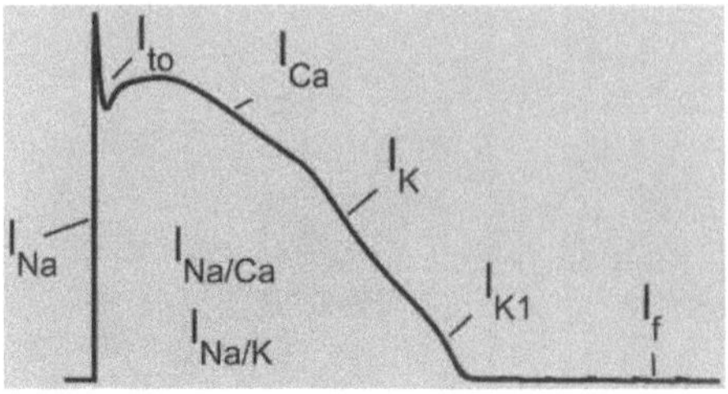

Fig. 3. Schematic diagram of important ionic currents determining the human ventricular action potential. *INa* Inward sodium current; *Ito* Transient outward K-current; *Ica* L-type calcium current; *IK* Delayed rectifier K-current; *IK1* Inward rectifier K-current; *If* Pacemaker current; *INa/Ca* Na/Ca exchange current; *INa/K* Na/K pump current.

Table 2. Alteration of action potential duration (APD) and K currents (*Ito* transient outward K-current; *IK1* inward rectifier K-current) in heart failure

Author	Species	Model details	ADP	I_{to}	I_{K1}
Wettwer et al. (1993)	human	terminal heart failure		=	
Beuckelmann et al. (1993)	human	terminal heart failure	↑	↓	(↓)
Wettwer et al. (1994)	human	terminal heart failure		subendocardial ↓	
Näbauer et al. (1996)	human	terminal heart failure		subepicardial ↓	
Käab et al. (1996)	dog	pacing-induced failure	↑	↓↓	(↓)
Thuringer et al. (1996)	hamster	hereditary CMP	↑	↓↓	
Rozanski et al. (1997)	rabbit	pacing-induced failure	↑	↓↓	=

Pacemaker current I_f in heart failure

The hyperpolarization-activated inward current (I_f) is thought to be the main depolarizing current during spontaneous diastolic depolarization in pacemaker cells underlying physiological automaticity [14]. In the last few years, this current has been extensively characterized in human atrial and ventricular myocytes [11, 27, 28]. Like in animal studies I_f activates slowly at hyperpolarization pulses and is blocked by extracellular cesium in both cell groups. In addition, the dependence of the current density on the extracellular potassium concentration and the selectivity of I_f for Na^+ and K^+ was found to be similar in atrial and ventricular human myocytes. There is a great difference in the voltage at which I_f activates between sino-atrial cells from animals and human working myocytes. In sino-atrial cells I_f activates at a more positive potential level (–40 mV) [19] compared to human atrial and ventricular myocytes (–80 mV).

Hoppe et al. [27, 28] have shown that I_f is expressed at significant levels in ventricular cells of the human working myocardium and that isoproterenol shifts the activation curve of I_f to more positive potentials (+10.3±0.3 mV) (Fig. 4). The expression in myocytes from patients with dilated cardiomyopathy (–1.37±0.12 pA/pF) and ischemic cardiomyopathy (1.39±0.24 pA/pF) at –130 mV was increased compared to non-failing controls (1.18±0.21 pA/pF), although this difference did not reach statistical significance (Fig. 5).

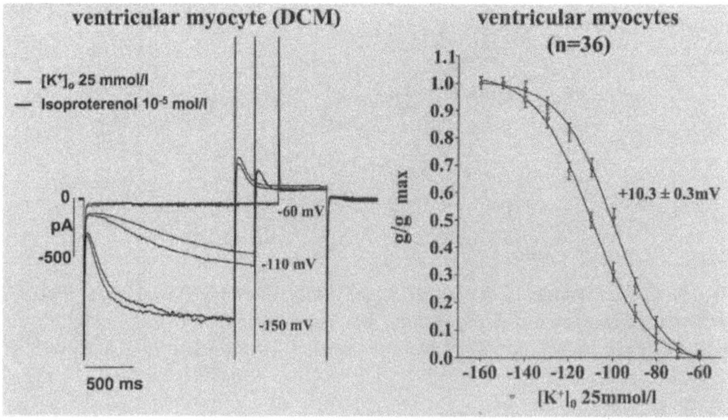

Fig. 4. Experimental traces of the hyperpolarization-activated inward current (I_f) in a human ventricular myocyte at 25 mmol/l extracellular potassium in the absence and in the presence of 10^{-5} M isoproterenol upon hyperpolarization to the various voltages indicated. Isoproterenol causes a shift of the activation curve to positive potentials.

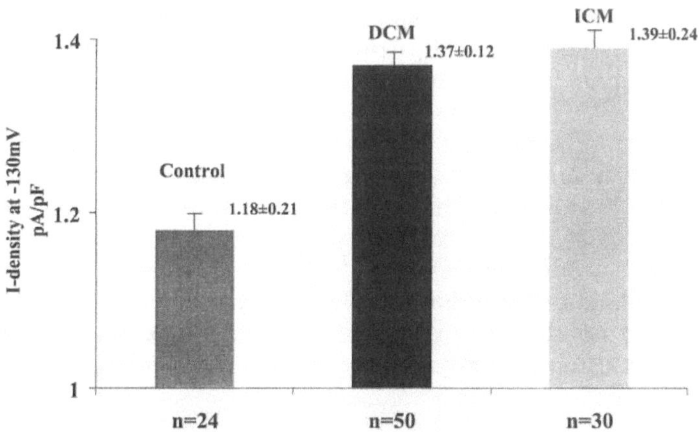

Fig. 5. Current density of the pacemaker current (I_f) in human ventricular myocytes from patients with terminal heart failure (*DCM* dilated cardiomyopathy; *ICM* ischemic cardiomyopathy) and non-failing controls.

Unlike in pacemaker cells, the impact of I_f on the diastolic phase of the action potential and thereby for automaticity in working myocardial cells remains unclear. Because of its small current density and its activation at very negative potentials, I_f may play a functional role during the diastolic phase only under pathological conditions.

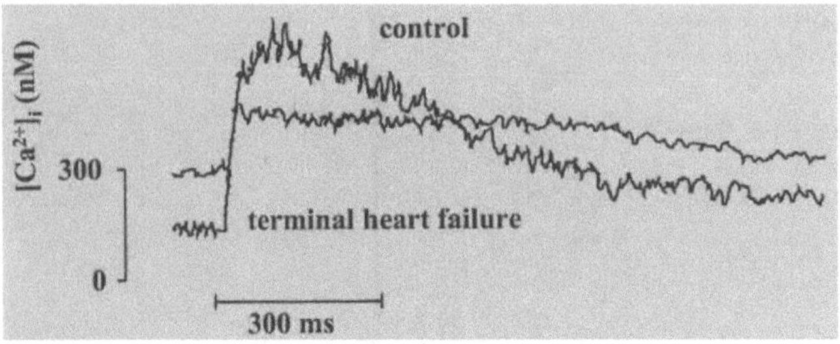

Fig. 6. $[Ca^{2+}]_i$ transients during external stimulation. Myopathic and control cells stimulated externally at a frequency of 0.5 Hz. Resting $[Ca^{2+}]_i$ in diseased cells was significantly higher than in control cells. Peak $[Ca^{2+}]_i$ transients were smaller and the decline of $[Ca^{2+}]_i$ was significantly slower.

Intracellular $[Ca^{2+}]_i$ handling in heart failure

A prominent feature of the single myocyte of the failing heart is an alteration of intracellular $[Ca^{2+}]_i$ handling [6, 20] and an enhanced activity of the Na^+-Ca^{2+} exchanger [17, 48]. Gwathmey et al. [20] were the first to describe an abnormal intracellular $[Ca^{2+}]_i$ handling in human cardiac contractile failure. Their experiments were performed in papillary muscles from patients with terminal heart failure using the bioluminescent photoprotein aequorin as a $[Ca^{2+}]_i$ indicator. From their experiments these authors postulated a combined defect of $[Ca^{2+}]_i$ handling by the sarcolemma and sarcoplasmic reticulum (SR). Studies in isolated ventricular myocytes have shown that in cells from patients with severe heart failure diastolic $[Ca^{2+}]_i$ is increased, systolic $[Ca^{2+}]_i$ transients are markedly reduced, and that the decay of $[Ca^{2+}]_i$ during diastole is prolonged (Fig. 6). The mechanisms underlying these alterations are predominantly caused by a reduced uptake of $[Ca^{2+}]_i$ into the SR. It has been postulated that these abnormalities may give rise to arrhythmias in heart failure, but proof for this hypothesis is lacking.

Mathematical model of the human ventricular action potential

Mathematical models of the cellular action potential and its underlying ionic currents may help to elucidate possible arrhythmogenic mechanisms on a cellular level. For this purpose a model of the ventricular action potential was developed based on Hodgkin-Huxley formalisms [26]. Selected depolarizing and repolarizing ionic currents and the intracellular $[Ca^{2+}]_i$ handling incorporated into this model were based on quantitative measurements in single ventricular myocytes isolated from non-failing and terminally failing human hearts.

Using this model we evaluated which ionic currents may effect the action potential in human myocardium and which cellular abnormalities in human ventricular myocytes from failing hearts may contribute to arrhythmogenesis in heart failure [47].

A variety of ionic currents and electrogenic ion pumps and exchangers that have been described in animals have not been sufficiently characterized in human ventricular myocytes. Therefore, these currents were calculated by equations used in an action potential model developed for guinea pig ventricular myocytes (LR model) [34, 35]. However, the major ionic currents, the L-type Ca^{2+} current (I_{Ca}), the transient outward K^+ current (I_{to}), the delayed rectifier K^+ current (I_K) with its two components (I_{Kr}+I_{Ks}) and the inward K^+ current (I_{K1}) were based on human data. In addition, the intracellular $[Ca^{2+}]_i$ transients in human myocytes and their alterations in failing myocytes observed experimentally [6] were simulated by this model. The other currents included in the model, a fast Na^+ current (I_{Na}), a Na^+-Ca^{2+} exchanger current (I_{NaCa}) and a Na^+-K^+ pump current (I_{NaK}), had to be adopted from the LR model and modulated in such a way that simulations were consistent with available human data.

Voltage clamp data for I_{Ca}, I_{to} and I_{K1} and calcium measurements were used as previously published [4–6, 40, 41].

Under space-clamp conditions, the differential equation describing the time-dependent changes in membrane potential (V) is

$$dV/dt = -(1/C_m)(I_{Na}+I_{Ca}+I_{to}+I_{Kr}+I_{Ks}+I_{K1}+I_{NaCa}+I_{NaK}+I_{Na,b} + I_{Ca,b}+I_{st}) \quad (1)$$

where C_m is the membrane capacitance and I_{st} is an externally applied stimulus current. The ionic currents I_X were calculated by ionic gates using Hodgkin-Huxley-type formalisms. All ionic currents were computed for 1 pF of cell membrane capacitance.

L-type Ca^{2+} current. The kinetics of I_{Ca} have been shown to be unaltered in myocytes from failing hearts [5, 37, 45]. Therefore, for calculating I_{Ca} the same gating parameters were used in both groups. In animal and human studies, it could be clearly demonstrated that the inactivation of I_{Ca} is voltage dependent. In addition, there is experimental evidence that inactivation of I_{Ca} is also calcium dependent [13, 55]. This type of regulation of I_{Ca} seems also to exist in human ventricular myocytes [12]. Consequently, we integrated a proportional factor, f_{Ca}, into the equation of I_{Ca} which was formulated as follows: $f_{Ca}=(1+([Ca^{2+}]_i/600\ nM))^{-1}$. Fitting of experimental I_{Ca} was performed with simulated $[Ca^{2+}]_i$ transients formulated as $A\cdot(\exp(-t/\tau_1)-\exp(-t/\tau_2))+R$. A indicates a proportional factor, τ_1 and τ_2 are time constants and R is the basal calcium level.

Transient outward K^+ current. No significant alterations of the kinetics of I_{to} have been found in failing myocytes compared to controls [58]. Therefore, the same gating parameters for simulating I_{to} are used in both groups. Based on experimental data [41] the current density of I_{to} was assumed to be 64% of the value measured in non-failing myocytes.

Delayed rectifier K^+ current. The existence of two components of the delayed rectifier, a rapidly activating (I_{Kr}) and a slowly activating component (I_{Ks}), has been documented by Li et al. [33]. Based on their data both currents were incorporated into the model. The method for simulating I_{Kr} in human ventricular myocytes was the same as that used by Sanguinetti et al. [49] in guinea pig myocytes. For simplification the slow inactivation of I_{Kr} during depolarization at +50 mV observed experimentally [33] was not considered. Quantitative values of I_{Ks} were calculated by fitting the experimental voltage clamp traces recorded in this study to a single exponential function. Upon depolarization the activation of I_{Ks} in human ventricular myocytes follows a sigmoidal time course like in guinea pig ventricular myocytes [49]. This strong sigmoidal activation was also found in wild-type I_{Ks} [56]. Therefore, the second power of activation in the Hodgkin-Huxley formalism of I_{Ks} was used to obtain an adequate fit to the measured traces. We did not consider a calcium-dependent regulation of I_{Ks} and I_{Kr} in our model. At the present time, the properties of I_{Kr} and I_{Ks} in heart failure are unknown. Therefore, we assumed that I_{Ks} and I_{Kr} are unchanged in heart failure.

Inward rectifier K^+ current. The simulated current density of I_{K1} was assumed to be reduced by 25% at −70 mV in the failing myocyte compared to controls based on results of experimental studies [4, 32]. Since the time-dependent inactivation of I_{K1} can only be observed at voltages more negative than −110 mV, I_{K1} was assumed to be time-independent. As in animal ventricular myocytes, I_{K1} is also almost solely carried by potassium ions in human ventricular myocytes. Therefore, the reversal potential of I_{K1} (E_{K1}) was calculated by using the Nernst equation.

Na^+-Ca^{2+} exchanger current. The Na^+-Ca^{2+} exchanger current (I_{NaCa}) was integrated into the model using values from the LR model because data in human ventricular myocytes are not available at present. To compute I_{NaCa} in a non-failing myocyte only the scaling factor of I_{NaCa}, k_{NaCa}, was changed to 50% of the value used in the LR model taking into account the smaller activity of I_{NaCa} in human myocytes compared to other animal species [53]. With such a value of k_{NaCa}, I_{NaCa} simulated in a non-failing myocyte with the same protocol as in the experiments by Sham et al. was in the range of the experimental data (model: 0.50 pA/pF; experiment: 0.54±0.1 pA/pF). In a failing myocyte, we assumed a 65% higher Na^+-Ca^{2+} exchanger activity than in a non-failing myocyte. This assumption was based on the observation of an increase of the Na^+-Ca^{2+} exchanger activity in myocardium from patients with heart failure [48].

Na^+-K^+ pump current. For simulation of the Na^+-K^+ pump current we used the equation of the LR model. The magnitude of I_{NaK} was chosen in such a way that APD in a non-failing myocyte at a stimulation frequency of 1 Hz was in the range as measured experimentally in a single human cell from non-failing hearts by our group (unpublished data) and by Peeters et al. [46]. There is a report which suggests that the concentration of the Na^+-K^+ ATPase is decreased by as much as 42% in failing hearts [54]. This alteration is assumed to represent a proportional decrease in I_{NaK}. Therefore, a 42% reduction in I_{NaK} of a failing myocyte was incorporated into the model.

Intracellular $[Ca^{2+}]_i$-transient. To simulate the $[Ca^{2+}]_i$ transients in both groups the approach of the LR model was chosen [35]. In some equations for calculating the calcium homeostasis the parameters were changed in such a way that simulated $[Ca^{2+}]_i$ transients closely resembled those measured in non-failing and failing human ventricular myocytes [4].

CICR by the SR: The threshold for the calcium-induced calcium release from the cardiac SR (CICR) was reduced from 0.18 to 0.005 μmol/l because of the smaller size of the peak L-type calcium current in human compared to animal myocytes. The time constants for the activation (τ_{on}) and deactivation (τ_{off}) of the release process was set to 4 ms. Experimental studies revealed that the function and number of the ryanodine channels are widely unaltered in heart failure [51]. Therefore, the CICR mechanism was assumed to be equal in non-failing and failing myocytes.

Calcium buffers in the myoplasm and the SR: There are reports that the affinity of troponin C to Ca^{2+} is unaltered in heart failure [21]. Consequently, because of the great contribution of troponin C to the total myoplasmic calcium buffer capacity, we used equal myoplasmic buffer concentrations in non-failing and failing myocytes. For simulating the calcium buffering in the JSR (calsequestrin), we adopted the values of the LR model for our model. There is no evidence for differences in the level of calsequestrin in heart failure. Therefore, equal concentrations of calsequestrin were used in both cell groups. With the approach of Hilgemann and Noble [25], we computed the steady-state buffering process numerically by using Newton's iterative method.

Ca^{2+} uptake and leakage by the NSR: Reduction of the activity of Ca^{2+} ATPase of the SR in heart failure, as shown in experimental studies [23, 52], were integrated into the model. To obtain the characteristic calcium transients in both cell groups the scaling factor for Ca^{2+} uptake, $\bar{I}_{up}$, was set to 0.0045 mmol/(l*ms) in non-failing and 0.0015 mmol/(l·ms) in failing myocytes. The rate of Ca^{2+} leakage out of the NSR (K_{leak}) in both cell groups was chosen in such a way that Ca^{2+} leakage out of the NSR is equal to the Ca^{2+} uptake in the NSR at basal $[Ca^{2+}]_i$ (non-failing: $K_{leak} = 0.00026\ ms^{-1}$; failing: $K_{leak} = 0.00017\ ms^{-1}$).

Table 3. Summary of alterations of various ionic currents in ventricular myocytes from patients with severe heart failure

I_{Na}	↔
I_{to}	↓
I_{Ca}	↔
I_{K}	↔
I_{K1}	↓
I_{f}	(↑)
$I_{Na/Ca}$	↑
$I_{Na/K}$	↓

$[Ca^{2+}]_i$ handling: diastolic $[Ca^{2+}]_i$ ↑, systolic $[Ca^{2+}]_i$, ↓ diastolic $[Ca^{2+}]_i$ delay ↔

Sarcolemmal calcium pump: The contribution of the sarcolemmal calcium pump to the extrusion of Ca^{2+} out of the cell has been shown to be very small [7]. Therefore, we did not consider this pump in our model.

Background currents. First, a linear Ca^{2+} background current ($I_{Ca,b}$) was incorporated into the model for balancing the Ca^{2+} extrusion through I_{NaCa} at resting potential in both cell groups. By this mechanism, the resting level of $[Ca^{2+}]_i$ was maintained at 0.12 µmol/l in a non-failing myocyte and at 0.15 µmol/l in a failing myocyte.

Second, a linear Na^+ background current ($I_{Na,b}$) was also incorporated into the model of a non-failing myocyte for maintaining the resting level of $[Na^+]_i$ (10 mmol/l in both cell groups). In a failing myocyte, Na^+ ion extrusion by I_{NaK} balanced the Na^+ ion entry by I_{NaCa} so that incorporation of $I_{Na,b}$ into this model was not necessary in that cell.

Changes of various currents and transport systems that have been described in heart failure and that have been implemented into this model are summarized in Table 3.

The model was written in Pascal and tested using a Turbo-Pascal compiler (Borland International) on an IBM-compatible computer. A fourth-order Runge-Kutta method with fixed time intervals is used for numerical integration of differential equations.

Results

To test the validity of this action potential model we simulated the ionic currents I_{Ca}, I_{to}, I_{Kr}, I_{Ks} and I_{K1} under voltage-clamp conditions using pulse protocols similar to those used in the experiments previously performed.

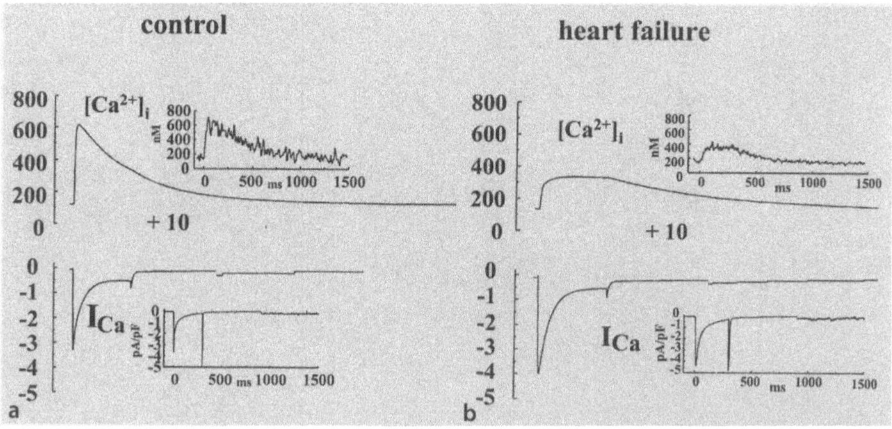

Fig. 7. Calcium current through L-type calcium channels (I_{Ca}) and intracellular $[Ca^{2+}]_i$ transients ($[Ca^{2+}]_i$) of a non-failing (**a**) and failing myocyte (**b**) upon depolarization to +10 mV in the model and in the experiment (insets). Holding potential: –40 mV. Like in the experimental study I_{NaCa} is present in these simulations. Intracellular sodium concentration: 5 mM.

$[Ca^{2+}]_i$ transients

Fig. 7 shows I_{Ca} and intracellular $[Ca^{2+}]_i$ transients in a non-failing and failing myocyte upon depolarization to +10 mV, respectively. Experimental data are shown as insets. Simulations of $[Ca^{2+}]_i$ transients at various depolarizations are started with $[Ca^{2+}]_{NSR} = [Ca^{2+}]_{JSR} = 2.5$ mM in a non-failing myocyte and $[Ca^{2+}]_{NSR} = [Ca^{2+}]_{JSR} = 1$ mM in a failing myocyte based on experimental data. Under these conditions, simulated and experimentally found I_{Ca} and intracellular $[Ca^{2+}]_i$ transients are similar in both cell groups. In particular, values of resting and peak $[Ca^{2+}]_i$ at +10 mV are in the range of experimental data.

The simulated action potential is prolonged in heart failure – effects of I_{to} inhibition

The action potential duration at 90% repolarization (APD_{90}) was significantly longer in a failing than in a non-failing myocyte (548.8 vs. 374.0 ms, respectively) (Fig. 8). In contrast to this, differences in the action potential duration at 25% and 50% repolarization between both cell groups were smaller (APD_{25}: non-failing: 262.9 ms, failing: 305.7 ms; APD_{50}: non-failing 310.2 ms, failing 374.5 ms). Therefore, the prolongation of AP in heart failure is mainly due to the slower rate of repolarization in the late phase of AP in a failing compared to a non-failing myocyte which was also found in an experimental study on human myocardium.

4-Aminopyridine is known to prolong the AP. From this result it has been postulated that reduction of I_{to} may prolong the action potential in cardiac myocytes [30]. However, there are additional effects of 4-aminopyr-

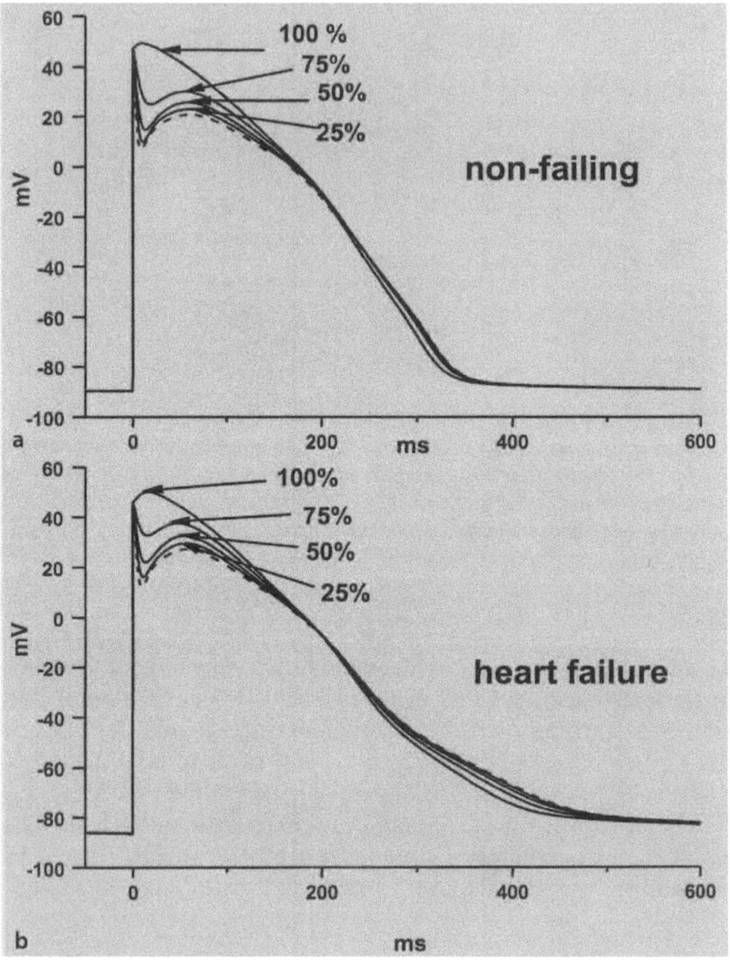

Fig. 8. Effect of inhibition of the transient outward K^+ current (I_{to}) on the action potential duration. Action potentials are simulated at various degrees of inhibition of I_{to} in a non-failing (**a**) and in a failing myocyte (**b**). These simulations imply that I_{to} has only a small effect on the action potential duration in human myocardium.

idine on other currents, especially on I_{Ca} [2] and I_K [42]. With our model we investigated the possible contribution of I_{to} to the APD in human ventricular myocytes. To assess the effect of I_{to} on APD we simulated the action potentials in both cell groups under conditions of various degrees of I_{to} inhibition (25%, 50%, 75% and 100%). Simulations are preceded by ten stimulations to obtain steady-state conditions. The simulated action potentials shown in Fig. 8 demonstrate that inhibition of I_{to} does not significantly prolong the action potential in a non-failing nor in a failing myocyte.

I_{Kr} and I_{Ks} control repolarization in human myocardium

Despite their relative small current densities, I_{Kr} and I_{Ks} largely control repolarization of the action potential in human ventricular myocytes. Inhibition of I_{Kr}, the main mechanism of class III antiarrhythmic agents, has also been shown to prolong the action potential in *in vivo* mapping studies [24, 29].

Carlsson et al. have found a pronounced prolongation of the action potential in non-failing human ventricular muscles after inhibition of I_{Kr} by 10^{-6} H 234/09 (almokalant) [9]. At this concentration almokalant significantly blocks only I_{Kr}.

We tried to imitate this effect of I_{Kr} on APD in human myocardium by varying the maximal conductance of I_{Kr}, g_{max}, to 75%, 50%, 25% and 0% of its original value. To obtain steady state of the intracellular $[Ca^{2+}]_i$ transient, 20 action potentials were elicited. Fig. 9 shows the prolongation of the action potential in a non-failing cell by inhibition of I_{Kr} to various degrees (top). Like in the experimental study, increased inhibition of I_{Kr} results in a progressive prolongation of AP. At 100% inhibition of I_{Kr}, APD_{90} was lengthened from 374.0 to 689.4 ms which is in the same range measured by Carlsson et al. [9]. Inhibition of I_{Kr} also prolonged AP in a failing myocyte. In contrast to a non-failing myocyte, 50% inhibition of I_{Kr} results, however, in an incomplete repolarization of the cell membrane in a failing myocyte at 1.0 Hz. At 75% inhibition of I_{Kr}, even an early afterdepolarization develops after three stimulations. Therefore, a failing myocyte is more sensitive than a non-failing myocyte to I_{Kr} inhibition. Simulations with various degrees of inhibition of I_{Ks} indicate that this current also has a significant impact on APD in both cell groups. However, inhibition of I_{Kr} has an even greater effect. In a non-failing myocyte, 100% inhibition of I_{Ks} prolongs APD_{90} from 374.0 to 526.1 ms. In a failing myocyte, incomplete repolarization occurs at 100% inhibition of I_{Ks}.

Complete inhibition of I_{Kr} induces development of recurrent EADs in failing myocytes

The previous simulations reveal the critical role of I_{Kr} for repolarization and thereby for the electric stability of the cell membrane in a failing myocyte. Therefore, inhibition of I_{Kr} may facilitate the formation of EADs in failing myocytes. At 75% inhibition of I_{Kr}, we can observe an EAD after three stimulations (Fig. 9). To investigate if there are recurrent EADs in a failing myocyte without preconditioning stimulations, simulation of the action potential in a failing myocyte was performed assuming complete inhibition of I_{Kr}. It is obvious that 100% inhibition of I_{Kr} leads to recurrent early afterdepolarizations in a failing myocyte. It is also obvious that only in cells from patients with heart failure does inhibition of I_{Kr} facilitate the induction of early afterdepolarizations.

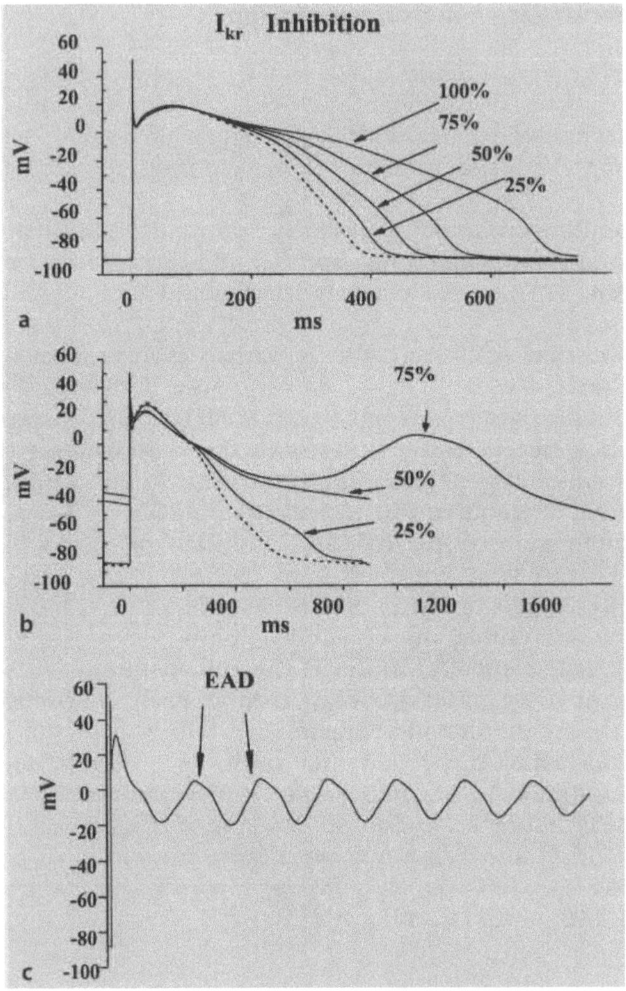

Fig. 9. Simulated action potentials under control conditions (dashed line) and when the maximum conductance of the rapidly activating component of the delayed rectifier K^+ current (I_{Kr}) is reduced by 25%, 50%, 75% or 100% in a non-failing (**a**) and in a failing myocyte (**b**, **c**). Generation of recurrent early afterdepolarizations (EADs) in a failing myocyte after complete inhibition of I_{Kr}.

The likelihood of premature action potentials is enhanced in a failing myocyte

Premature action potentials can be triggered by delayed afterdepolarizations (DAD) which are caused by a spontaneous calcium release from the sarcoplasmic reticulum (SR) [16, 18]. Since I_{NaCa} as a possible underlying current is enhanced in failing myocytes, it appears possible that premature action potentials may occur more frequently in these myocytes than in non-failing cells. However, the generation of DADs can only exert a proar-

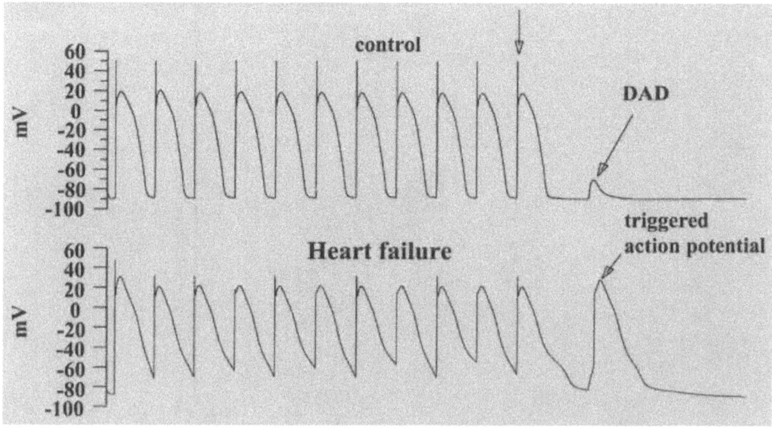

Fig. 10. Effect of spontaneous calcium release from the sarcoplasmic reticulum (SR) in a non-failing myocyte. Spontaneous calcium release from the SR is assumed to happen 250 ms after the last action potential (indicated by an arrow). Subsequently, the intracellular calcium concentration $[Ca^{2+}]_i$ increases quickly and then declines. This is linked to a generation of a delayed afterdepolarization (DAD).

rhythmogenic effect if depolarization reaches the threshold to open sodium channels and trigger a premature action potential. Consequently, we investigated whether the combined electrophysiological alterations in heart failure enhance the likelihood of premature action potentials. For this purpose, a spontaneous calcium release from the SR was simulated in both cell groups. As Luo and Rudy [36] have shown the recovery from the slow inactivation of sodium channels, named as factor j in their model, determines the recovery of the excitability after the action potential. To investigate the influence of I_{NaCa} on the generation of premature action potentials separately, the sodium channels should be completely recovered from their slow inactivation at the start of the spontaneous calcium release from the SR. Therefore, a spontaneous calcium release from the SR was assumed to occur at least 250 ms after 90% repolarization of the last action potential in both cell groups. After this diastolic time interval, the factor j = 1, e.g., the availability of sodium channels, was about 100% in both cell groups. We assumed an equal calcium-independent mechanism of the spontaneous calcium release from the SR in both cell groups. Simulations of spontaneous calcium release from the SR were preceded by a train of stimulations at 2.0 Hz for elevating the calcium content of the SR. After eleven stimulations, diastolic $[Ca^{2+}]_i$ was higher in a failing (275 nM) than in a non-failing myocyte (218 nM). $[Ca^{2+}]_{NSR}$ was increased from 2.9 to 3.4 mM in a non-failing and from 1.2 to 1.5 mM in a failing myocyte. As expected, the postulated spontaneous calcium release from the SR resulted in a greater increase of $[Ca^{2+}]_i$ in a non-failing (1394 nM) than in a failing myocyte (713 nM). A premature action potential was, however, generated only in a failing myocyte as the other repolarizing ionic currents, e.g., I_{K1} and I_{NaK}, were reduced in this cell (Fig. 10).

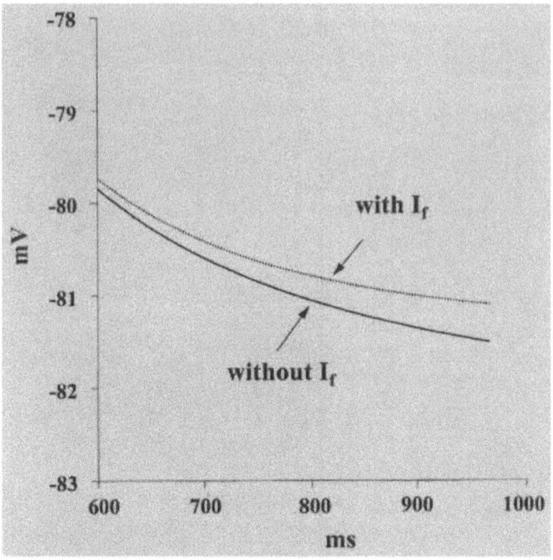

Fig. 11. Simulations of the action potential (AP) without (solid line) and with I_f (dashed line) during the terminal phase of the action potential.

Does spontaneous diastolic depolarization of ventricular myocytes play a role in arrhythmogenesis?

To assess the role of I_f on the diastolic phase of the action potential (AP) of ventricular myocytes, APs were simulated with and without I_f. Simulations of AP in undiseased (undiseased cells in both cell groups) and diseased myocytes are shown in Fig. 11. APs simulated without I_f (dashed line) were superimposed to those simulated with I_f (solid line). There was only a negligible difference between both APs in all cell groups. This small effect of I_f on AP was due to its very small current density during AP in comparison to that of I_{K1}. These simulations make clear that under physiological conditions the contribution of I_f to the diastolic phase of AP is very small in undiseased ventricular myocytes as well as in the case of altered electric cellular properties in heart failure.

Discussion

Results of simulations of ionic currents show that this model can reproduce important electrophysiological characteristics of human ventricular myocytes. Voltage-clamp simulations of the major ionic currents and the simulation of AP closely resemble experimental data obtained from human ventricular myocytes. Simulations of the ionic currents during the time course of the action potential and simulations of ionic current inhibition reveal the important role of I_{Kr} and I_{Ks} for repolarization in human ventricular myocytes. The influence of I_{Kr} and I_{Ks} on APD may be one reason for the wide range of measured APDs in different publications between 233 ms [12] and 650 ms [4] in single myocytes from non-failing hearts. Yue et al. [61] have demonstrated that the expression of I_K in cells isolated from canine heart is very dependent on the isolation technique.

Among other factors, different expression of I_{Kr} and I_{Ks} in single human myocytes possibly due to different isolation procedures could be a reason for this divergence of APD. However, the action potential simulated in a non-failing myocyte by our model very closely resembles the AP measured in single cells by us and by Peeters et al. [46]. Using the monophasic action potential technique in *in vivo* studies, the observed shape and duration of AP in human hearts are very similar to our simulations [3, 39]. Furthermore, simulations of ionic currents during the action potential demonstrate that I_{NaCa} is an important depolarizing current during the late phase of repolarization in a failing myocyte because of the enhanced activity of the Na^+-Ca^{2+} exchanger and the slow decay of $[Ca^{2+}]_i$ transient in this cell.

In studies of various animal models of heart failure or hypertrophy, a reduction of I_{to} has been found and this has been assumed to be an important factor causing action potential prolongation in heart failure. Our simulations of different degrees of inhibition of I_{to} suggest, however, that inhibition of I_{to} does not prolong AP in non-failing nor failing myocytes of human hearts. A reason for this discrepancy with experimental data could be that 4-aminopyridine used in that experimental study also blocked I_{Ks} and I_{Kr} which would lengthen the action potential. Considering this problem in experimental conditions, we conclude from the simulations of our model that the influence of I_{to} on APD is small in human myocardium. Of course, this model cannot prove that I_{to} does not alter APD, but it strongly suggests that reduction of the current density of I_{to} found in failing myocytes of human hearts does not seem to contribute significantly to the APD prolongation in heart failure.

Conclusions from the simulated action potentials for arrhythmogenesis in heart failure

From the results shown in Figs. 8 and 9, we conclude that in heart failure one important mechanism for triggered arrhythmias could be DADs. In our model, DADs are initiated by a postulated spontaneous calcium release from the SR. The resulting $[Ca^{2+}]_i$ increase depolarizes the cell membrane through I_{NaCa} in both cell groups. Therefore, like in animal myocytes, this indicates that I_{NaCa} may also significantly contribute to the generation of DADs in human myocytes. Although the activity of the Na^+-Ca^{2+} exchanger is enhanced in failing myocytes, I_{NaCa} is slightly larger in a non-failing than in a failing myocyte as the intracellular $[Ca^{2+}]_i$ increase is much higher in this cell. Nevertheless, a premature action potential can be triggered only in a failing myocyte as the repolarizing ionic currents, I_{K1} and I_{NaK}, are reduced in this cell. This indicates that a reduction of repolarizing currents (I_{K1} and I_{NaK}) rather than an increase of the depolarizing current

(I_{NaCa}) seems to be responsible for the enhanced likelihood of triggered action potentials in failing myocytes. At present, the mechanism of the spontaneous calcium release from the SR is unknown. Experiments in animal studies demonstrated that DADs and triggered action potentials were observed more frequently in failing or hypertrophied animal myocytes [1, 57]. The simulations clearly show that spontaneous calcium release leads to a triggered action potential only in a failing myocyte. From these triggered action potentials triggered arrhythmias may arise.

The conclusion about the role of I_{NaCa} for DADs and triggered action potentials does not mean that calcium-dependent nonspecific cation channels have no role in the arrhythmogenesis in heart failure. In animal studies, there is evidence for their contribution in generating delayed afterdepolarizations [8, 15]. However, Koester et al. [31] have shown that a nonspecific cation channel is only expressed in human atrial but not in ventricular myocardium. Therefore, a calcium-dependent nonspecific cation channel cannot carry transient inward currents underlying DADs in human ventricular myocytes.

Early afterdepolarizations are triggered during the plateau phase of an action potential and are thought to be caused by reactivation of the L-type calcium current [43, 60]. The membrane potential has to remain at voltages more positive than -35 mV until the L-type calcium channels are able to recover from their inactivation and can open again. Nordin and Ming showed that current-induced early afterdepolarizations in guinea pig ventricular myocytes are mainly due to the L-type calcium channel window current. In various preparations, specific block of I_{Kr} has been found to result in EADs in non-failing animal myocytes. However, EADs are not generated by inhibition of I_{Kr} block in a non-failing myocyte in this model (Fig. 9a). In contrast to this, 75% inhibition of I_{Kr} can lead to an EAD in a failing myocyte (Fig. 9b, 75%). When the inhibition of I_{Kr} is 100% even recurrent EADs develop in this myocyte (Fig. 9c). In conclusion, our results indicate that EADs are difficult to induce in human compared to animal myocytes. They can be generated only in failing myocytes after blocking I_{Kr} by at least 75%. This discrepancy in EAD formation between animal and this model is supported by experimental data. Vermeulen et al. [57] have observed that early afterdepolarizations occur only in papillary muscles of rabbit hearts, but never in human papillary muscles. Further studies are required to assess the role of EADs for arrhythmias in human ventricular myocytes.

The model clearly indicates that the pacemaker current I_f in ventricular myocytes does not play a significant role in cellular mechanisms of arrhythmias. Even under the assumption of a maximally activated β-adrenoceptor with shift of the activation curve by +10 mV does this current not induce a significant depolarization even at low stimulation frequencies, probably due to the large inward rectifier current.

Although the present model has the advantage of being based partially on human data it also has several limitations. Significant uncertainty remains concerning the magnitude of I_{NaCa}. At present, voltage clamp data of this current in human ventricular myocytes are not available. Comparison of I_{NaCa} incorporated in the model to the measured data in the human atrium suggests that the magnitude of the simulated I_{NaCa} has been well estimated. Nevertheless, it should be pointed out that some results have to be interpreted with caution because of their dependence on I_{NaCa}. However, the simulations indicate that increase of I_{NaCa} could play an important role in the arrhythmogenesis in heart failure and that its quantification in human ventricular myocytes is desirable. Another assumption of the model which has not been investigated is that I_{Kr} and I_{Ks} are unaltered in heart failure. At present, there are no experimental studies addressing this issue. In animal models of heart hypertrophy and of heart failure, the majority of authors could not find any changes in I_K [22]. Based on this, we assumed unchanged I_{Kr} and I_{Ks} in failing myocytes.

In conclusion experimental data and the mathematical model presented here indicate that delayed afterdepolarizations and, though to a lesser degree, early afterdepolarization may be important mechanisms triggering arrhythmias in patients with severe heart failure. Spontaneous depolarizations due to I_f activation do not play a significant role in this context. One theory as to why these alterations of ion transport mechanisms and ionic channel remodeling occur in heart failure is that prolongation of the action potential and increased activity of the Na^+/Ca^{2+} exchanger are mechanisms to increase inotropy, prevent elevated diastolic Ca^{2+} levels, but that this comes at the price of labile repolarization. Experimental proof of this theory, however, is still lacking.

Acknowledgments. This study was supported by the Deutsche Forschungsgemeinschaft (Be 1113/2-3), (Ho 2146/1-1) and the Bundesministerium für Bildung, Wissenschaft, Forschung und Technologie (01 KS 9502).

References

1. Aronson RS (1981) Afterdepolarizations and triggered activity in hypertrophied myocardium from rats with renal hypertension. Circ Res 48:720–727
2. Bénitah JP, Bailly P, D'Agrosa MC, Da P, Delgado C, Lorente P (1992) Slow inward current in single myocytes isolated from adult human ventricles. Pflugers Arch 421:176–187
3. Berger F, Borchard U, Hafner D, Kammer T, Weis T (1995) Modulation of action potential duration by inhibition of the transient outward current in sheep cardiac Purkinje fibers. Basis Res Cardiol 90:185–191
4. Beuckelmann DJ, Näbauer M, Erdmann E (1993) Alterations of K^+ currents in isolated human ventricular myocytes from patients with terminal heart failure. Circ Res 73:379–385
5. Beuckelmann DJ, Näbauer M, Erdmann E (1991) Characteristics of calcium-current in isolated human ventricular myocytes from patients with terminal heart failure. J Mol Cell Cardiol 23:929–937

6. Beuckelmann DJ, Näbauer M, Erdmann E (1992) Intracellular calcium handling in isolated ventricular myocytes from patients with terminal heart failure. Circulation 85:1046–1055
7. Beuckelmann DJ, Näbauer M, Krüger C, Erdmann E (1995) Altered diastolic $[Ca^{2+}]_i$ handling in human ventricular myocytes from patients with terminal heart failure. Am Heart J 129:684–689
8. Cannell MB, Lederer WJ (1986) The arrhythmogenic current I_{ti} in the absence of electrogenic sodium-calcium exchange in sheep cardiac Purkinje fibres. J Physiol (Lond) 374:201–219
9. Carlsson L, Abrahamsson C, Almgren O, Lundberg C, Duker G (1991) Prolonged action potential duration and positive inotropy induced by the novel class III antiarrhythmic agent H 234/09 (almokalant) in isolated human ventricular muscle. J Cardiovasc Pharmacol 18:882–887
10. Cerbai E, Barbieri M, Li Q, Mugelli A (1994) Ionic basis of action potential prolongation of hypertrophied cardiac myocytes isolated from hypertensive rats of different ages. Cardiovasc Res 28:1180–1187
11. Cerbai E, Pino R, Porciatti F, Sani G, Toscano M, Maccherini M, Giunti G (1997) Characterization of the hyperpolarization-activated current, I(f), in ventricular myocytes from human failing heart. Circulation 95:568–571
12. Cohen NM, Lederer WJ (1993) Calcium current in single human cardiac myocytes. J Cardiovasc Electrophysiol 4:422–437
13. De Leon M, Wang Y, Jones L, Perez-Reyes E, Wei X, Wah Soong T, Snutch TP, Yue DT (1995) Essential Ca^{2+}-binding motif for Ca^{2+}-sensitive inactivation of L-type Ca^{2+} channels. Science 270:1502–1505
14. DiFrancesco D (1991) The contribution of the 'pacemaker' current (I_f) to generation of spontaneous activity in rabbit sino-atrial node myocytes. J Physiol Lond 434:23–40
15. Ehara T, Noma A, Ono K (1988) Calcium-activated non-selective cation channels in ventricular cells isolated from adult guinea-pig hearts. J Physiol (Lond) 403:117–133
16. Fedida D, Noble D, Rankin AC, Spindler AJ (1987) The arrhythmogenic transient inward current I_{ti} and related contraction in isolated guinea-pig ventricular myocytes. J Physiol (Lond) 392:523–542
17. Flesch M, Schwinger RHG, Schiffer F, Frank K, Südkamp M, Kuhn-Regnier F, Arnold G, Böhm M (1996) Evidence for functional relevance of an enhanced expression of the Na^+-Ca^{2+} exchanger in failing human myocardium. Circulation 94:992–1002
18. Giles W, Shimoni Y (1989) Comparison of sodium-calcium exchanger and transient inward currents in single cells from rabbit ventricle. J Physiol (Lond) 417:465–481
19. Ginneken ACG, Giles W (1991) Voltage clamp measurements of the hyperpolarization-activated inward current I_f in single cells from rabbit sino-atrial node. J Physiol 434:57–83
20. Gwathmey JK, Copelas L, MacKinnon R, Schoen FJ, Feldman MD, Grossman W, Morgan JP (1987) Abnormal intracellular calcium handling in myocardium from patients with end-stage heart failure. Circ Res 61:70–76
21. Gwathmey JK, Hajjar RJ (1990) Relation between steady-state force and intracellular $[Ca^{2+}]_i$ in intact human myocardium. Index of myofibrillar responsiveness to Ca^{2+}. Circulation 82:1266–1278
22. Hart G (1994) Cellular electrophysiology in cardiac hypertrophy and failure. Cardiovasc Res 28:933–946
23. Hasenfuss G, Reinecke H, Studer R, Meyer M, Pieske B, Holtz J, Holubarsch C, Posival H, Just H, Drexler H (1994) Relation between myocardial function and ex-

pression of sarcoplasmic reticulum Ca^{2+}-ATPase in failing and nonfailing human myocardium. Circ Res 75:434–442
24. Hayward RP, Taggart P (1986) Effect of sotalol on human atrial action potential duration and refractoriness: cycle length dependency of class III activity. Cardiovasc Res 20:100–107
25. Hilgemann DW, Noble D (1987) Excitation-contraction coupling and extracellular calcium transients in rabbit atrium: reconstruction of basic cellular mechanism. Proc R Soc Lond 230:163–205
26. Hodgkin AL, Huxley AF (1952) A quantitative description of membrane current and its application to conduction and excitation in nerve. J Physiol 117:500–544
27. Hoppe UC, Beuckelmann DJ (1998) Characterization of the hyperpolarization-activated inward current in isolated human atrial myocytes. Cardiovasc Res 38:788–801
28. Hoppe UC, Jansen E, Sudkamp M, Beuckelmann DJ (1998) Hyperpolarization-activated inward current in ventricular myocytes from normal and failing human hearts. Circulation 97:55–65
29. Huikuri HV, Yli-Mayry S (1992) Frequency dependent effects of d-sotalol and amiodarone on the action potential duration of the human right ventricle. PACE 15:2103–2107
30. Kääb S, Nuss HB, Chiamvimonvat N, O'Rourke B, Pak PH, Kass DA, Marban E, Tomaselli GF (1996) Ionic mechanism of action potential prolongation in ventricular myocytes from dogs with pacing-induced heart failure. Circ Res 78:262–273
31. Köster O, Szigeti GP, Beuckelmann DJ (1999) Characterisation of a $[Ca^{2+}]_i$-dependent current in human atrial and ventricular myocytes in the absence of Na^+ and K^+. Cardiovasc Res 41:175–187
32. Koumi S, Backer CL, Arentzen CE (1995) Characterization of inwardly rectifying K^+ channel in human cardiac myocytes. Alterations in channel behavior in myocytes isolated from patients with idiopathic dilated cardiomyopathy. Circulation 92:164–174
33. Li GR, Feng J, Yue L, Carrier M, Nattel S (1996) Evidence for two components of delayed rectifier K^+ current in human ventricular myocytes. Circ Res 78:689–696
34. Luo CH, Rudy Y (1994) A dynamic model of the cardiac ventricular action potential. I. Simulations of ionic currents and concentration changes. Circ Res 74:1071–1096
35. Luo CH, Rudy Y (1994) A dynamic model of the cardiac ventricular action potential. II. Afterdepolarizations, triggered activity, and potentiation. Circ Res 74:1097–1113
36. Luo CH, Rudy Y (1991) A model of the ventricular cardiac action potential. Depolarization, repolarization, and their interaction. Circ Res 68:1501–1526
37. Mewes T, Ravens U (1994) L-type calcium currents of human myocytes from ventricle of non-failing and failing hearts and from atrium. J Mol Cell Cardiol 26:1307–1320
38. Meyer M, Schillinger W, Pieske B, Holubarsch C, Heilmann C, Posival H, Kuwajima G, Mikoshiba K, Just H, Hasenfuss G (1995) Alterations of sarcoplasmic reticulum proteins in failing human dilated cardiomyopathy. Circulation 92:778–784
39. Morgan JM, Cunningham D, Rowland E (1992) Electrical restitution in the endocardium of the intact human right ventricle. Br Heart J 67:42–46
40. Näbauer M, Beuckelmann DJ, Erdmann E (1993) Characteristics of transient outward current in human ventricular myocytes from patients with terminal heart failure. Circ Res 73:386–394
41. Näbauer M, Beuckelmann DJ, Überfuhr P, Steinbeck G (1996) Regional differences in current density and rate-dependent properties of the transient outward current in subepicardial and subendocardial myocytes of human left ventricle. Circulation 93:168–177

42. Navarro-Polanco RA, Sanchez-Chapula JA (1997) 4-Aminopyridine activates potassium currents by activation of a muscarinic receptor in feline atrial myocytes. J Physiol 498.3:663–678
43. Nordin C, Gilat E, Aronson RS (1985) Delayed afterdepolarizations and triggered activity in ventricular muscle from rats with streptozotocin-induced diabetes. Circ Res 57:28–34
44. Nordin C, Ming Z (1995) Computer model of current-induced early afterdepolarizations in guinea pig ventricular myocytes. Am J Physiol 268:H2440–2459
45. Ouadid H, Albat B, Nargeot J (1995) Calcium currents in diseased human cardiac myocytes. J Cardiovasc Pharmacol 25:282–291
46. Peeters GA, Sanguinetti MC, Eki Y, Konarzewska H, Renlund DG, Karwande SV, Barry WH (1995) Method for isolation of human ventricular myocytes from single endocardial and epicardial biopsies. Am J Physiol 268:H1757–1764
47. Priebe L, Beuckelmann DJ (1998) Simulation study of cellular electric properties in heart failure. Circ Res 82:1206–1223
48. Reinecke H, Studer R, Vetter R, Holtz J, Drexler H (1996) Cardiac Na^+/Ca^{2+} exchange activity in patients with end-stage heart failure. Cardiovasc Res 31:48–54
49. Sanguinetti MC, Jurkiewicz NK (1990) Two components of cardiac delayed rectifier K^+ current. Differential sensitivity to block by class III antiarrhythmic agents. J Gen Physiol 96:195–215
50. Sanguinetti MC, Jurkiewicz NK (1992) Role of external Ca^{2+} and K^+ in gating of cardiac delayed rectifier K^+ currents. Pflugers Arch 420:180–186
51. Schumacher C, Konigs B, Sigmund M, Kohne B, Schondube F, Vob M, Stein B, Weil J, Hanrath P (1995) The ryanodine binding sarcoplasmic reticulum calcium release channel in nonfailing and in failing human myocardium. Naunyn Schmiedebergs Arch Pharmacol 353:80–85
52. Schwinger RH, Böhm M, Schmidt U, Karczewski P, Bavendiek U, Flesch M, Krause EG, Erdmann E (1995) Unchanged protein levels of SERCA II and phospholamban but reduced Ca^{2+} uptake and Ca^{2+}-ATPase activity of cardiac sarcoplasmic reticulum from dilated cardiomyopathy patients compared with patients with nonfailing hearts. Circulation 92:3220–3228
53. Sham JSK, Hatem SN, Morad M (1995) Species differences in the activity of the Na^+-Ca^{2+} exchanger in mammalian cardiac myocytes. J Physiol 488.3:623–631
54. Shamraj OI, Grupp IL, Grupp G, Melvin D, Gradoux N, Kremers W, Lingrel JB, De Pover A (1993) Characterisation of Na/K-ATPase, its isoforms, and the inotropic response to ouabain in isolated failing human hearts. Cardiovasc Res. 27:2229–2237
55. Sipido KR, Callewaert G, Carmeliet E (1995) Inhibition and rapid recovery of Ca^{2+} current during Ca^{2+} release from sarcoplasmic reticulum in guinea pig ventricular myocytes. Circ Res 76:102–109
56. Splawski I, Tristani-Firouzi M, Lehmann MH, Sanguinetti MC, Keating MT (1997) Mutations in the hmink gene cause long QT syndrome and suppress I_{Ks} function. Nature Genet 17:338–340
57. Vermeulen JT, McGuire MA, Opthof T, Coronel R, de Bakker JMT, Klöpping C, Janse MJ (1994) Triggered activity and automaticity in ventricular trabeculae of failing human and rabbit hearts. Cardiovasc Res 28:1547–1554
58. Wettwer E, Amos G, Gath J, Zerkowski HR, Reidemeister JC, Ravens U (1993) Transient outward current in human and rat ventricular myocytes. Cardiovasc Res 27:1662–1669
59. Wettwer E, Grundke M, Ravens U (1992) Differential effects of the new class III antiarrhythmic agents almokalant, E-4031 and D-sotalol, and of quinidine, on delayed rectifier currents in guinea pig ventricular myocytes. Cardiovasc Res 26:1145–1152

60. Wiederhold KF, Nilius B (1986) Increased sensitivity of ventricular myocardium to intracellular calcium overload in Syrian cardiomyopathic hamster. Biomed Biochim Acta 45:1333–1337
61. Yue L, Feng J, Li GR, Nattel S (1996) Transient outward and delayed rectifier currents in canine atrium: properties and role of isolation methods. Am J Physiol 270:H2157–2168

CHAPTER 13

Potassium channel overexpression

U.C. HOPPE, H.B. NUSS, B. O'ROURKE, E. MARBÁN, D.C. JOHNS

Section of Molecular and Cellular Cardiology, Division of Cardiology, Johns Hopkins University School of Medicine, Baltimore, MD, USA

Introduction

Ion channels in the plasma membrane play a critical role in cellular function. These proteins are the gatekeepers that control ion homeostasis and shape excitability. Excitable cells use a variety of different ion channels to fashion their hallmark electrical signal, the action potential. Advances in molecular electrophysiology have led to the identification of more ion channel genes than there are identified membrane currents. This excess is particularly striking with potassium channels, where the wide diversity of genes is compounded by variable levels of hetero-multimerization, alternative splicing and post-translational modification. The classical methods of studying the roles of each gene rely either on exogenous expresison in frog oocytes or pharmacological manipulation of native currents. While these techniques have yielded a wealth of information concerning ion channel structure and function, they have come up short in linking individual genes and their products to physiology and disease.

Defects in ion channels have been linked to a number of inherited diseases including epilepsy, periodic paralysis, cystic fibrosis and long QT syndrome. In addition, changes in cellular excitability are associated with several common disease states including drug addiction, depression, and heart failure [14, 30, 39]. Finally, an enormous number of pharmaceutical agents either directly or indirectly affect cellular excitability. This may be by design, as in the case of local anesthetic block of sodium channels, or as an unwanted side effect which limits the potential usefulness of the agent, such as erythromycin-induced block of cardiac potassium channels leading to fatal arrhythmias.

While the ability to modify cellular excitability genetically has broad applications in the study of neurons and muscle cells, we have principally targeted the cardiac cell for these studies. In particular, we have focused on reversing the pathological changes that lead to an increased susceptibility to arrhythmias. Sudden death from lethal arrhythmias remains the single largest cause of death in the United States [44]. Many of these arrhythmias arise from abnormalities of repolarization, originating from prolonged action potentials [25]. The cardiac action potential has a characteristic waveform that is the result of several ion channels working in concert. Figure 1 shows a normal

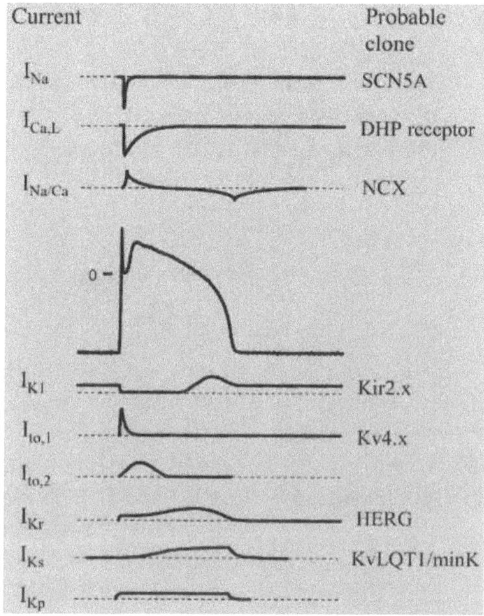

Fig. 1. Cardiac action potential and the currents that shape it

cardiac action potential and the various ionic currents which contribute to excitation (on the left; time courses of currents and action potential in the middle; predominant gene encoding each current is listed on the right). Changes in the action potential waveform are associated with congenital long QT syndrome, heart failure and hypertrophy, and account for the high rate of sudden death in these populations [27]. Treatment for these conditions has been difficult, relying on antiarrhythmic drugs or implantable defibrillators, both of which have significant limitations [38]. Experimental techniques that enable molecular dissection of the action potential waveform would greatly enhance our understanding of these lethal diseases. The goal of this research is to develop appropriate modern techniques and to use them to probe excitability and manipulate it genetically, laying the groundwork for potential gene therapy of ion channel diseases.

In preliminary work, we showed that the use of adenoviral vectors to express ion channels in isolated heart cells was efficient in modifying the action potential waveform [19]. Using this approach, we were able to reverse the salient phenotypic changes which occur in an animal model of heart failure [33]. However, the reversal was often accompanied by an excessive abbreviation of the action potential waveform, which could be arrhythmogenic or at the very least could compromise contractile function.

This suggested two areas for improvement:
- tighter control of the amount of channel expressed, and
- screening of other channels whose ionic-flux properties may provide a more physiological modification of the action potential waveform with less potential for excessive abbreviation.

In order to address the latter, we next focused our attention on two currents which have been demonstrated to be dynamically regulated in disease states, the calcium-independent transient outward potassium current (I_{to1}) and the human *ether-a-go-go*-related gene (*Herg*) product, thought to comprise the rapid component of delayed rectifier current (I_{kr}). I_{to1} has been shown to be down-regulated in heart failure [5, 20]; in addition *Herg* has been shown to be mutated (with loss of function) in inherited long QT syndrome [8, 21].

Genetic suppression of I_{to1}

A necessary first step was to determine the molecular identity of I_{to1}. Various members of two separate potassium channel gene families have been implicated in the formation of I_{to1}. The first was Kv1.4, a member of the *Shaker* family which, when expressed in oocytes, exhibits roughly appropriate kinetics (fast activation and fast inactivation) during single depolarizing voltage stimuli [35, 36]. However, the recovery kinetics of the heterologously-expressed Kv1.4 channel are much slower than those of I_{to1} in native heart cells, and there is no correlation between the amount of current and the message levels for Kv1.4 [9]. More recently, Kv4.2 and Kv4.3 have emerged as stronger candidates [4, 10]. When expressed alone, these members of the *Shal* family exhibit plausible kinetics (although, again, the match with native cells is imperfect) [40]. These genes are richly expressed in ventricular myocytes and in neurons which express I_{to1} [4, 24, 40, 41, 45]; furthermore, antisense oligonucleotides targeting Kv4.2 suppress I_{to1} in rat ventricular myocytes [11]. Nevertheless, there is a paucity of evidence at the protein level that Kv4 genes underlie I_{to1}. The picture is further confused by the fact that many tissues express both Kv4.2 and Kv4.3 [9, 10, 40], which differ when expressed individually but which are thought to be capable of forming heteromultimers that obscure such differences.

Selective gene suppression has become an attractive method for elucidating protein function experimentally. The two most commonly used strategies to accomplish this include antisense methodologies [49] and dominant negative constructs [13]. Both have been used to manipulate functional expression of ion channels [7, 11], but the latter has proven to be particularly useful in manipulating potassium channels due to the fact that they form multimers in the cell membrane [3, 6, 16, 22, 23, 34, 43, 46, 47]. One dysfunctional K channel subunit (e.g., with a missense mutation in the pore region) can suffice to cripple an otherwise normal tetrameric complex; indeed, such dominant-negative interactions underlie various forms of the inherited long QT syndrome [21, 42]. The introduction of a dominant-negative ion channel construct into native cells also has been used to map the levels of specific channel families in neurons from *Xenopus* embryos [37]. Unfortunately, such a technique is generally not applicable to mammalian systems without manipulating the germline.

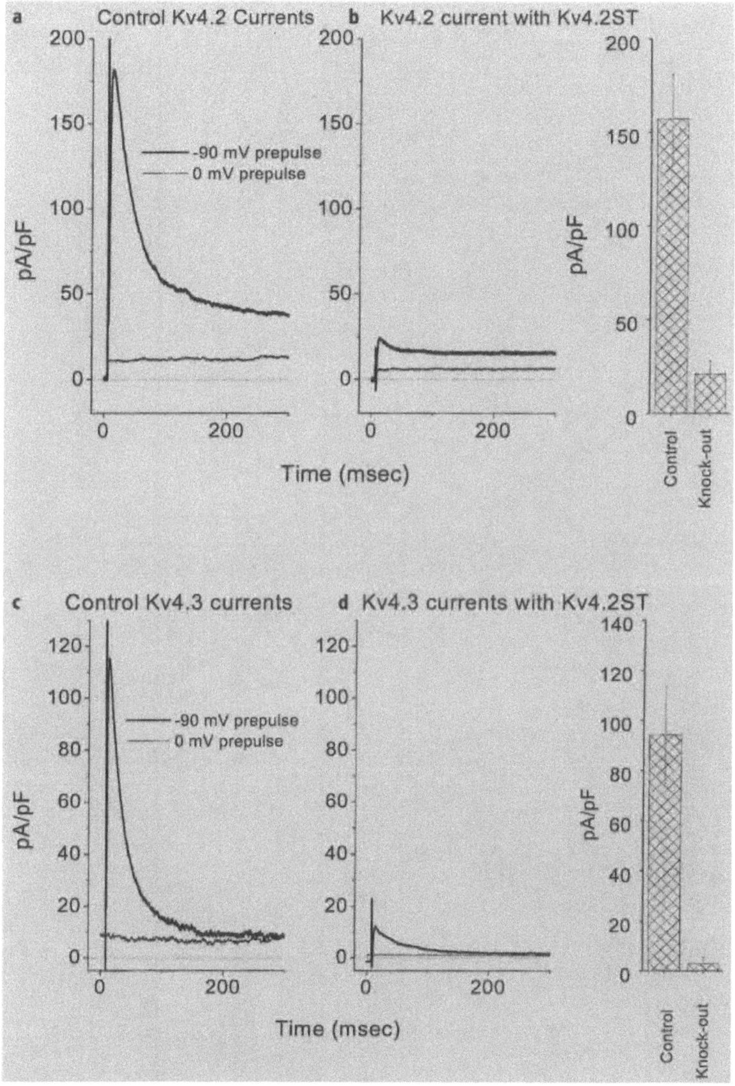

Fig. 2. Suppression of Kv4 family genes with Kv4.2ST. Cells transfected with wild-type Kv4.2 or Kv4.3 and control plasmids (**a**, **c** respectively) or Kv4.2 or Kv4.3 and Kv4.2ST (**b**, **d**). Reprinted by permission from J Biol Chem 272(50):31598–31603, 1997.

We have used somatic gene transfer methods to introduce dominant-negative Kv4 constructs into various cell types [17]. We first demonstrated that a truncated version of Kv4.2 (Kv4.2ST) acts to suppress currents encoded by either Kv4.2 or Kv4.3 in CHO-K1 cells (Fig. 2). This effect was specific, as it did not suppress currents encoded by Kv1.4, Kv1.5 or Kir2.1 (see [17]). For gene delivery into myocytes and neurons, which are resis-

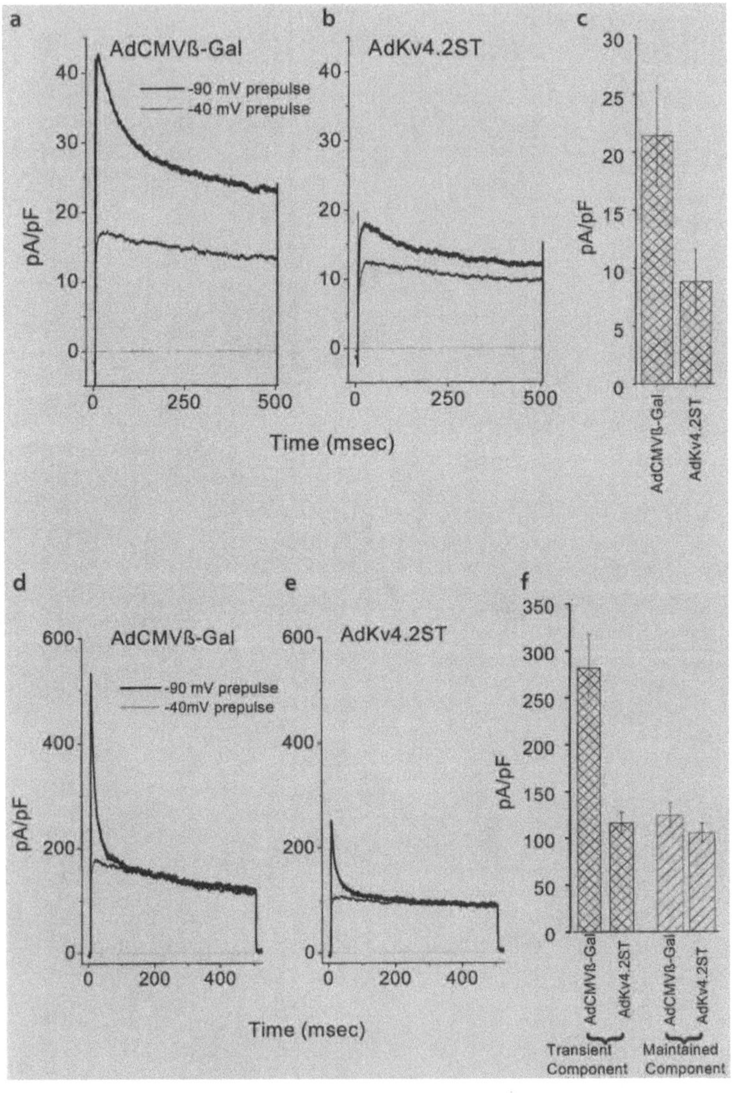

Fig. 3. Suppression of native currents with AdKv4.2ST. Primary adult rat ventricular myocytes were infected with a control virus (**a**) or AdKv4.2ST (**b**). The summary data (**c**) reveal a 60% reduction in the transient outward component. Likewise, cerebellar granule neurons were infected with a control virus (**d**) or AdKv4.2ST (**e**) also resulting in a significant decrease in the size of the I_{to} (**f**). Reprinted by permission from J Biol Chem 272(50):31598–31603, 1997.

tant to conventional transfection methods, we engineered a recombinant adenovirus which overexpresses Kv4.2ST (AdKv4.2ST). Infection with AdKv4.2ST significantly suppressed the transient outward component in both adult rat cardiomyocytes and rat cerebellar granule neurons (Fig. 3). This suppression was also specific as shown by the lack of suppression of the maintained component of the outward current. Our results support the idea that *Shal* (Kv4 family) potassium channels represent the major constituents of the A-type current in neuronal cells and of I_{to} in adult cardiac myocytes.

Delivery of functional ion channels by cell fusion

Our preliminary studies and those of others have described phenotypic changes that occur in the action potential of cardiac myocytes with time in culture [26, 33]. In general, there is an increase in the action potential duration, particularly the time to 90% repolarization (APD_{90}), presumably due to altered expression of various ion channel genes. To avoid these changes we sought to develop an alternative approach for genetic modification which would not require that the cells be maintained for several days in primary culture. We adapted protocols for creating heterokaryons via polyethylene glycol (PEG)-mediated cell fusion [1, 12, 15, 48] to fuse freshly isolated cardiac myocytes and CHO-K1 cells expressing a channel of choice. Transfer of fluorescence from the CHO cell expressing GFP to the myocyte cytoplasm allowed us to identify heterokaryons. To study the role of I_{to1} on repolarization of the cardiac action potential, guinea pig myocytes (which physiologically lack I_{to1}) were fused to CHO cells expressing Kv4.3 (CHO-Kv4.3 cells). As controls, nontransfected CHO cells were fused to myocytes using the same protocol. Cell fusion itself did not affect the basal electrophysiology of guinea pig myocytes. Figure 4 shows that myocytes fused with CHO-Kv4.3 cells (Fig. 4c, e, g) exhibited a robust I_{to1} that ranged from 1.9 to 44.2 pA/pF at 40 mV (mean 16.5±2.6 pA/pF; 37 °C, n = 19), whereas control cells had no transient outward current (Fig. 4a). Action potentials from heterokaryons demonstrated that the introduction of I_{to1} substantially changed the waveform (Fig. 4d, f, h) compared with myocytes fused to control CHO cells (Fig. 4b). I_{to1} accelerated the initial repolarization velocity and suppressed the voltage of the plateau phase of guinea pig myocytes. Both effects became more pronounced as I_{to1} density increased. The introduction of I_{to1} into guinea pig ventriculocytes also shortened the overall action potential duration both at 50% and 90% repolarization in a current density-dependent manner. Although the rapid inactivation of Kv4.3 makes a direct contribution to the late phase of repolarization unlikely, the observed changes in the action potential duration may be due to indirect effects on other currents secondary to changes in the early plateau potential [2, 28]. Extremely large I_{to1} densities resulted in a spike-like configuration of the action potential reminiscent of that recorded in normal rat ventriculocytes (Fig. 4h).

Since the space constant of myocardial tissue is much larger (~10×) than the length of an isolated myocyte [50], punctate delivery of current into a myocyte will electrically affect the entire cell. Thus, the observed changes of the action potential waveform of guinea pig myocytes fused to

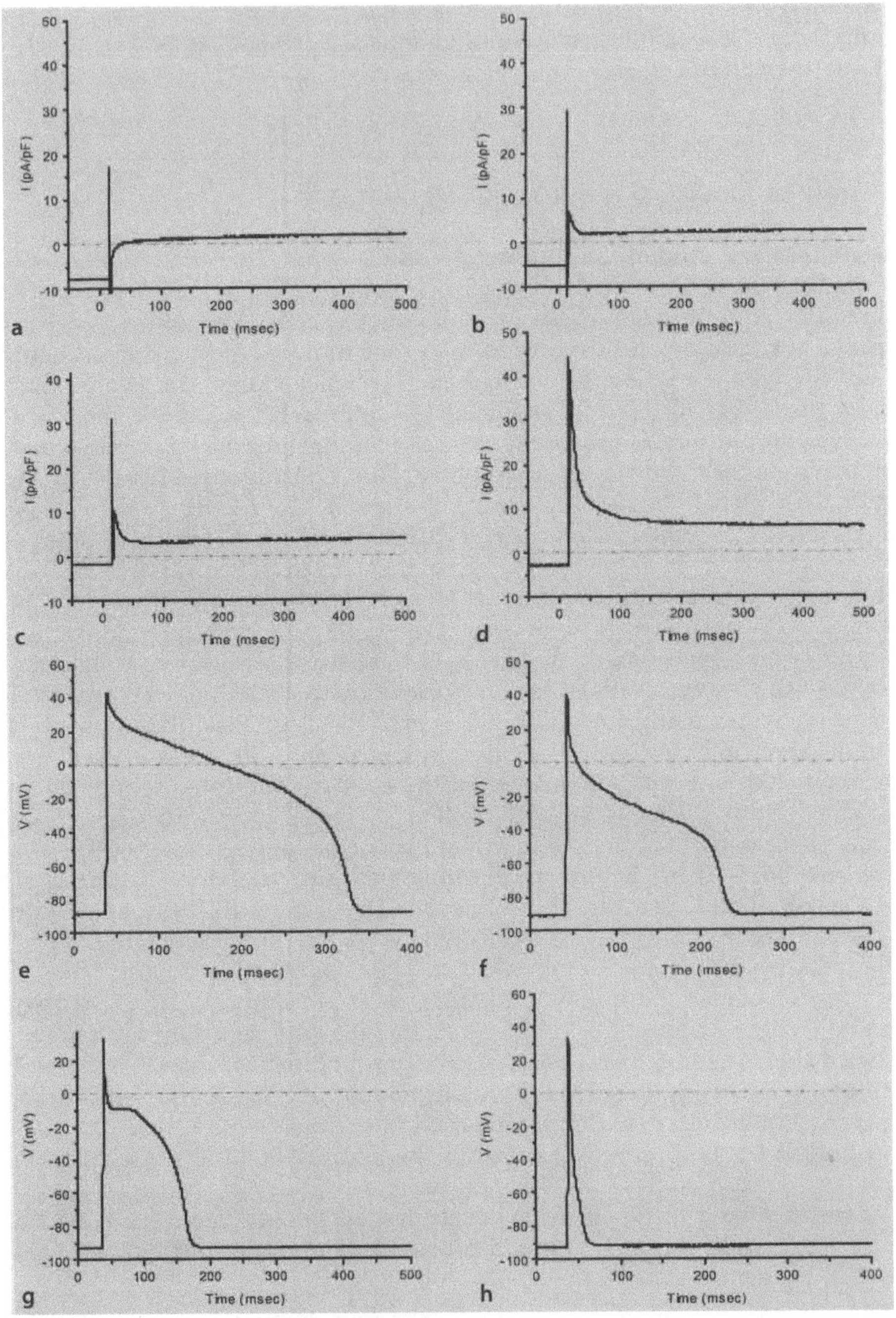

Fig. 4 a–h

CHO-Kv4.3 cells would be readily explained even if the Kv4.3 channels remained localized in the CHO cell membrane. Nevertheless, fusion of myocytes with CHO cells transiently expressing GFP and CD8 demonstrated that there is not only prompt cytosolic exchange, but also eventual redistribution of membrane proteins between fused cells (Fig. 5, p. 188). Thus, cell fusion not only represents an attractive method of screening the effects of different ion channels on the action potential in freshly isolated myocytes, but also enables further applications to introduce premade proteins into cardiomyocytes and to study their interaction with the endogenous myocyte membrane.

HERG suppresses EADs

The identification of mutations in the human *ether-a-go-go*-related gene (*Herg*) underlying congenital long QT syndrome (LQT) makes exogenous expression of the wild-type *Herg* gene a logical strategy for prevention of arrhythmias. *Herg* is particularly attractive because its ion flux is greatest during repolarization, so that it may not interfere with normal excitation. To test the effects of exogenous expression of the *Herg* channel in cardiac myocytes, we engineered an adenovirus containing the gene under the control of the Rous sarcoma virus promoter. This virus directed high-level expression of *Herg* currents when infected into CHO-K1 cells [32].

The aforementioned changes that occur when heart cells are cultured recapitulate many of the changes that have been noted in heart failure. In particular, there is a much enhanced frequency of occurrence of spontaneous early afterdepolarizations (EADs) in cultured rabbit myocytes (Fig. 6a, p. 189). Early afterdepolarizations are the cellular basis of long QT arrhythmias. We have used the cultured cells as a model system to test the hypothesis that *Herg* expression would suppress EADs without dramatically affecting the action potential waveform. Indeed, there was a marked suppression in the frequency of EADs (61% of AdGFP-infected cells vs. 11% AdHerg-infected cells; $P<0.02$) without significant changes in the waveform or duration (Fig. 6b, p. 189) as compared to freshly isolated cells (Fig. 6c, p. 189). These results show that exogenous expression of *Herg* (or pharmacologic agonists of the channel) may have therapeutic value for suppres-

Fig. 4. Transient outward currents and action potentials of myocytes fused with CHO-Kv4.3 cells and non-transfected CHO cells ($I_{to1}=0$ pA/pF). In myocytes fused with non-transfected CHO cells no I_{to1} could be recorded (**a**). Introduction of I_{to1} into guinea pig myocytes (**c**, **e**, **g**) substantially changed the action potential waveform (**d**, **f**, **h**) compared to myocytes fused with non-transfected CHO cells (**b**). These changes became more pronounced with increasing densities of transient outward currents, resulting in a suppression of the plateau potential and abbreviation of the overall action potential duration. Introduction of very large I_{to1} densities (**g**) caused a spike-like action potential (**h**). Reprinted by permission from Circ Res 84:964–972, 1999.

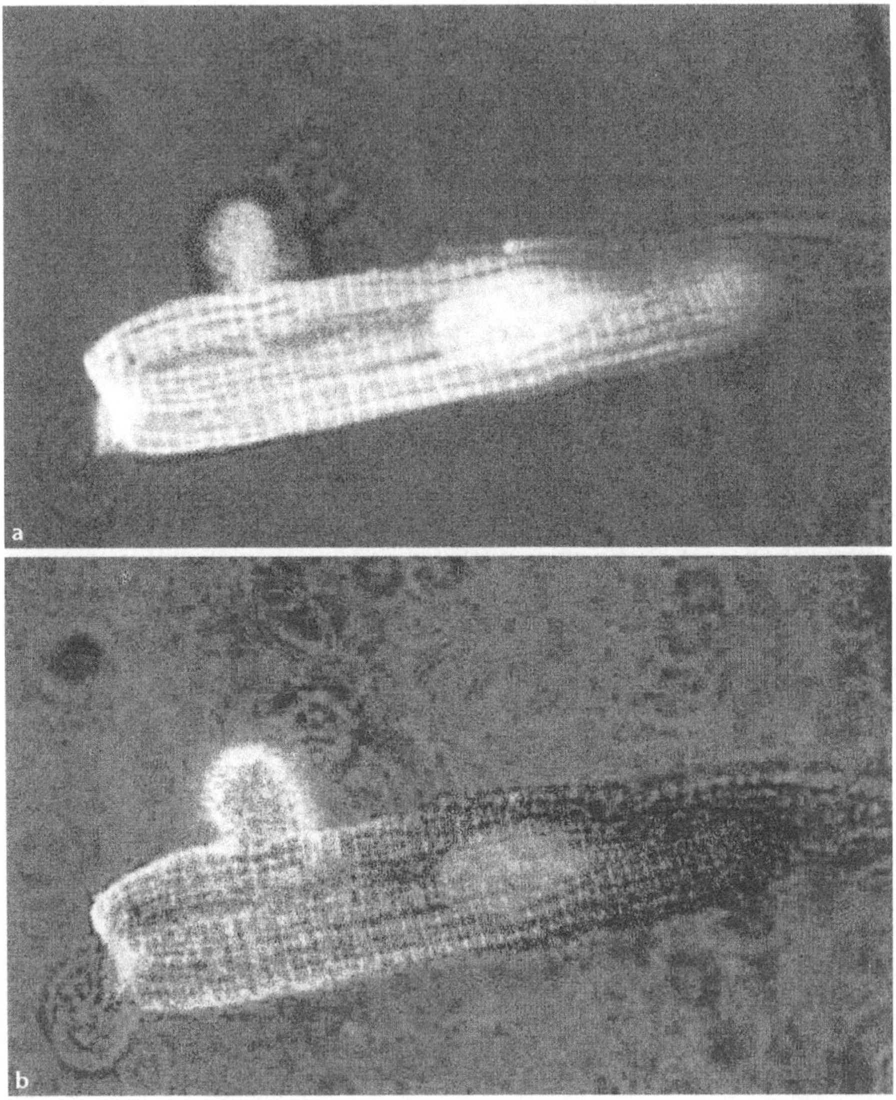

Fig. 5. Confocal images of heterokaryons. CHO cells were transiently transfected with GFP and CD8. After cell fusion, cells were fixed and CD8 was visualized with R-phycoerythrin-conjugated monoclonal CD8 antibodies. **a** Green fluorescence image: green fluorescence of the myocyte indicates transfer of cytosolic GFP from the fused CHO cell. **b** Red fluorescence image: red staining of the surface membrane and of t-tubular structures of the myocyte verifies that CD8 from the CHO cell membrane mixed with the membranes of the myocyte (cells were fixed 2 h after cell fusion). Cell fusion had no obvious effects on myocyte morphology, except at the site of fusion itself. Reprinted by permission from Circ Res 84:964–972, 1999.

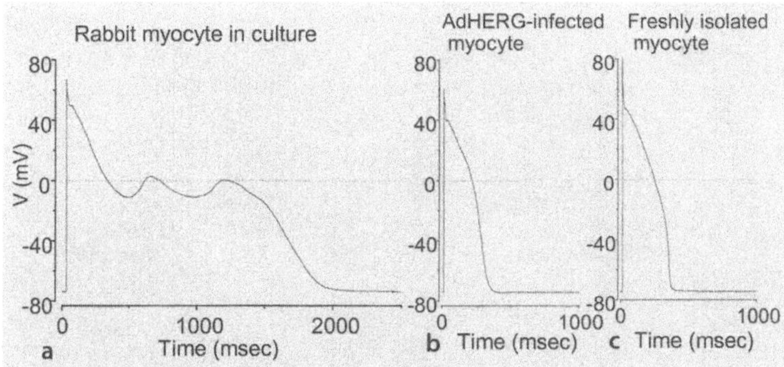

Fig. 6. Suppression of EADs by AdHERG. Cultured rabbit ventricular myocytes have prolonged action potentials which have frequent EADs (**a**). Infection with AdHERG blocks or reverses these changes (**b**) resulting in action potentials which are very similar to freshly isolated action potentials (**c**). Reprinted by permission from J Clin Invest 103:889–896, 1999.

sing long QT-related arrhythmias including those that cause sudden death in heart failure patients.

Inducible suppression of neuronal excitability

A fundamental point which the previous experiments have uncovered is the need to be able to control or titrate the levels of ion channels delivered to the target cell. In another study [18] we chose to implement two strategies to do that. The use of an internal ribosome entry site (IRES) limits the efficiency of translation of the ion channel genes. This may be a mechanism of regulation of ion channel genes in nature, and at least one ion channel has been shown to contain an IRES in its five prime untranslated region [29]. The second means of regulation that we have used is transcriptional regulation using an inducible promoter. The ecdysone-inducible system [31] was chosen for this purpose due to its demonstrated tight control of expression. We felt this would be of importance in working with ion channels which are normally expressed at much lower levels than ubiquitously expressed house keeping genes. Figure 7 shows a schematic of the viral-based ecdsyone vectors we used to first demonstrate the utility of this system. The inwardly rectifying potassium channel, Kir2.1, was chosen based on our prediction that expressing this channel would suppress excitability. For proof-of-principle experiments, superior cervical ganglion (SCG) neurons were chosen as a convenient model of excitable cells exhibiting spontaneous activity. Figure 8 shows infected SCG neurons which were either treated with vehicle (ethanol; a) or the ecdysone analog, muristerone A (b). The inclusion of GFP prior to the IRES in the viral vector made it easy not only to detect infected cells but also made it possible to determine the amount of the transgene being expressed by simple visual

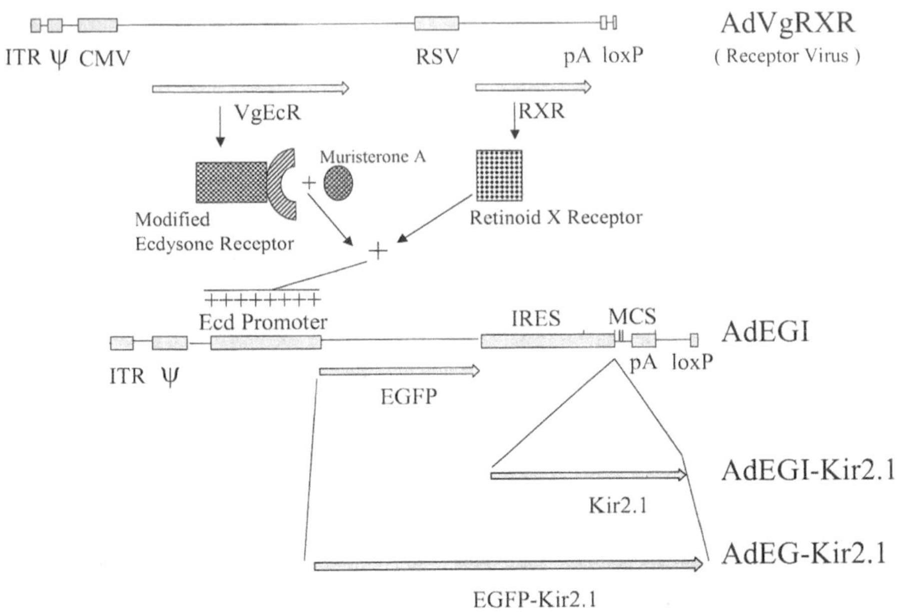

Fig. 7. Schematic representation of the basis for the ecdysone-nducible adenovirus vectors. *VgECR* modified ecdysone receptor, *RXR* retinoid X receptor, *ITR* inverted terminal repeat, *ψ* packaging signal, *ECD promoter* ecdysone-inducible promoter, *IRES* internal ribosome entry site, *pA* SV40 poly-adenylation signal, *MCS* multiple cloning site. The receptor virus (AdVgRXR) directs expression of the ecdysone receptor components which upon ligand addition stimulate expression from one of the target viruses (AdEGI, AdEGI-Kir2.1, AdEG-Kir2.1). Reprinted by permission from J Neurosci 19:1691–1697, 1999.

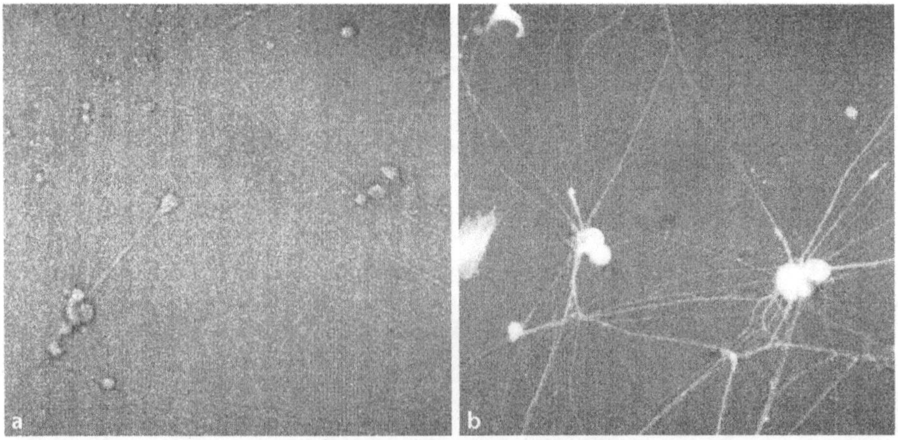

Fig. 8. Infection of SCG neurons with inducible adenovirus constructs. Confocal images of SCG neurons infected with AdEGI-Kir2.1 and AdVgRXR in the absence (**a**) and presence (**b**) of muristerone A. Reprinted by permission from J Neurosci 19:1691–1697, 1999.

inspection. The electrical effects of expressing Kir2.1 in these neurons are displayed in Figs. 9 and 10. The two parameters used to illustrate this are the amount of current needed to reach threshold (Fig. 9a–f) and the effect on spontaneous activity (Fig. 9g–i). In both of these cases we use low concentrations (50 μM) barium (Ba^{2+}) to specifically block Kir2.1. The summary data shown in Fig. 10 reveal that expression of Kir2.1 causes a hyperpolarization of the resting membrane potential (a) and a graded increase in the size of stimulus needed to trigger an action potential (b). This last point is of particular interest from a therapeutic point because it suggests the potential that, by titrating the amount of channel, one could reverse hyperexcitability while preserving normal excitability.

Summary

Sudden death is a major killer in the United States. Lamentably little is known about the molecular basis of this disease. We have used molecular genetic approaches to dissect several aspects of the cardiac action potential. The effects of the dominant-negative Kv4.2 construct define the molecular identity of I_{to1} as being principally due to a *Shal* family gene. Introduction of this current into cardiac myocytes which lack I_{to1} demonstrates that this current can modify the action potential waveform. This modification may be too dramatic for practical therapeutic use. Exogenous expression of the *Herg* potassium channel results in a marked suppression in EAD frequency, without a significant change in the action potential waveform. Investigation of the use of *Herg* expression as an antiarrhythmic principle is warranted. We have constructed new viral vectors which promise to be useful in modulating excitability both *in vitro* and *in vivo* in a controllable and reversible fashion. We have demonstrated the utility of these vectors by suppressing evoked and spontaneous electrical activity in primary sympathetic neurons. Lastly, the lessons learned here will aid in the design of new experiments aimed at further elucidating the molecular basis of cellular excitability in both normal and diseased muscle and neuronal cells.

Acknowledgments. This study was supported by a grant from NIH (P50 HL52370 to E.M.), a Research Career Development Award from the CARE Foundation (to D.C.J.), and a fellowship from the Deutsche Forschungsgemeinschaft (to U.C.H.), a scientist development grant from the American Heart Association (to H.B.N.), a grant from the NIH (RO1 H61711 to B.O.R.). E.M. was the recipient of the Michel Mirowski, M.D. Professorship in Cardiology of The Johns Hopkins University.

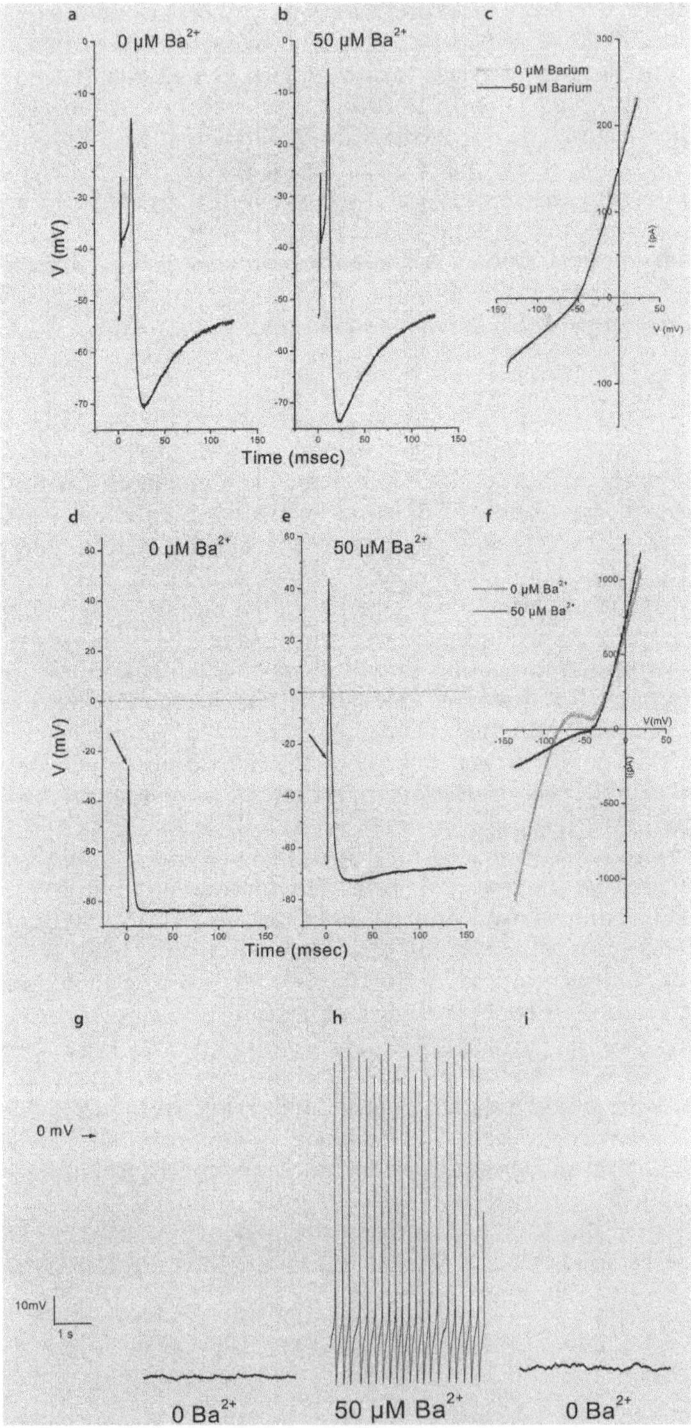
a
b
c
0 μM Ba2+
50 μM Ba2+
0 μM Barium
50 μM Barium
V (mV)
Time (msec)
I (pA)
V (mV)
d
e
f
0 μM Ba2+
50 μM Ba2+
0 μM Ba2+
50 μM Ba2+
V (mV)
Time (msec)
V(mV)
I(pA)
g
h
i
0 mV
10mV
1 s
0 Ba2+
50 μM Ba2+
0 Ba2+

Fig. 9 a–i

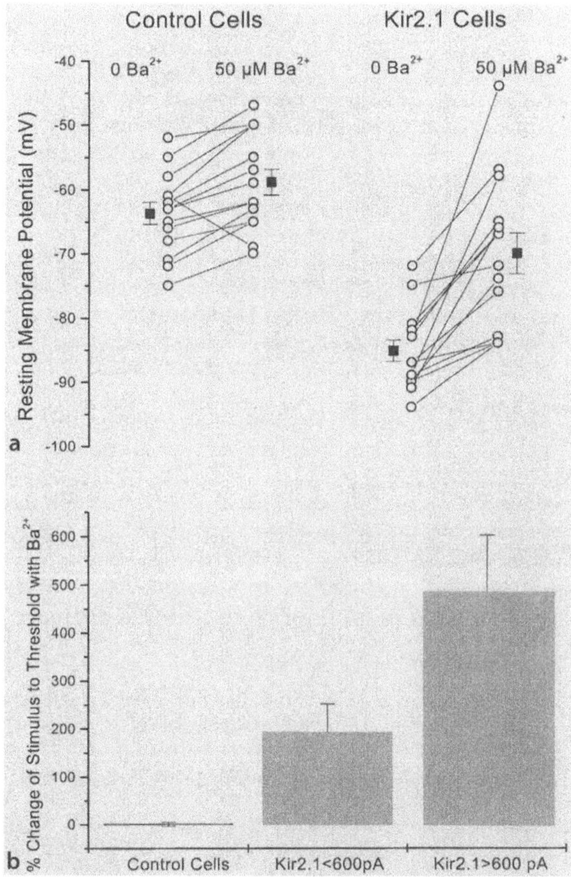

Fig. 10. Cumulative effects of exogenous expression of Kir2.1. Cells expressing Kir2.1 are hyperpolarized with respect to control cells. This effect is reversed upon blocking the Kir2.1 channels (**a**). Increasing amounts of Kir2.1 current increase the size of the stimulus needed to fire an action potential (**b**). Reprinted by permission from J Neurosci 19:1691–1697, 1999.

Fig. 9. Exogenous expression of Kir2.1 suppresses excitability. The effects of a supra-threshold stimulus on a control cell do not change with the addition of barium (**a**, **b**). The membrane current recorded from the same cell under these conditions using a ramp protocol from −138 mV to +22 mV over 500 ms (**c**). The addition of barium had little or no detectable effect on the outwardly rectifying I–V curves in control cells. The response to a sub-threshold stimulus on a Kir2.1-infected cell (**d**) is markedly changed by the addition of barium (**e**); in both panels, the arrow indicates the cessation of the applied stimulus. The I–V curve for this cell is much different upon addition of barium (**f**). Membrane current recordings from a Kir2.1-infected cell shown in normal saline (**g**), upon superfusion with saline containing barium (**h**) and upon washout (**i**). Reprinted by permission from J Neurosci 19:1691–1697, 1999.

References

1. Ahkong QF, et al (1987) Movements of fluorescent probes in the mechanism of cell fusion induced by poly(ethylene glycol). J Cell Sci 88 (Pt 3):389–398
2. Antzelevitch C, et al (1991) Heterogeneity within the ventricular wall. Electrophysiology and pharmacology of epicardial, endocardial, and M cells. Circ Res 69(6):1427–1449
3. Babila T, et al (1994) Assembly of mammalian voltage-gated potassium channels: evidence for an important role of the first transmembrane segment. Neuron 12(3):615–626
4. Barry DM, et al. (1995) Differential expression of voltage-gated K^+ channel subunits in adult rat heart. Relation to functional K^+ channels? Circ Res 77(2):361–369
5. Beukelman DJ, Näbauer M, Erdmann E (1993) Alterations of K^+ currents in isolated human ventricular myocytes from patients with terminal heart failure. Circ Res 73:386–394
6. Chen ML, Hoshi T, Wu CF (1996) Heteromultimeric interactions among K+ channel subunits from Shaker and eag famillies in Xenopus oocytes. Neuron 17(3):535–542
7. Chung S, Saal DB, Kaczmarek KL (1995) Elimination of potassium channel expression by antisense oligonucleotides in a pituitary cell line. Proc Natl Acad Sci USA 92:5955–5959
8. Curran ME, et al (1995) A molecular basis for cardiac arrhythmia: HERG mutations cause long QT syndrome. Cell 80(5):795–803
9. Dixon JE, McKinnon D (1994) Quantitative analysis of potassium channel mRNA expression in atrial and ventricular muscle of rats. Circ Res 75(2):252–260
10. Dixon JE, et al (1996) Role of the Kv4.3 K^+ channel in ventricular muscle. A molecular correlate for the transient outward current. Circ Res 79(4):659–668
11. Fiset C, Clark RB, Shimoni Y, Giles WR (1997) Shal-type channels contribute to the Ca-independent transient outward K current in rat ventricle. J Physiol 500(1):51–64
12. Goshima K, et al (1984) Beating activity of heterokaryons between myocardial and non-myocardial cells in culture. Exp Cell Res 151(1):148–159
13. Herskowitz I (1987) Functional inactivation of genes by dominant negative mutations. Nature 329:219–222
14. Hoffman PL, Tabakoff B (1994) The role of the NMDA receptor in ethanol withdrawal. Exs 71:61–70
15. Hoppe UC, et al (1999) Manipulation of cellular excitability by cell fusion: effects of rapid introduction of transient outward K^+ current on the guinea pig action potential. Circ Res 84(8):964–972
16. Isacoff EY, Jan YN, Jan LY (1990) Evidence for the formation of heteromultimetric potassium channels in Xenopus oocytes. Nature 345:530–534
17. Johns DC, Nuss HB, Marban E (1997) Suppression of neuronal and cardiac transient outward currents by viral gene transfer of dominant-negative Kv4.2 constructs. J Biol Chem 272(50):31598–31603
18. Johns DC, et al (1999) Inducible genetic suppression of neuronal excitability. J Neurosci 19(5):1691–1697
19. Johns DC, et al (1995) Adenovirus-mediated expression of a voltage-gated potassium channel in vitro (rat cardiac myocytes) and in vivo (rat liver). A novel strategy for modifying excitability. J Clin Invest 96(2):1152–1158
20. Kaab S, et al (1996) Ionic mechanism of action potential prolongation in ventricular myocytes from dogs with pacing-induced heart failure. Circ Res 78(2):262–273

21. Kass RS, Davies MP (1996) The role of ion channels in an inherited heart disease: molecular genetics of the long QT syndrome. Cardiovasc Res 32:443–454
22. Lee TE, et al (1994) Structural determinant for assembly of mammalian K^+ channels. Biophys J 66(Pt 1):667–673
23. Li M, Jan YN, Jan LY (1992) Specification of subunit assembly by the hydrophilic amino-terminal domain of the Shaker potassium channel. Science 257(5074): 1225–1230
24. Maletic-Savatic M, Lenn NJ, Trimmer JS (1995) Differential spatiotemporal expression of K+ channel polypeptides in rat hippocampal neurons developing in situ and in vitro. J Neurosci 15 (Pt 2):3840–3851
25. Marban E (1999) Heart failure: the electrophysiologic connection. J Cardiovasc Electrophysiol 10(10):1425–1428
26. Mitcheson JS, Hancox JC, Levi AJ (1996) Action potentials, ion channel currents, and transverse tubule density in adult rabbit ventricular myocytes maintained for 6 days in cell culture. Pflugers Arch Eur J Physiol 431:814–827
27. Myerburg RJ, Castellanos A (1988) Cardiac arrest and sudden cardiac death. In: Braunwald E (ed) Heart Disease: The Textbook of Cardiovascular Medicine. Saunders, Philadelphia, pp 742–777
28. Näbauer M, et al (1996) Regional differences in current density and rate-dependent properties of the transient outward current in subepicardial and subendocardial myocytes of human left ventricle. Circulation 93(1):168–177
29. Negulescu D, et al (1998) Translation initiation of a cardiac voltage-gated potassium channel by internal ribosome entry. J Biol Chem 273(32):20109–20113
30. Nestler EJ, Berhow MT, Brodkin ES (1996) Molecular mechanisms of drug addiction – adaptations in signal transduction pathways. Molecular Psychiatry 1(3):190–199
31. No D, Yao T-P, Evans RM (1996) Ecdysone-inducible gene expression in mammalian celsl and transgenic mice. Proc Natl Acad Sci USA 93:3346–3351
32. Nuss HB, Marban E, Johns DC (1999) Overexpression of a human potassium channel suppresses cardiac hyperexcitability in rabbit ventricular myocytes. J Clin Invest 103(6):889–896
33. Nuss HB, et al (1996) Reversal of potassium channel deficiency in cells from failing hearts by adenoviral gene transfer: a prototype for gene therapy for disorders of cardiac excitability and contractility. Gene Therapy 3(10):900–912
34. Panyi G, Deutsch C (1996) Assembly and suppression of endogenous Kv1.3 channels in human T cells. J Gen Physiol 107(3):409–420
35. Po S, et al (1993) Heteromultimeric assembly of human potassium channels. Molecular basis of a transient outward current? Circ Res 72(6):1326–1336
36. Po S, et al (1992) Functional expression of an inactivating potassium channel cloned from human heart. Circ Res 71(3):732–736
37. Ribera AB (1996) Homogenous development of electrical excitability via heterogenous ion channel expression. J Neurosci 16(3):1123–1130
38. Roden DM (1994) Risks and benefits of antiarrhythmic therapy. N Engl J Med 331:785–791
39. Sanguinetti MC, et al (1995) A mechanistic link between an inherited and an acquired cardiac arrhythmia: HERG encodes the IKr potassium channel. Cell 81(2):299–307
40. Serodio P, Vega-Saenz De Miera E, Rudy B (1996) Cloning of a novel component of A-type K^+ channels operating at subthreshold potentials with unique expression in heart and brain. J Neurophys 75(5):2174–2179
41. Sheng M, et al (1992) Subcellular segregation of two A-type K^+ channel proteins in rat central neurons. Neuron 9(2):271–284

42. Spector PS, et al (1996) Fast inactivation causes rectification of the I^{kr} channel. J Gen Physiol 107:611–619
43. Tinker A, Jan YN, Jan LY (1996) Regions responsible for the assembly of inwardly rectifying potassium channels. Cell 87(5):857–868
44. Tomaselli GF, et al (1994) Sudden cardiac death in heart failure. The role of abnormal repolarization (76 refs). Circulation 90(5): 2534–2539
45. Tsaur ML, et al (1992) Differential expression of K^+ channel mRNAs in the rat brain and down-regulation in the hippocampus following seizures. Neuron 8(6): 1055–1067
46. Tu L, Santarelli V, Deutsch C (1995) Truncated K^+ channel DNA sequences specifically suppress lymphocyte K^+ channel gene expression. Biophys J 68(1):147–156
47. Tu L et al (1996) Voltage-gated K+ channels contain multiple intersubunit association sites. J Biol Chem 271(31):18904–18911
48. Uchida T (1988) Introduction of macromolecules into mammalian cells by cell fusion. Exp Cell Res 178(1):1–17
49. Wagner RW (1995) The state of the art in antisense research. Nature Medicine 1:1116–1118
50. Weidmann S (1970) Electrical constants of trabecular muscle from mammalian heart. J Physiol (Lond) 210(4):1041–1054

CHAPTER 14

Mechanisms and relevance of apoptosis

J. HOLTZ, M. TOSTLEBE, D. DARMER
Institute of Pathophysiology, Halle, Germany

Introduction

In recent years, we have witnessed an explosion in published research on apoptosis, the genetically predetermined intrinsic program of active cellular self destruction. Although this program of cell suicide originally was considered as highly ritualized and rather uniform, recent progress revealed an extreme variability in modifications of the program, with a plethora of molecules involved in induction, execution or inhibition of this program and with great differences in the program in different tissues. As in any organ of multicellular organisms, activation of the program contributes to the adjustment of cellular stoichiometry of the myocardium in mammals during embryogenesis [81], and it is more or less activated in all forms of postnatal cardiac pathologies [2, 4, 14, 29, 71, 82–84, 123, 160]. In spite of this abundance of published data on activated apoptosis in cardiomyocytes and in other cells of the heart, there is no consensus with regard to the importance of this cardiac apoptosis. Neither the relevance of the activated program for the progression of cardiac diseases, nor the therapeutic potential of anti-apoptotic interventions can be considered as established. Here, we will summarize our present view in this still controversial field together with some expectations on its future development.

Relevance of myocardial apoptosis

Conclusions concerning the relevance of apoptosis in the heart can be derived from two approaches: quantitative analyses may show how many cells in an organ are dying in a certain cardiac disease, while the analyses of functional consequences of anti-apoptotic interventions can be applied in experimental models of cardiac diseases. This latter approach documented a substantial contribution of activated apoptosis to myocyte losses in ischemic heart disease, although morphological analyses showed mixed forms of necrotic and apoptotic cell death in ischemic or postischemic, reperfused myocardium (for reviews see [4, 17, 83]). In the overloaded, nonischemic myocardium, however, conclusions on the relevance of the apoptotic process are largely dependent on quantitative analyses.

Quantitative aspects: nuclear apoptosis vs. "cytosolic pre-apoptosis"

For hearts confronted with chronic hemodynamic overload, the critical transition from compensated cardiac hypertrophy to failure has been speculated to result from distension-induced apoptosis of cardiomyocytes [7]. And indeed, distension-induced myocyte apoptosis has been demonstrated in isolated papillary muscle, albeit with a degree of stretch which can hardly occur in vivo [24]. However, in support of this speculative proposal, myocytes with apoptotic nuclei have been observed in hearts with infarctions, localized in the nonischemic, overloaded wall remote from the infarction [23, 112, 158, 183], in myocardium of animals with chronic pressure overload [43, 69, 113, 209] and in terminally failing, explanted myocardium from patients with terminal heart failure [5, 147, 157, 182, 186, 190]. Furthermore, the hemodynamic unloading by implanted ventricular assist devices in patients with terminal heart failure has been shown to reduce myocardial apoptosis in these failing, mechanically unloaded hearts [5].

Stretching of cardiomyocytes cultured on distensable membranes has been used to analyze cellular mechanisms in distension-induced apoptosis and have implicated the local renin-angiotensin system in this reaction [106, 107]. The relevance of these in vitro observations for the overloaded myocardium in vivo is still debatable, since isolated, cultured cardiomyocytes have an extremely high basal rate of apoptosis even prior to the application of the distending stretch, probably as a result of the isolation process. However, the occurrence of apoptotic myocytes in overloaded, decompensated failing myocardium, previously predicted by speculation [7], can now be considered as an established fact. With regard to the clinical relevance of this cardiomyocyte apoptosis in overloaded, nonischemic myocardium, the discussion centers around quantitative issues: is the "melting rate" of apoptotic myocardium high enough to account for the impairment of pump function and for the detrimental progression of the dysfunction in terminal failure?

Myocardial apoptosis is normally analyzed by the biochemical and histological demonstration of nuclear DNA cleavage. Unfortunately, quantitative assessments of myocardial apoptosis by the histologic TUNEL technique yield highly variable results. In explanted ventricles from patients with terminal heart failure, the reported extreme values for apoptotic myocyte nuclei differed between 45 per one million [186] and 182000 per one million myocyte nuclei [147]. Plausible values, based on efforts to standardize the technique [183], are between 0.1 to 0.2% of TUNEL-positive myocyte nuclei in explanted human ventricles with terminal failure, with higher values in patients with rapid progression of the disease immediately prior to heart transplantation and somewhat lower values from patients, who were more stable before the operation [157, 182, 235].

However, many myocyte nuclei might appear TUNEL-positive in overloaded myocardium because of activated DNA repair processes [91] and not only because of apoptotic DNA cleavage. Furthermore, it is not possible to calculate an "apoptotic melting rate" for failing myocardium from a value of 0.1–0.2% TUNEL-positive nuclei: the duration of the TUNEL-positive process of apoptotic DNA cleavage in the nucleus is unknown. Furthermore, myocyte losses in failing myocardium can also occur with a necrotic type of DNA lysis [66]. Finally, some myocyte losses might be replaced by myocyte proliferation: myocyte mitoses have been unequivocally documented in human ventricular myocardium [3, 89]. This is in contrast to the classic concept of adult mammalian cardiomyocytes as terminally differentiated, postmitotic cells. In normal ventricular myocardium of donor hearts, both apoptotic and mitotic myocyte nuclei are extremely rare, around ten per one million [89, 157]. In terminal heart failure, this frequency is enhanced tenfold for mitotic nuclei, but more than a hundredfold for TUNEL-positive nuclei [89, 157]. This suggests that the overall balance between apoptotic myocyte losses and proliferative myocyte replacement in the failing heart appears shifted towards myocyte losses. However, it does not tell us whether this myocyte loss, visible in some 0.1% TUNEL-positive myocyte nuclei and in nucleosome-sized DNA fragmentation in myocardial extracts [5, 190], is an interesting, but neglectable epiphenomenon or a critical determinant of failure progression.

Probably, analyses of earlier steps in the apoptotic program prior to the nuclear DNA degradation tell us more about the functional relevance of apoptosis for the failing heart. Release of cytochrome c from the mitochondria is an important part of the apoptotic program (see section Caspase activation by mitochondria). In failing human ventricles, this cytochrome c release affects more than 50% of the myocytes and more than 60% of the total myocardial cytochrome c [148]. This massive release causes activation of cytosolic caspases, indicated by massive cleavage of the terminal effector caspase 3 [148] and cleavage of cytosolic caspase substrates in the majority of myocytes, such as protein kinase δ and troponin-C [67]. On the other hand, however, cleavage of the nuclear caspase substrate PARP (poly ADP-ribose polymerase, an established indicator of nuclear apoptosis [47]) is not yet demonstrable [148] and TUNEL-positive nuclear DNA cleavage is only detectable in some 0.2% of the myocytes [157, 182].

This substantial activation of cytosolic elements of the program in the majority of myocytes in the presence of only minimal nuclear apoptosis means that there must be some postmitochondrial retardation of the program in failing human myocardium. Potential mechanisms of this retardation will be considered in the section Postmitochondrial retardation of myocardial apoptosis. Furthermore, this apoptotic release of cytochrome c is a reversible event in neurons [128] and probably in cardiomyocytes [92], suggesting that mitochondrial cytochrome c release and activation of cytosolic caspases is also a potentially reversible state of cytosolic pre-apoptosis in cardiomyocytes. Presently ongoing research tries to visualize this cytosolic, potentially reversible pre-apoptosis by a noninvasive approach, based on annexin-V binding to the membranes of myocytes with the cytosolic activation of the program [188]. Annexin-V binds to phosphatidyl serine, which is translocated to the external leaflet of the cell membrane early in the apoptotic process [38].

However, what does it mean for the function of terminally failing hearts that the proteolytic cascade of cytosolic caspases is strongly activated and that more than 50% of the mitochondrial cytochrome c in the entire tissue is located extra-mitochondrially? Mitochondria from most mammalian cells have no excess reserve of cytochrome c oxidase or cytochrome c relative to the respiratory chain capacity [225]. This suggests that a massive loss of cytochrome c may cause a drastic decrease in respiratory capacity or cytochrome-c oxidase activity [88]. Such decrements in respiratory capacity have been previously observed in failing myocardium [115, 116, 133, 171, 178], although other alterations in addition to cytochrome c release might have contributed to these decrements. Caspase-mediated cleavage of troponin C in failing myocardium [67] should directly reduce myocardial contractility [114]. Furthermore, activated caspase-mediated cytosolic substrate cleavage may initiate degradation of myocyte organelles. In failing myocardium, massive cytoplasmic proteolysis in cardiomyocytes without nuclear apoptosis [235] and substantial losses of myofibrils and mitochondria have been observed [56, 185, 192], which might be a consequence of sustained cytosolic caspase activation.

Presently, the functional relevance of cytosolic pre-apoptosis in failing myocytes cannot yet be quantified exactly. However, the sheer degree of this cytosolic activation suggests that the major relevance of myocyte apoptosis for the failing heart lies more in the cytosolic part of the program and not in its final nuclear execution.

Experimental interventions with the apoptotic program

Several inhibitors of caspases, which have been shown to inhibit or retard the execution of apoptosis in many cellular models [27, 151, 154, 191, 211, 224], are available. Furthermore, apoptosis can be attenuated or prevented in many cellular models by experimental overexpression of anti-apoptotic members of the Bcl-2 family or of components of survival pathways (see section Mitochondrial dysfunction as a consequence of cytosolic pre-apoptosis). Many of these approaches have been used in various experimental models of myocardial ischemia in vivo, in isolated perfused hearts or in myocyte cultures with simulated ischemia, with or without reperfusion or reoxygenation [for overview see 4, 17, 83]. From these experiments it has to be concluded that the apoptotic program is activated in ischemia-jeopardized cardiomyocytes, that inhibition of this program temporarily attenuates myocyte losses and deterioration of myocardial function in experimental ischemia, and that myocyte losses in myocardial infarction are due to mixed forms of cell death with activation of the apoptotic program as well as with necrotic collapse of cellular compartmentation and regulation. While these experiments with inhibitors of apoptosis clearly illustrate the relevance of the program for myocardial ischemia, they do not indicate that inhibition of apoptosis shall be a preventive option against the myocardial consequences of coronary heart disease (see section Therapeutic inhibition of apoptosis for cardioprotection?).

While these experiments with inhibitors clearly show the relevance of apoptosis for myocardial ischemia, similar experiments illustrating the relevance of apoptosis in overload-induced heart failure are not available. In this case, speculations on the pathological relevance of the process must be derived from quantitative analyses of the cytosolic components of the program (see above).

Endogenous regulation of apoptosis

Phases of the apoptotic program

The activation of a cascade of cysteine-containing aspartic acid proteases or "caspases" is considered as the central component of the apoptotic program [154, 191, 211]. However, rare examples of programmed cell death independent from caspase activation do exist, and activated caspases may also mediate other cellular reactions besides apoptosis [51]. Within the cascade of caspases, the "terminal caspases" (e.g., caspase-3) mediate the various steps of the "execution phase" of the apoptosis, including nuclear condensation, DNA degradation with internucleosomal cleavage and lysis of the nuclear scaffold, cell membrane alterations with translocation of an asymmetrically distributed membrane phospholipid (phosphatidylserine) to the outer leaflet of the lipid bilayer, alterations of the cellular cytoskeleton, shrinkage of cellular volume and degradation of cytosol. The proteolytic cascade of caspases is initiated by "initiator caspases", and the autoactivation of such initiator caspases arises from activated death receptors (see section Caspase activation by death receptors) or from mitochondria (see section Caspase activation by mitochondria). In most cell types, a mitochondrial amplification step is required for full activation of the apoptotic cascade, even if the initiation started from death receptors.

Because of the central role of mitochondria in the apoptosis of most cells, the apoptotic program is divided into premitochondrial and postmitochondrial cytosolic phases and a terminal phase with nuclear manifestations. The activation of effector caspases is clearly a postmitochondrial event. However, activated effector caspases can act on those mitochondria of a cell which have not yet contributed to cytochrome c release and can induce the release reaction, acting in a positive feedback mode from activated caspases on mitochondria, triggering further activation (see section Intermitochondrial amplification).

Caspases as executioners of apoptosis

Activated caspases are considered as the central mediators of the cell death machinery, since cells can usually be rescued from apoptosis by caspase inhibitors [for review see 224]. Under certain special conditions, cell death can be induced by apoptotic stimuli in the presence of caspase inhibitors [105, 134]. Therefore, the possibility of caspase-independent apoptosis cannot be excluded, but will not be considered here. At present, 14 different caspases have been identified in mammals. Some caspases contain large prodomains and are initiators of cell death (caspases-8, -9, -10); others have small prodomains (caspase 3, 6, 7) and are mostly involved in the execution of cell death.

Although a high number of targets of activated effector caspases has been identified [32, 202], it is not quite clear how the activated caspase cascade mediates the final steps of the apoptotic program. Recently, in erythroblasts it has been shown that the caspase-mediated cleavage of the transcription factor GATA-1 is the critical step, to which the programs of apoptosis and cellular differentiation converge [34]. GATA-1 strongly induces and stabilizes the expression of the anti-apoptotic protein Bcl-x_L [64, 159], which is also downregulated in the failing myocardium [5]. However, it is very doubtful, whether in all cells a similar single step, such as cleavage of GATA-1 in erythroblasts, functions as the critical bottle neck of the program.

Caspase activation by death receptors

Death receptors are transmembrane proteins and are a subgroup of the NGF/TNF-receptor superfamily, with a so-called "death domain" in the cytosolic part of the receptor molecule [74]. This death domain is necessary for binding of cytosolic adapter molecules to activated death receptors, and this binding transduces the "death signal" to the apoptotic effector machinery of the cell. Activation of these receptors by ligand binding results in trimerization of the receptors, thereby facilitating aggregation of adaptor molecules to the cytosolic part of the receptors with formation of DISCs (death- inducing signaling complexes). Initiator procaspases are included in these signaling complexes, and their aggregation facilitates proteolytic autoactivation of the procaspases with subsequent activation of the effector caspases. In many cells, involvement of a mitochondrial enforcement step (see section Caspase activation by mitochondria) of the activating cascade is necessary for death induction by death receptor activation. However, various reactions and not only apoptosis can arise from the DISCs of activated death receptors, which partially explains the extreme diversity of cellular reactions associated with those receptors in different cell types. Ligands of the death receptors are certain cytokines, occurring as transmembrane proteins in the membranes of immune cells and other cells, and as soluble extracellular molecules after proteolytic cleavage of the extracellular part of the ligand [74].

Within the group of death receptor-activating cytokines, candidate mediators of the "cytokine hypothesis of heart failure" [194] are TNF, activating the death receptor TNF-receptor type I or TNF-RI (TNF-RII is not a death receptor), and Fas-ligand or FasL, activating Fas, while nothing is known on a pathophysiologic role of other death receptors in the myocardium [74].

Circulating levels of TNF are elevated in severe chronic heart failure [108, 213], cardiac TNF expression is enhanced in terminal heart failure and this enhancement is attenuated by hemodynamic unloading of failing hearts by ventricular assist devices [215]. TNF receptors are expressed in cardiomyocytes [214], TNF induces apoptosis in isolated cultured cardiomyocytes [101], and cardiac-specific overexpression of TNFα causes dilative cardiomyopathy with signs of myocyte nuclear apoptosis [102, 103]. Furthermore, chronic TNF infusion into rats caused progressing cardiac dysfunction, dilatory remodeling and enhanced TUNEL labeling of cardiomyocyte nuclei [13]. Remarkably, these failure-typical changes were induced by a TNF dose resulting in plasma levels, which are reported in heart failure patients [13]. In spite of this impressive experimental support for the cytokine hypothesis of heart failure, it is not clear whether TNF acted by inducing caspase activation in this model of experimental cardiac failure. The authors compared TUNEL labeling of myocytes with another technique for histologic identification of apoptotic DNA fragmentation [41], which demonstrated no nuclear labeling in the TNF-treated rat hearts [13], illustrating the limited reliability of histologic quantification of nuclear apoptosis (see section Quantitative aspects: nuclear apoptosis vs. "cytosolic pre-apoptosis"). The TNF infusion caused reduction of ventricular fractional shortening in vivo and attenuated in vitro shortening of cardiomyocytes isolated from TNF-treated hearts, and these effects were reversible by stopping the TNF infusion or with the application of a TNF antagonist [13]. While all this is consistent with the assumption of cytosolic caspase activation and caspase-mediated impairment of cardiomyocyte function, cytosolic pre-apoptosis has not been analyzed in this failure model, and several negative inotropic effects of TNF have been identified [57, 90, 144, 145]. Thus, the relevance of TNF-mediated caspase activation in severe heart failure remains unresolved.

The death receptor Fas is expressed in cardiomyocytes, and this expression is enhanced by hypoxia [208] and by severe overstretching of myocardium in vitro [24]. In severe heart failure, the soluble circulating Fas ligand is enhanced [153, 234]. In the healthy human heart, soluble Fas isoforms due to alternative splicing of the primary Fas transcript are expressed in addition to the Fas receptor [190], and these soluble Fas isoforms can act as Fas antagonists [19, 20, 164]. In terminal heart failure, the expression of these Fas antagonists is reduced, and this reduction is renormalized during VAD-induced hemodynamic unloading [5, 190]. While Fas-mediated alterations in cardiomyocyte Ca^{2+}-homeostasis [54] and myocardial transcription factor AP-1 activation [231] have been demonstrated, Fas-induced cardiomyocyte apoptosis remains to be shown. Caspase activation by TNF or FasL probably exerts a pathophysiological role in cardiac failure or cardiac ischemia/reperfusion only in combination with other cytokines and/or with an endotoxin [58, 145].

Caspase activation by mitochondria

A crucial event in the initiation of apoptosis is the release of cytochrome c from the intermembrane space of mitochondria [95, 96, 117], which results in the activation of procaspase-9. The critical adaptor in this cytochrome c-mediated caspase activation is APAF-1 (apoptosis protease-activating factor) [10, 199, 242, 243]. In resting cells without apoptotic activation, APAF-1 is fixed to the outer surface of the mitochondria by anti-apoptotic proteins of the Bcl-2-family (e.g., Bcl-x_L or Bcl-2) and cytochrome c is within the intermembrane space, serving as a shuttle for electrons between complex III and complex IV of the mitochondrial respiratory chain. An apoptotic signal results in the translocation of proapoptotic Bcl-2 family proteins from the cytosol to the mitochondria (e.g. Bak, Bax, BAD), which triggers release of cytochrome c, detachment of APAF-1 from anti-apoptotic Bcl, alteration of APAF-1 conformation by cytochrome c and ATP, and oligomerization of APAF-1 with several procaspase-9 molecules, facilitating autoactivation of this initiator caspase [155, 167, 219, 220]. In situations without sufficient ATP available extramitochondrially, this process results in cell death with necrotic features instead of classical apoptosis [152, 218]. Concomitantly with cytochrome c, AIF (apoptosis-inducing factor), another factor important for apoptotic nuclear DNA degradation [120, 204], is released together with several procaspases [181, 203] and many other mitochondrial proteins [166]. However, the critical initiator of the apoptotic caspase cascade appears to be the extramitochondrially located cytochrome c, which alone can activate the whole process [240].

The detailed mechanism of release of cytochrome c and other soluble intermembrane space molecules from the mitochondria is not yet clear. At least five different models have been delineated for altering the protein permeability of the outer mitochondrial membrane, and some of these different mechanisms might occur in the same cell concomitantly or in response to different apoptotic stimuli. With the release of soluble intermembrane proteins from the mitochondria, a dramatic decline of the inner membrane potential is associated and, finally, the "permeability transition pore", which allows exchange of solute molecules between matrix and the cytosol [100, 237, 241], is opened. However, collapse of the mitochondrial inner membrane potential and loss of barrier function of mitochondrial membranes are not prerequisites for release of cytochrome c [63, 223]; they appear to represent late events of the mitochondrial involvement in the apoptotic process.

Proteins of the large Bcl-2 family, from which presently more than 20 members are known, are critical regulators of outer membrane permeability, inner membrane potential loss, and apoptosis-associated translocation processes to the mitochondria and/or the nucleus [1, 172, 173, 220, 223]. They are grouped into three categories:

anti-apoptotic proteins with Bcl-x_L and Bcl-2 as the best characterized members; all of which inhibit apoptotic activation and share sequence homologies in BH (from Bcl-2 homology) domains BH1 to BH4 (although the BH4 domain is lacking in some proteins of this group);

proteins of this group stabilize membranes and prevent release of intermembrane proteins and intracellular translocation of apoptotic signals;
pro-apoptotic proteins with BH1 to BH4 domains, such as Bax, Bak, BAD, Mtd and others, and some proteins of this subgroup also lack a BH4 domain; proteins of this group antagonize the protective effects of the first group.
pro-apoptotic "BH3"-only proteins, e.g., Bik, Bid, Bim, Hrk, Bnip3, which share sequence homology only in the BH3 domain, by which they induce apoptotic cytochrome c release.

Proteins of the first two groups can form ion channels in artificial membranes, but the relevance of such channel formation for the pro- or anti-apoptotic role of these proteins is unknown. Many signals regulating death or survival appear to converge at mitochondria via various members of this large family, and the activity of these proteins is modified by phosphorylation/dephosphorylation reactions, translocation between cellular compartments, homo- and heterodimerization with other Bcl-2 proteins, complexation with other proteins, and/or proteolytic modification. It should be remembered that anti-apoptotic Bcl-2 proteins are not only inserted in the mitochondrial membrane, but also in nuclear and endoplasmic reticulum membranes, although scarcely anything is known about the function of Bcl-2 proteins at these non-mitochondrial membranes [for reviews see 1, 172, 173, 220, 223].

In the heart, Bcl-x_L and Bcl-2 are the most important anti-apoptotic members of this family, and Bcl-x_L is downregulated in terminal heart failure and is reinduced during VAD-induced hemodynamic unloading of failing hearts [5].

Intermitochondrial amplification of caspase activation

In the program sequence of apoptotic steps, the activation of the cascade of caspases is clearly a postmitochondrial event [63]. However, once caspases are activated in the cytosol, they are able to induce the release of caspase-activating cytochrome c (and other pro-apoptotic signals) from further mitochondria, thereby amplifying the apoptotic avalanche by an intermitochondrial effect [11, 16, 104, 129]. This intermitochondrial amplification requires the action of caspases on cytosolic substrates [11, 104]. Intermitochondrial amplification appears to play a decisive role in the execution of the apoptotic program: cells with overexpression of the anti-apoptotic protein Bcl-x_L do not undergo apoptosis, although cytosolic caspase activation is induced by stimulated Fas receptors [9, 184, 222]. This means that a pro-apoptotic effect of activated caspases on mitochondria is necessary for full activation of the program in most cell types.

Two molecular mechanisms of intermitochondrial amplification have been identified (but more mechanisms might exist): first, caspase-mediated cleavage of the cytosolic protein Bid into an active fragment with a BH3 domain, which binds to the protein Bax, thereby enhancing the pro-apoptotic efficacy of Bax causing cytochrome c release [39, 65, 110, 122]. Second, activated caspases can cleave the anti-apoptotic Bcl-x_L, which is anchored in the outer mitochondrial membrane, and by this cleavage convert Bcl-x_L into a pro-apoptotic, cytochrome c-releasing molecule [22, 26, 30]. On the other hand, overexpression of Bcl-x_L can prevent the intermitochondrial amplification (see section Caspase activation by mitochondria). Therefore, a critical balance between the amount of activated caspases and the level of anti-apoptotic Bcl-proteins determines whether the intermitochondrial amplification proceeds, converting Bcl-x_L into a pro-apoptotic factor and transducing the process into the nucleus. Thus, in the failing myocardium, factors attenuating the activity of cytosolic caspases might contribute to the postmitochondrial retardation of nuclear myocyte apoptosis by attenuating intermitochondrial amplification (see section Postmitochondrial retardation).

Transduction from activated caspases to nuclear apoptosis

The classical nuclear hallmarks of apoptosis are pyknosis (i.e., shrinkage of nuclei with condensed, clumped chromatin), karyorrhexis (i.e., fragmentation of the nucleus) and DNA cleavage to nucleosome-sized fragments [233]. Only recently have several mechanisms been identified, which contribute to the transduction of the apoptotic signal from the activated caspases to the nucleus (Table 1). Presently, it appears unlikely that all these mechanisms have to be activated simultaneously for mediating the canonical degradation of the nucleus in an apoptotic cell. Organ differences in the expression of these effectors have been reported, with a substantial expression of CAD (DFF40) in the heart [142]. It is not yet clear which combination of nuclear apoptosis effectors must be activated in a certain cell type or in response to a certain apoptotic stimulus. For the failing myocardium, with the strong cytosolic pre-apoptosis (see section Quantitative aspects), the transduction of this cytosolic activation to the myocyte nuclei must be under the influence of retarding mechanisms (see section Postmitochondrial retardation). However, neither the transducing nor the retarding mechanisms in the overloaded cardiomyocyte can be delineated precisely.

Postmitochondrial retardation of myocardial apoptosis

Parallel to the first description of cytosolic pre-apoptosis in the failing human myocardium [148], it was speculated that a number of unidentified mechanisms may inhibit apoptosis downstream of mitochondrial cytochrome c release in largely postreplicative cells such as adult cardiomyocytes and differentiated neurons [174]. These unidentified inhibiting mechanisms in the failing heart must interfere with the transmission of the apoptotic signal from the mitochondrially driven caspase activation in the cytosol to the nucleus (see section Phases of the apoptotic program).

Obviously, major distances between cytochrome c-releasing mitochondria and the nucleus in such large cells may cause some postmitochondrial retar-

Table 1. Effectors of nuclear apoptosis

Effector	Mode of activation	Nuclear effect	Refs.
CAD (caspase-activated DNase) = CPAN (caspase-activated nuclease) = DFF40 (DNA fragmentation factor-40)	Caspase cleavage of the cytosolic CAD inhibitor ICAD (or DFF45) liberates CAD for import into nucleus	Cleavage of DNA between nucleosomes into 200 base pairs (or multiples thereof)	119, 52, 180, 142, 68, 118
AIF (apoptosis-inducing factor)	Release from mitochondrial intermembrane space and import into nucleus	Chromatin condensation to nuclear periphery and partial DNA fragmentation	204
ACINUS (apoptotic chromatin condensation inducer in the nucleus)	Intranuclear cleavage by imported caspase-3 and another protease into active fragment	Chromatin condensation by active acinus fragment via unknown mechanism	179
L-DNase II	Acid-dependent modification of serpin-like LEI (leukocyte elastase inhibitor) and import into nucleus	Chromatin condensation+ DNA cleavage into nucleosome-sized fragments	216
Cathepsin B	Release from lysosomes and import into nucleus	Chromatin condensation+ DNA cleavage into nucleosome-sized fragments	221
Activated caspases-3 and -6	Cleavage of lamin-B and of gelsolin	Disruption of interior structure of nucleus	206, 161

dation in the execution of the apoptotic program. However, cardiomyocytes probably have the highest cytosolic density of mitochondria, distributed almost evenly over the entire normal myocyte. Although substantial functional differences between inner and outer mitochondria of cardiomyocytes do occur [60], it is not easy to envisage functional constellations in the overloaded myocyte, which render outer mitochondria more susceptible to cytochrome c-releasing stimuli, while inner mitochondria, located more closely to the nucleus, remain resistant to such stimuli. Cytokine-activated death receptors in the cell membrane do activate caspases and induce mitochondrial release of apoptogenic signals (see above). Cytokines might contribute to the induction of myocyte apoptosis (see section Postmitochondrial retardation). Therefore, this process might affect superficial mitochondria more easily than inner, perinuclear mitochondria. Furthermore, enlarged myocytes from hearts with chronic heart failure may contain large intracellular spaces without myofibrils and mitochondria, probably a result of degradation processes [185, 192]. Such spaces would attenuate the propagation of the apoptotic signal from the remaining mitochondria to the nucleus. However, more detailed morphological analyses are required to learn whether intracellular heteroge-

Table 2. Postmitochondrial retardation of myocardial apoptosis: candidate inhibitors associated with cardioprotection

Inhibitor	Mode of action	Association with cardioprotection	Refs.
Hsp70	Anti-apoptosis downstream of activated caspases	Hsp70 inducible by transient ischemia; Hsp70 overexpressing myocardium partially protected against ischemia	80, 137, 138, 217
HO1	Anti-apoptosis by promoting iron efflux and lowering non-ferritin iron	Enhanced HO1 expression and CO formation in ischemic preconditioning HO1 overexpression enhances cardiac xenograft survival	55, 195, 131, 132, 130, 198
ARC	Inhibitory interaction with death receptor-activated caspases	Expression restricted to cardiac and skeletal muscle	99
NOS	Caspase inhibition by S-nitrosylation of cysteine in the active center	Treatment by ACE inhibitors up-regulates cardiac NOS-III expression in normal and failing myocardium	45, 127, 111, 126, 62, 140
Akt-kinase in survival pathways	Caspase-9 inactivation by phosphorylation	Attenuated survival signaling promotes decompensation in cardiac overload (see section Mitochondrial dysfunction and Table 3)	18

Hsp70 heat shock protein 70; *HO1* heme oxygenase-1; *ARC* *a*poptosis *r*epressor with *c*aspase recruitment domain; *NOS* nitric oxide synthase; *ACE* angiotensin-converting enzyme

neities and enhanced intracellular distances do really contribute to the post-mitochondrial retardation of apoptosis in the failing heart.

In addition to intracellular distances, several regulatory mechanisms with an apoptosis-retarding potential at or downstream to the mitochondria can be considered as potential candidates, which may also contribute to the retardation between mitochondrial cytochrome c release and nuclear degradation in the failing myocardium (Table 2). Interestingly, all these mechanisms have been associated previously with cardioprotection under certain conditions.

The best candidate for this retardation is Hsp70, since it has been shown to inhibit nuclear apoptotic alterations downstream of the effector caspases, such as caspase-3 [80, 141]. This is similar to the situation in the failing heart with substantial cytosolic caspase activation, but only marginal nuclear apoptotic alterations [148]. The cardioprotective action of overexpressed Hsp70 has been analyzed against ischemic myocardial damage [138, 217], but not against overload-associated apoptosis. Unfortunately, the localization of cytochrome c and the status of cytosolic caspases has not yet been analyzed in Hsp70-protected, ischemia-stressed myocardium. Furthermore, the mechanism of this Hsp70-mediated inhibition of nuclear apoptosis is still enigmatic, and it is unclear whether this protection can be mediated by the basal myocardial Hsp70 levels in the failing heart. Therefore, the proposed role of Hsp70 as a mediator of postmitochondrial retardation of apoptosis in the failing heart is still speculative.

Heme oxygenase-1 (HO1) is also known as Hsp32 [93]. Similarly to Hsp70 and other heat shock proteins, it is induced rapidly following exposure to a number of stressful stimuli [25]. In the myocardium, its expression is enhanced by short, transient ischemias, and it has been implicated in cardioprotection by ischemic preconditioning [130–132, 195]. The stress-inducible HO1 and the constitutive HO2 catalyze the degradation of heme to bilirubin, carbon monoxide (CO) and iron [124], and HO1 protects cells from damage by oxidative stress [170]. The antioxidant properties of bilirubin [200], the induction of cytoprotective ferritin by free iron [49], and the vascular relaxation by CO-mediated cGMP formation [201] have been considered as mediators of this cytoprotection. Furthermore, HO1 stimulates iron efflux from cells, thereby facilitating iron reutilization [169] and preventing apoptosis by lowering intracellular iron levels [55]. Free intracellular iron is assumed to give rise to cytosolic oxidative stress by radical formation [135], thereby triggering the release of mitochondrial apoptogenic signals. Thus, an anti-apoptotic function of myocardial HO1 is clear, but the protective mechanism appears to be mainly mitochondrial and relevant for ischemic myocardium. The contribution of HO1 to the postmitochondrial retardation of the program in failing myocardium might consist in a retardation of the "intermitochondrial amplification" of the death program from superficial, death receptor-activated mitochondria to more centrally located mitochondria.

ARC, the "*a*poptosis *r*epressor with *c*aspase recruitment domain", is an inhibitor of caspases, which is expressed primarily in skeletal muscle and in myocardium [99]. The inhibition by ARC is specific for caspases-8 and -2, which are involved in the apoptosis induced by activated death domain receptors. However, caspase-9, the initiator caspase activated primarily by mitochondrial release of cytochrome c, is not inhibited [99]. Therefore, the myocardial ARC might be a reason for the partial resistance of healthy myocardium against the induction of apoptosis by TNF, FasL or other death receptor ligands. In overload-associated heart failure, myocardial apoptosis is mainly triggered by the mitochondria, but some systemic inflammatory activation is assumed to contribute [48, 212]. This contribution may be attenuated by ARC, retarding the progression of the program. However, this retardation is not specifically postmitochondrial, but attenuates also cytochrome c release [50] and therefore may not be important for the postmitochondrial retardation in the failing myocardium.

Similar to ARC, several caspases are also inhibited by mammalian homologues to viral IAPs (*i*nhibitors of *ap*optosis) such as baculovirus p35 [31] and cowpox virus CrmA [210]. These mammalian caspase inhibitors, expressed in most cell types, are XIAP, c-IAP1 and c-IAP2 [40, 177]. However, it is not yet known whether these mammalian IAPs are induced in the stressed or failing myocardium, or whether the basal myocardial expression is sufficient for some retardation of cardiac apoptosis. Similar to HO1, endogenous caspase inhibitors like ARC and IAPs might contribute to the attenuation of intermitochondrial amplification in the failing heart.

Caspase-3, the terminal effector caspase of mitochondrially induced apoptosis, can be inhibited by nitric oxide via S-nitrosylation of a cysteine residue at the active center of the enzyme [45, 111, 126, 127]. For this anti-apoptotic protection by NO, low levels of the signal produced by the NOS-III isoform of the enzyme are relevant, while high NO levels resulting from the inflammation-associated inducible NOS-I can act pro-apoptotic and cytotoxic. Interestingly, NOS-III expression in myocardium and large arteries is enhanced by chronic ACE inhibitor treatment with clinically relevant dosages [62, 140]. Thus, the ACE inhibitor treatment of patients with terminal heart failure may retard the progression of apoptosis by lowering caspase-3 activity. A similar attenuation of mitochondrially induced apoptosis is obtained by phosphorylation and inhibition of caspase-9 [18]. This inhibitory phosphorylation is induced by the kinase Akt, which is an important element of the survival receptor pathways discussed in the section Mitochondrial dysfunction. Activation of these pathways contributes to the cardiac adaptation to overload and appears necessary for maintaining the compensated state of overload-induced cardiac hypertrophy (see section Mitochondrial dysfunction).

Thus, a combination of intracellular spatial heterogeneities, postmitochondrial inhibition of apoptosis by Hsp70, and retardation of "intermitochondrial amplification" at the level of effector caspases might contribute to the discrepancy between strongly activated cytosolic apoptosis and minimal nuclear apoptosis in the failing myocardium.

Activation of cytosolic pre-apoptosis in myocardium

The two cardiac pathologies, in which detailed analyses of myocyte apoptosis have been obtained, are myocardial damage due to ischemia/reperfusion and terminal heart failure of chronically overloaded myocardium. In both conditions, there is evidence for the contribution of mitochondrial cytochrome c release and subsequent caspase activation to the apoptotic process. However, the exact mechanisms causing the release of cytochrome c and the activation of the cytosolic pre-apoptosis under either condition have not yet been identified.

Mitochondrial release of cytochrome c and activation of the terminal effector caspase-3 have been shown after myocardial ischemia and reperfusion in vivo, in hypoxic adult ventricular myocytes in vitro, and in cultured neonatal rat cardiomyocytes [8, 35, 125]. Furthermore, the attenuation of myocyte apoptosis in experimental models of ischemia and reperfusion by caspase inhibitors indirectly suggests that this sequence of mechanisms was operative [156, 236]. In isolated mitochondria, reactive oxygen species as well as calcium overload of the mitochondrial matrix have been identified as inducers of permeability transition pore opening, outer membrane rupture and cytochrome c release, but the nature of the cytochrome c releasing mechanism in the ischemic and postischemic cardiomyocyte is unknown.

In terminal overload-associated heart failure, cytosolic pre-apoptosis with massive release of mitochondrial cytochrome c has been demonstrated (see section Quantitative aspects). Enhanced neuroendocrine activation, overload-induced myocyte distension and inflammatory activation are considered as factors contributing to the progression of failure, and they are potential causes for the activation of apoptosis.

Activation of apoptosis in terminal heart failure might result from TNFα-induced activation of myocardial TNF type I receptors, in agreement with the cytokine hypothesis of cardiac failure (see section Caspase activation by death receptors). However, as discussed previously, it is not clear whether TNF (or other failure-activated cytokines) do contribute to mitochondrial cytochrome c release and cytosolic pre-apoptosis or whether they act by other negative inotropic mechanisms (see section Caspase activation by death receptors).

Myocyte apoptosis due to overload-induced myocyte distension is generally assumed to occur, but has been demonstrated directly in isolated papillary muscle in vitro under a degree of overstretching, which cannot occur in vivo [24]. Recently, load-induced myocardial apoptosis with caspase activation has been demonstrated in long-term incubation of working papillary muscles under pathophysiologically relevant degrees of mechanical loading [85–87]. However, cytochrome c release in this model and a mechanism for transferring the mechanical load to the mitochondria remains to be shown. Components of the cytoskeleton appear as candidates for such a transfer. The Wnt/Frizzled signaling system is an attractive candidate for involvement in mechanosensitive apoptosis regulation [136, 230]. In overloaded myocardium with activated apoptosis, the expression of Wnt-antagonistic soluble frizzled-related proteins is enhanced [189], and β-catenin as important component of Wnt-signaling and of cytoskeletal anchorage might modulate Bcl-protein expression, but this remains to be documented in myocardium.

Neuroendocrine overstimulation has been evaluated extensively as a potential inductor of myocyte apoptosis. Catecholamines, angiotensin II and ANF (atrial natriuretic factor) have all been proposed as contributors to myocyte apoptosis in terminal heart failure, mainly on the basis of cell culture data or of experiments with overexpression. Surprisingly, however, these data do not yet establish the role of neuroendocrine mediators for myocyte pre-apoptosis in the failing heart.

ANF has been shown to induce apoptosis in neonatal rat cardiomyocytes in culture, suggesting a pathological autocrine role of enhanced cardiac ANF formation in cardiac overload [232]. However, in intact animals, enhancement of circulating ANF by inhibition of its degradation does not induce myocardial apoptosis, although an autocrine ANF effect on myocardial cGMP formation is demonstrable in vivo (Heinrich et al., unpublished observation from our laboratory).

Catecholamines have been shown to induce β-adrenoceptor-mediated apoptosis in cultured cardiomyocytes [28, 77]. Cardiac overexpression of β_1-adrenoceptors induces augmented cardiac contractility in young mice, but dilative cardiomyopathy with depressed contractility and myocyte apoptosis in older animals [53, 196], and a dilated cardiomyopathy with signs of nuclear myocyte apoptosis is also observed in mice overexpressing $G\alpha_s$ [61, 78, 79] and in several $G\alpha_q$ overexpressing transgenic mice (see [196]). Activation of mitogen-activated kinase cascades are considered as mediators of these catecholamine-associated apoptotic activations [196], but it is very difficult to derive any conclusions on the relevance of adrenoceptor-mediated activation of apoptosis or cytochrome c release in hearts with downregulated β-adrenoceptor signal transduction.

Angiotensin II has been shown as a mediator of stretch-induced myocyte apoptosis in vitro by AT_1-receptor activation [106] and cardiospecific overexpression of AT_1 receptors induces cardiac hypertrophy with age-dependent accumulation of interstitial and replacement fibrosis, but apoptosis was not evaluated in this model [165].

Although several experimental arguments and observations suggest that overload-induced distension, enhanced neuroendocrine overstimulation and inflammatory activation may contribute to the induction of myocardial apoptosis in failing myocardium, none of these stimuli can be identified as the culprit causing the substantial cytochrome c release and cytosolic pre-apoptosis visible in terminal heart failure.

Mitochondrial dysfunction as a consequence of cytosolic pre-apoptosis

What is the function of mitochondria in overloaded, distended cardiomyocytes, which have released a large fraction of their cytochrome c content from their intermembrane space? The physiological role of cytochrome c in this space is to act as a diffusible electron transfer shuttle from complex III to complex IV. Therefore, mitochondria with cytochrome c deficiency should have impaired function of complex III, and this is exactly what has been observed recently in human myocardium from patients with dilative and/or ischemic cardiomyopathy: a significant, selective decline in complex III activity/citrate synthase activity [88]. Unfortunately, no effort was made in this study to correlate this depression of complex III activity with cytochrome c content [88]. This depression of normalized complex III activity resulted in a significant reduction in overall mitochondrial cytochrome c oxidase activity in these failing hearts [88]. A much quoted concept predicts that impairments within the respiratory chain would result in enhanced unpaired electron transfer (i.e., radical formation) in respiratory chain complexes proximal to the impairment in the presence of high pO_2 [12, 21, 197]. In agreement with the predictions of this concept, enhanced mitochondrial superoxide anion formation mainly in complex I, and subsequent hydroxyl radical production was shown in freeze-clamped tissue homogenates from failing hearts using ESR techniques [75, 76], which correlated with the impairment of contractile function observed in vivo. Again, no correlation with cytochrome c depletion was considered, and the superoxide anion formation in complex I might not exclusively be due to this depletion. Probably, the enhanced expression of catalase in terminally failing hearts [42] is a reaction to this enhanced mitochondrial radical formation in myocardium with massive cytosolic pre-apoptosis and cytochrome c translocation.

The reduction in normalized complex III activity mentioned above [88] might underestimate the actual impairment of mitochondrial respiratory function in failing myocardium for two reasons: first, normalization was obtained by relation to matrix enzyme activity (citrate synthase), which also tended to be lowered [88]; this tendency might be explained by mitochondrial destruction demonstrated previously by electron microscopy in terminal heart failure [56, 185, 192]. Secondly, deficiencies in myocardial creatine transporter and creatine content may add to the impairment of mitochondrial function in the failing heart [149, 150].

Mitochondrial dysfunction is probably not only a consequence of cytosolic pre-apoptosis of terminal heart failure with substantial relevance for the contractile performance of the failing heart. Mitochondrial dysfunction might also act as a starting signal for the initiation of cytosolic pre-apoptosis: with increasing age, mutations and deletions in myocardial mitochondrial DNA accumulate, and it has been repeatedly speculated that this accumulation might contribute to accumulating mitochondrial impairments and enhanced cardiac susceptibility for cytosolic pre-apoptosis in the senescent heart. However, consideration of this problem is beyond the scope of this text.

Anti-apoptotic cardioprotection by survival receptors

In many cell systems, several growth stimuli will result in apoptosis unless survival signals are concomitantly activated, allowing a proliferative response of the stimulated cells. A similar balance of the growth stimulus "hemodynamic overload" and of activated survival signals appears necessary in the ventricular myocardium of adult mammals. Activation of survival signals appears mandatory to avoid or to delay the overload-induced myocyte apoptosis and to allow the hypertrophic growth response of the myocytes (Table 3). The three examples in that table indicate that defects in different survival signals are at least associated with myocardial apoptosis and cardiac failure in overloaded myocardium. All three survival signal systems from the Table 3 have been shown to suppress apoptosis and to modulate cell proliferation and differentiation in various cellular models.

The first analyses of molecular mechanisms of the survival pathways identified an important role of the pro-apoptotic, "BH3 only" Bcl-2 protein BAD [239]. BAD is a cytosolic protein without a transmembrane-anchoring domain, which has probably no direct, cytochrome c releasing effect on mito-

Table 3. Attenuated survival signal activation associated with myocyte apoptosis in cardiac overload

Model	Modified survival signal	Cardiac effects	Refs.
Mice: pressure overload by aortic banding	Ventricular restricted conditional knockout of gp130	Rapid chamber dilation, massive apoptosis and premature mortality; Yet: gp130-deficient hearts without pressure overload remain normal	73
Rats: pressure overload by aortic banding	Ventricular expression of erbB2 & erbB4 receptors depressed in late phase of overload, but normal in early compensated phase	Depressed systolic function and signs of failure in late phase but not in early compensated phase	175
Rats: hypertension due to chronic NO-synthase inhibition	Less LV expression of IGF-I and of IGF-IR than in any other rat model of hypertension	No increase in LV mass and reduced number of LV myocytes; LV apoptosis suppressible by hemodynamically neutral IGF-I substitution	229 207 143

NO nitric oxide; *erbB(s)* neuregulin receptor(s); *LV* left ventricular; *IGF* insulin-like growth factor; *IGF-IR* IGF-I receptor type 1

chondria [46]: BAD binds the anti-apoptotic proteins Bcl-2 and Bcl-x_L, which protect mitochondria by complexing pro-apoptotic Bax-like proteins and by other, less well understood mechanisms (see section Caspase activation by mitochondria). Binding by BAD abolishes the protective efficacy of Bcl-2 or Bcl-x_L, and phosphorylation of BAD at critical serine residues causes binding of phosphorylated BAD to cytosolic 14-3-3 proteins (14-3-3 is a protein domain motif, which binds several phosphoproteins), thereby liberating Bcl-2/Bcl-x_L from their inhibitory complex with BAD and re-establishing their protective efficacy [239]. The first kinase identified as mediating the critical serine-phosphorylation of BAD was the protein kinase B (PKB), also called Akt [33, 37]. However, PKB/Akt is not the only kinase inhibiting the pro-apoptotic effect of BAD; this inhibitory BAD phosphorylation is also obtained from a cAMP-activated kinase (PKA) [70, 239], by a kinase controlled by mitochondrially targeted Raf [228], and by a MAP kinase in the interleukin-4 pathway [187]. When BAD is complexed with Bcl-2 or Bcl-x_L, a mitochondria-specific AKAP (= A kinase-anchoring protein) is necessary for the phosphorylation of BAD, which liberates Bcl-2/Bcl-x_L [70]. Phosphorylated, 14-3-3-complexed, inactivated BAD can be dephosphorylated by the Ca^{2+}-activated phosphatase calcineurin [227]. However, calcineurin can not only act pro-apoptotic by dephosphorylating BAD, but calcineurin is also an element of hypertrophic signaling in cardiac and skeletal myocytes [139, 146, 193, 205], illustrating the close and complex interaction of trophic and apoptotic pathways. Cardiac-specific calcineurin overexpression causes cardiomyocyte hypertrophy together with protection against ischemia/reperfusion- associated apoptosis in vitro and in vivo [36]. The mechanism of this surprising protection is not quite clear, but calcineurin overexpression appears to be associated with massive activation of PKB/Akt [36], and this activation, promoting BAD phosphorylation/inactivation, may overcome the BAD-dephosphorylating effect of augmented calcineurin in the myocardium. In other cell types, calcineurin can both promote or inhibit apoptosis depending on the interaction with other signals [121].

Although the critical role of BAD in survival regulation is now intensively being analyzed, it is highly likely that other proteins of the Bcl-2 family will soon turn out to have similarly critical roles in the decision between survival and apoptosis around the mitochondria.

The "survival kinase" PKB/Akt mediates its protective role not only by phosphorylation of BAD, but other PKB/Akt targets are probably much more important and cells without BAD expression can be protected effectively by PKB/Akt [94]. PKB/Akt phosphorylates transcription factors of the "forkhead" family, which can induce pro-apoptotic signals such as FasL, and this PKB/Akt-mediated phosphorylation sequesters these transcription factors in the cytosol by binding to 14-3-3 proteins, thereby preventing their import into the nucleus [15, 98]. Furthermore, Akt can induce protective gene transcription via the NF-κB pathway [163, 176]. NF-κB promotes the expression of several anti-apoptotic genes and is normally kept inactive by cytosolic binding to the inhibitor I-κB [226]. Phosphorylation of I-κB by PKB/Akt causes degradation of I-κB and liberates NF-κB for nuclear import and for the induction of anti-apoptotic genes [163, 176]. NF-κB activation by mitogen-activated phosphorylation cascades also confers anti-apoptotic protection in myocardium [238]. However, this important protective regulator function of NF-κB in the pathway of survival signals can be overridden by caspase-mediated cleavage of NF-κB, which generates a transcriptionally inactive p65 fragment of NF-κB with apoptosis promoting, NF-κB-inhibiting properties [109]. Thus, the balance between apoptotic and survival signaling is regulated at several steps under the influence of PKB/Akt. At the level of caspases, PKB/Akt also protects cells from apoptosis by phosphorylating and inhibiting caspase-9 [18] (see also Table 2) and by activating the constitutive NO synthase III [44, 59]. Activated NO synthase III allows NO-mediated inactivation of caspases by S-nitrosylation (see Table 2).

It has been repeatedly discussed that the protective potency of PKB/Akt should be exploited therapeutically in chronic heart failure, suppressing the ongoing apoptosis by PKB/Akt-activating drugs. However, any strategy for preventing heart failure by chronically activating anti-apoptotic pathways has to consider the tumorigenic risk of chronic overactivation of survival signaling!

Therapeutic inhibition of apoptosis for cardioprotection?

As mentioned above, inhibition of ischemia/reperfusion- associated apoptosis has been repeatedly tried with the application of pharmacological caspase inhibition, and this treatment resulted in decreased numbers of apoptotic nuclei in jeopardized cardiac areas and short-term improvements of contractile function [see 4, 17], suggesting that an apoptotic component contributes to ischemia-associated cardiomyocyte losses, although clear features of necrotic or "oncotic" myocyte death dominate in coronary heart disease.

However, most of the initial experiments in this field had not evaluated the long-term fate of ischemic myocardium of caspase inhibitor-treated hearts, and this has probably not improved. In a rabbit model of ischemia (30 min) and reperfusion (6 h), caspase inhibition prior to ischemia substantially attenuated TUNEL staining of myocyte nuclei, DNA ladder fragmentation and enhancement of caspase-3 activity in the myocardial area at risk. Nevertheless, infarct size was not reduced [156]. Infarct size was determined by TTC staining of viable cardiomyocytes, which labels the NADH in the mitochondria, and this staining as well as electron microscopic signs of mitochondrial swelling, rupture and disintegration could not be improved by caspase inhibitor pretreatment [156]. This is in contrast to the protection obtained by ischemic preconditioning, assessed by similar techniques in similar models [168].

This negative result appears understandable, given the fact that caspase inhibition should not be able to modify the primary mechanisms of mitochondrial damage; at best it can retard secondary damages resulting from the caspase-mediated intermitochondrial amplification of cytochrome c release (see section Intermitochondrial amplification). Such retardation of the process might explain controversial observations obtained with different protocols of caspase inhibitor application in similar ischemia/reperfusion models [236]. However, the main problem remains regardless of minor literature discrepancies: once mitochondrial function is damaged to a major extent, attenuation of subsequent caspase activation might retard the resulting myocyte death, but, in longer consequence, the picture of cellular demise should only shift from an apoptotic/necrotic mixture to a purely necrotic form of death due to the lack of sufficient ATP to perform ATP-requiring steps of the program. Therefore, apoptosis inhibition might be at best an adjuvant strategy in ischemic heart disease, aiming to prolong the time window for the application of causal therapy. Whether such adjuvant caspase inhibition is really able to improve the results of acute revascularizations may be difficult to prove.

Probably, similar skepticism should be formulated against anti-apoptotic therapy in overload-associated, terminal heart failure, although this skepticism is not an argument against the pathophysiological relevance of apoptotic activation in this condition.

Caspase inhibition appears not as a promising option in terminal heart failure. The failing cardiomyocyte without caspase inhibition is a cell with substantial cytochrome c released and cytosolic pre-apoptosis, but a strong, largely unexplained retardation in the postmitochondrial progression of this process to the nucleus (see section Postmitochondrial retardation). Yet, this pre-apoptotic myocyte is failing, partially because of mitochondrial problems. Caspase inhibition cannot alleviate these mitochondrial problems, it might retard their progression by attenuating the intermitochondrial amplification, and it might retard the disintegration of myofibrils due to caspase-mediated cleavage of troponin C [67]. However, is it really an advantage for a myocyte with cytochrome c-depleted mitochondria to maintain ATP-consuming myofibrils in function? One might speculate that depressing cellular contractile function by caspase-mediated troponin C cleavage is a survival strategy for the myocyte with cytosolic pre-apoptosis. Only therapy removing the primary stimulus for cytochrome c release, such as hemodynamic unloading and attenuation of neuroendocrine and inflammatory overstimulation (e.g., TNFα-antagonists) might have the potential of attenuating pre-apoptosis, but such therapy certainly lacks specificity against apoptosis alone. It should be stressed that this skepticism concerning caspase inhibitor therapy is not based on experimental observations, it is pure speculation regardless of its plausibility.

Approaches with enhanced activation of survival pathways have the theoretical potential of a premitochondrial mode of action. However, this approach in chronic application would require absolute restriction to the myocardium because of its tumorigenic potential [6] and because of the physiological role of apoptosis in normal cell turnover, in the immune system and in spermatogenesis [97]. Furthermore, premitochondrial regulation of apoptosis is very complex (see the dual role of calcineurin as a potential inhibitor and potential inductor of apoptosis [121]) and its role in the myocardium is not understood [72] (see also section Activation of cytosolic pre-apoptosis).

Direct targeting of the mitochondria by interventions aiming to attenuate oxidative stress is a rather unspecific intervention. Although positive results with this approach have been published in experimental cardiac overload failure [162], its therapeutic potential cannot yet be estimated realistically. A similar approach (i.e., directly targeting mitochondria) would be the cardiac-specific overexpression of anti-apoptotic Bcl-2 or Bcl-x_L. This approach has been used in short-term experiments to attenuate nuclear DNA fragmentation in jeopardized myocardium of myocardial ischemia/reperfusion models (see section Experimental interventions). Provided that such an approach could be applied chronically, it might interfere with the physiological turnover of myocardial mitochondria, and this may cause long-term difficulties due to enhanced accumulation of damaged mitochondrial DNA.

Therefore, we conclude that anti-apoptotic therapy in cardiac pathologies appears to be attractive because of the large pathophysiological relevance of cytosolic, mitochondria-associated pre-apoptosis, but promising approaches to this conceptually attractive goal are not yet at hand.

References

1. Adams JM, Cory S (1998) The Bcl-2 protein family: arbiters of cell survival. Science 281:1322–1325
2. Anversa P, Kajstura J (1998) Myocyte cell death in the diseased heart. Circ Res 82:1231–1233
3. Anversa P, Kajstura J (1998) Ventricular myocytes are not terminally differentiated in the adult mammalian heart. Circ Res 83:1–14
4. Bartling B, Holtz J, Darmer D (1998) Contribution of myocyte apoptosis to myocardial infarction? Basic Res Cardiol 93:71–84
5. Bartling B, Milting H, Schumann H, Darmer D, Arusoglu L, Koerner MM, El-Banayosy A, Koerfer R, Holtz J, Zerkowski HR (1999) Myocardial gene expression of regulators of myocyte apoptosis and myocyte calcium homeostasis during hemodynamic unloading by ventricular assist devices in patients with end-stage heart failure. Circulation 100 (suppl II):II216–II223
6. Baserga R, Hongo A, Rubini M, Prisco M, Valentinis B (1997) The IGF-I receptor in cell growth, transformation and apoptosis. Biochim Biophys Acta 1332:F105–F126
7. Bing OHL (1994) Hypothesis: apoptosis may be a mechanism for the transition to heart failure with chronic pressure overload. J Mol Cell Cardiol 26:943–948
8. Black SC, Huang JQ, Rezaiefar P, Radinovic S, Eberhart A, Nicholson DW, Rodger IW (1998) Co-localization of the cysteine protease caspase-3 with apoptotic myocytes after in vivo myocardial ischemia and reperfusion in the rat. J Mol Cell Cardiol 30:733–742
9. Boise TH, Thompson CB (1997) Bcl-xL, can inhibit apoptosis in cells that have undergone Fas-induced protease activation. Proc Natl Acad Sci 94:3759–3764
10. Boldin MP, Varfolomeev EE, Pancer Z, Mett IL, Camonis JH, Wallach D (1995) A novel protein that interacts with the death domain of Fas/APO1 contains a sequence motif related to the death domain. J Biol Chem 270:7795–7798
11. Bossy-Wetzel E, Green DR (1999) Caspases induce cytochrome c release from mitochondria by activating cytosolic factors. J Biol Chem 274:17484–17490
12. Boveris A, Chance B (1973) The mitochondrial generation of hydrogen peroxide: general properties and effect of hyperbaric oxygen. Biochem J 134:707–716
13. Bozkurt B, Kribbs SB, Clubb FJ, Michael LH, Didenko VV, Hornsby PJ, Seta Y, Oral H, Spinale FG, Mann DL (1998) Pathophysiologically relevant concentrations of tumor necrosis factor-α promote progressive left ventricular dysfunction and remodeling in rats. Circulation 97:1382–1391
14. Broemme HJ, Holtz J (1996) Apoptosis in the heart: when and why? Molecular and Cellular Biochemistry 163/164:261–275
15. Brunet A, Bonni A, Zigmont MJ, Lin MZ, Juo P, Hu LS, Anderson MJ, Arden KC, Blenis J, Greenberg ME (1999) Akt promotes cell survival by phosphorylating and inhibiting a Forkhead transcription factor. Cell 96:857–868
16. Brustugun OT, Fladmark KE, Doskeland SO, Orrenius S, Zhivotovsky B (1998) Apoptosis induced by microinjection of cytochrome c is caspase-dependent and is inhibited by Bcl-2. Cell Death Differ 5:660–668
17. Buja LM, Entman ML (1998) Modes of myocardial cell injury and cell death in ischemic heart disease. Circulation 98:1355–1357
18. Cardone MH, Roy N, Stennicke HR, Salvesen GS, Franke TF, Stanbridge E, Frisch S, Reed JC (1998) Regulation of cell death protease caspase-9 by phosphorylation. Science 282:1318–1321
19. Cascino I, Fiucci G, Papoff G, Ruberti G (1995) Three functional soluble forms of the human apoptosis-inducing Fas molecule are produced by alternative splicing. J Immunol 154:2706–2713

20. Cascino I, Papoff G, De Maria R, Testi R, Ruberti G (1996) Fas/Apo-1 (CD95) receptor lacking the intracytoplasmic signaling domain protects tumor cells from Fas-mediated apoptosis. J Immunol 156:13–17
21. Chance B, Sies H, Boveris A (1979) Hydroperoxide metabolism in mammalian organs. Physiol Rev 59:527–603
22. Cheng EHY, Kirsch DG, Clem RJ, Ravi R, Kastan MB, Bedi A, Ueno K, Hardwick JM (1997) Conversion of Bcl-2 to a Bax-like effector by caspases. Science 278:1966–1968
23. Cheng W, Kajstura J, Nitahara JA, Li B, Reiss K, Liu Y, Clark WA, Krajewski S, Reed JC, Olivetti G, Anversa P (1996) Programmed myocyte cell death affects viable myocardium after infarction in rats. Exp Cell Res 226:316–327
24. Cheng W, Li B, Kajstura J, Li P, Wolin MS, Sonnenblick EH, Hintze TH, Olivetti G, Anversa P (1995) Stretch induced programmed myocyte cell death. J Clin Invest 96:2247–2259
25. Choi AM, Alam J (1996) Heme oxygenase-1: function, regulation, and implication of a novel stress-inducible protein in oxidant-induced lung injury. Am J Respir Cell Mol Biol 15:9–19
26. Clem RJ, Cheng EHY, Karp CL, Kirsch DG, Ueno K, Takahashi A, Kastan MB, Griffin DE, Earnshaw WC, Veliuona MA, Hardwick JM (1998) Modulation of cell death by bcl-x_L through caspase interaction. Proc Natl Acad Sci 95:554–559
27. Cohen GM (1997) Caspases: the executioners of apoptosis. Biochem 326:1–16
28. Communal C, Singh K, Pimentel DR, Colucci WS (1998) Norepinephrine stimulates apoptosis in adult rat ventricular myocytes by activation of the beta-adrenergic pathway. Circulation 98:1329–1334
29. Cook SA, Poole-Wilson PA (1999) Cardiac myocyte apoptosis. Eur Heart J 28:1619–1629
30. Cosulich SC, Worall V, Hege PJ, Grenn S, Clarke PR (1997) Regulation of apoptosis by BH3 domains in a cell-free system. Curr Biol 12:913–920
31. Crook NE, Clem RJ, Miller LK (1993) An apoptosis-inhibiting baculovirus gene with a zinc finger-like motif. J Virol 67:2168–2174
32. Cryns V, Yuan J (1998) Proteases to die for. Genes Dev 12:1551–1556
33. Datta SR, Dudek H, Tao X, Masters S, Fu H, Gotoh Y, Greenberg ME (1997) Akt phosphorylation of BAD couples survival signals to the cell-intrinsic death machinery. Cell 91:231–241
34. De Maria R, Zeuner A, Eramo A, Domenichelli C, Bonci D, Grignani F, Srinivasula SM, Alnemri ES, Testa U, Peschle C (1999) Negative regulation of erythropoiesis by caspase-mediated cleavage of GATA-1. Nature 401:489–493
35. De Moissac D, Gurevich RM, Zheng H, Singal PK, Kirshenbaum LA (2000) Caspase activation and mitochondrial cytochrome C release during hypoxia-mediated apoptosis of adult ventricular myocytes [in process citation]. J Mol Cell Cardiol 32:53–63
36. De Windt LJ, Lim HW, Taigen T, Wencker D, Condorelli G, Dorn GW 2nd, Kitsis RN, Molkentin JD (2000) Calcineurin-mediated hypertrophy protects cardiomyocytes from apoptosis in vitro and in vivo: an apoptosis-independent model of dilated heart failure. Circ Res 86:255–263
37. del Peso L, Gonzalez-Garcia M, Page C, Herrera R, Nunez G (1997) Interleukin-3-induced phosphorylation of BAD through the protein kinase Akt. Science 278:687–689
38. Denecker G, Dooms H, Van Loo G, Vercammen D, Grooten J, Fiers W, Declercq W, Vandenabeele P (2000) Phosphatidyl serine exposure during apoptosis precedes release of cytochrome c and decrease in mitochondrial transmembrane potential. FEBS Lett 465:47–52

39. Desagher S, Osen-Sand A, Nichols A, Eskes R, Montessuit S, Lauper S, Maundrell K, Antonsson B, Martinou JC (1999) Bid-induced conformational change of Bax is responsible for mitochondrial cytochrome c release during apoptosis. J Cell Biol 144:891–901
40. Deveraux QL, Takahashi R, Salvesen GS, Reed JC (1997) X-linked IAP is a direct inhibitor of cell-death proteases. Nature 388:300–304
41. Didenko VV, Hornby PJ (1996) Presence of double-stranded breaks with single-base 3' overhangs in cells undergoing apoptosis but not necrosis. J Cell Biol 135:1369–1376
42. Dieterich S, Bieligk U, Beulich K, Hasenfuss G, Prestle J (2000) Gene expression of antioxidative enzymes in the human heart: increased expression of catalase in the end-stage failing heart. Circulation 101:33–39
43. Díez J, Panizo A, Hernández M, Vega F, Sola I, Fortuno MA, Pardo J (1997) Cardiomyocyte apoptosis and cardiac angiotensin-converting enzyme in spontaneously hypertensive rats. Hypertension 30:1029–1034
44. Dimmeler S, Fleming I, Fisslthaler B, Hermann C, Busse R, Zeiher AM (1999) Activation of nitric oxide synthase in endothelial cells by Akt-dependent phosphorylation. Nature 399:601–605
45. Dimmeler S, Haendeler J, Nehls M, Zeiher AM (1997) Suppression of apoptosis by nitric oxide via inhibition of interleukin-1β-converting enzyme (ICE)-like and cysteine protease protein (CPP)-32-like proteases. J Exp Med 185:601–607
46. Downward J (1998) Mechanisms and consequences of activation of protein kinase B/Akt. Curr Opin Cell Biol 10:262–267
47. Duriez PJ, Shah GM (1997) Cleavage of poly(ADP-ribose) polymerase: a sensitive parameter to study cell death. Biochem Cell Biol 75:337–349
48. Dutka DP, Elborn JS, Delamere F, Shale DJ, Morris GK (1993) Tumor necrosis factor α in severe congestive cardiac failure. Br Heart J 70:41–143
49. Eisenstein RS, Garcia MD, Pettingell W, Munro HN (1991) Regulation of ferritin and heme oxygenase synthesis in rat fibroblasts by different forms of iron. Proc Natl Acad Sci 88:688–692
50. Ekhterae D, Lin Z, Lundberg MS, Crow MT, Brosius FC 3rd, Nunez G (1999) ARC inhibits cytochrome c release from mitochondria and protects against hypoxia-induced apoptosis in heart-derived H9c2 cells. Circ Res 85:e70–77
51. Elkon KB (1999) Caspases: multifunctional proteins. J Exp Med 190:1725–1727
52. Enari M, Sakahira H, Yokoyama H, Okawa K, Iwamatsu A, Nagata S (1998) A caspase-activated DNase that degrades DNA during apoptosis, and its inhibitor ICAD. Nature 391:43–50
53. Engelhardt S, Hein L, Wiesmann F, Lohse MJ (1999) Progressive hypertrophy and heart failure in beta1-adrenergic receptor transgenic mice. Proc Natl Acad Sci 96:7059–7064
54. Felzen B, Shilkrut M, Less H, Sarapov I, Maor G, Coleman R, Robinson RB, Berke G, Binah O (1998) Fas (CD95/Apo-1)-mediated damage to ventricular myocytes induced by cytotoxic T lymphocytes from perforin-deficient mice: a major role for inositol 1,4,5-triphosphate. Circ Res 82:438–450
55. Ferris CD, Jaffrey SR, Sawa A, Takahashi M, Brady SD, Barrow RK, Tysoe SA, Wolosker H, Baranano DE, Doré S, Poss KD, Snyder SH (1999) Haem oxygenase-1 prevents cell death by regulating cellular iron. Nature Cell Biol 1:152–157
56. Figulla HR, Rahlf G, Nieger M, Luig H, Kreuzer H (1985) Spontaneous hemodynamic improvement or stabilization and associated biopsy findings in patients with congestive cardiomyopathy. Circulation 71:1095–1104
57. Finkel MS, Oddis CV, Jacob TD, Watkins SC, Hattler BG, Simmons RL (1992) Negative inotropic effects of cytokines on the heart mediated by nitric oxide. Science 257:387–389

58. Frantz S, Kobzik L, Kim YD, Fukazawa R, Medzhitov R, Lee RT, Kelly RA (1999) Toll4 (TLR4) expression in cardiac myocytes in normal and failing myocardium. J Clin Invest 104:271–280
59. Fulton D, Gratton JP, McCabe TJ, Fontana J, Fujio Y, Walsh K, Franke TF, Papapetropoulos A, Sessa WC (1999) Regulation of endothelium-derived nitric oxide production by protein kinase Akt. Nature 399:597–601
60. Gallitelli MF, Schultz M, Isenberg G, Rudolf F (1999) Twitch-potentiation increases calcium in peripheral more than in central mitochondria of guinea-pig ventricular myocytes. J Physiol 518:433–447
61. Geng YJ, Ishikawa Y, Vatner DE, Wagner TE, Bishop SP, Vatner SF, Homcy CJ (1999) Apoptosis of cardiac myocytes in Gsalpha transgenic mice. Circ Res 84:34–42
62. Goetz RM, Holtz J (1999) Enhanced angiotensin-converting enzyme activity and impaired endothelium-dependent vasodilation in aortae from hypertensive rats: evidence for a causal link. Clin Sci 97:165–174
63. Green DR, Reed JC (1998) Mitochondria and apoptosis. Science 281:1309–1312
64. Gregory T, Yu C, Ma A, Orkin SH, Blobel GA, Weiss MJ (1999) GATA-1 and erythropoietin cooperate to promote erythroid cell survival by regulating bcl-x_L expression. Blood 94:87–96
65. Gross A, Yin XM, Wang K, Wei MC, Jockel J, Milliman C, Erdjument-Bromage H, Tempst P, Korsmeyer SJ (1999) Caspase cleaved BID targets mitochondria and is required for cytochrome c release, while BCL-XL prevents this release but not tumor necrosis-R1/Fas death. J Biol Chem 274:1156–1163
66. Guerra S, Leri A, Wang X, Finato N, Di Loreto C, Beltrami CA, Kajstura J, Anversa P (1999) Myocyte death in the failing human heart is gender dependent. Circ Res 85:856–866
67. Haider N, Kharbanda S, Chandrasekar Y, Srinivasula SM, Fitzpatrick JM, Anand I, Alnemri ES, Narula J (1999) Caspase-3 mediated cleavage of troponin-C at evolutionarily conserved calcium binding site: relevance of apoptosis in heart failure (abstr). Circulation 100 (suppl):I–283
68. Halenbeck R, MacDonald H, Roulston A, Chen TT, Conroy L, Williams LT (1998) CPAN, a human nuclease regulated by the caspase-sensitive inhibitor DFF45. Current Biol 8:537–540
69. Hamet P, Richard L, Dam TV, Teiger E, Orlov SN, Gaboury L, Gossard F, Tremblay J (1995) Apoptosis in target organs of hypertension. Hypertension 26:642–648
70. Harada H, Becknell B, Wilm M, Mann M, Huang LJ, Taylor SS, Scott JD, Korsmeyer SJ (1999) Phosphorylation and inactivation of BAD by mitochondria-anchored protein-kinase A. Mol Cell 3:413–422
71. Haunstetter A, Izumo S (1998) Apoptosis: basic mechanisms and implications for cardiovascular disease. Circ Res 82:1111–1129
72. Haunstetter A, Izumo S (2000) Toward antiapoptosis as a new treatment modality. Circ Res 86:371–376
73. Hirota H, Chen J, Betz U, Rajewsky K, Gu Y, Ross JJ, Muller W, Chien KR (1999) Loss of gp130 cardiac muscle cell survival pathway is a critical event in the onset of heart failure during biomechanical stress. Cell 97:189–198
74. Holtz J, Darmer D (2000) Death Receptors and Their Ligands. Kluwer Academic Publisher, pp 5–28
75. Ide T, Tsutsui H, Kinugawa S, Suematsu N, Hayashidani S, Ichikawa K, Utsumi H, Machida Y, Egashira K, Takeshita A (2000) Direct evidence for increased hydroxyl radicals originating from superoxide in the failing myocardium. Circ Res 86:152–157

76. Ide T, Tsutsui H, Kinugawa S, Utsumi H, Kang D, Hattori N, Uchida K, Arimura K, Egashira K, Takeshita A (1999) Mitochondrial electron transport complex I is a potential source of oxygen free radicals in the failing myocardium. Circ Res 85:357–363
77. Iwai-Kanai E, Hasegawa K, Araki M, Kakita T, Morimoto T, Sasayama S (1999) Alpha- and beta-adrenergic pathways differentially regulate cell type-specific apoptosis in rat cardiac myocytes. Circulation 100:305–311
78. Iwase M, Bishop SP, Uechi M, Vatner DE, Shannon RP, Kudej RK, Wight DC, Wagner TE, Ishikawa Y, Homcy CJ, Vatner SF (1996) Adverse effects of chronic endogenous sympathetic drive induced by cardiac GS alpha overexpression. Circ Res 78:517–524
79. Iwase M, Uechi M, Vatner DE, Asai K, Shannon RP, Kudej RK, Wagner TE, Wight DC, Patrick TA, Ishikawa Y, Homcy CJ, Vatner SF (1997) Cardiomyopathy induced by cardiac Gs alpha overexpression. Am J Physiol 272:H585–H589
80. Jäättelä M, Wissing D, Kokholm K, Kallunki T, Egeblad M (1998) Hsp70 exerts its anti-apoptotic function downstream of caspase-3-like proteases. EMBO J 17:6124–6134
81. James TN (1994) Normal and abnormal consequences of apoptosis in the human heart from postnatal morphogenesis to paroxysmal arrhythmias. Circulation 90:556–573
82. James TN (1997) Apoptosis in congenital heart disease. Coronary Art Dis 8:599–616
83. James TN (1997) Complex causes of fatal myocardial infarction. Circulation 96:1696–1700
84. James TN, Terasaki F, Pavlovich ER, Vikhert AM (1993) Apoptosis and pleomorphic mitochondriosis in the sinus nodes surgically excised from five patients with long QT syndrome. J Lab Clin Med 122:309–323
85. Janssen PML, Lehnart SE, Prestle J, Hasenfuss G (1999) Preservation of contractile characteristics of human myocardium in multi-day culture. J Mol Cell Cardiol 31:1419–1427
86. Janssen PML, Hasenfuss G, Zeitz O, Lehnart S, Darmer D, Holtz J, Schumann H (1999) Afterload-induced apoptosis in multicellular myocardial preparations in functional culture (abstr). Circulation 100(suppl):I–758
87. Janssen PML, Lehnart SE, Prestle J, Lynker JC, Salfeld P, Just H, Hasenfuss G (1998) The trabecula culture system: a novel technique to study contractile parameters over a multiday period. Am J Physiol 274:H1481–H1488
88. Jarreta D, Orus J, Barrietos A, Miro O, Roig E, Heras M, Moraes CT, Cardellach F, Casedemont J (2000) Mitochondrial function in heart muscle from patients with idiopathic dilated cardiomyopathy. Cardiovasc Res 45:860–865
89. Kajstura J, Leri A, Finato N, Di Loreto C, Beltrami CA, Anversa P (1998) Myocyte proliferation in end-stage cardiac failure in humans. Proc Natl Acad Sci 95:8801–8805
90. Kan H, Xie Z, Finkel MS (1999) TNF-alpha enhances cardiac myocyte NO production through MAP kinase-mediated NF-kappaB activation. Am J Physiol 277:H1641–1646
91. Kanoh M, Takemura G, Misao J, Hayakawa Y, Aoyama T, Nishigaki K, Noda T, Fujiwara T, Fukuda F, Minatoguchi S, Fujiwara H (1999) Significance of myocytes with positive DNA in situ nick end-labeling (TUNEL) in hearts with dilated cardiomyopathy: not apoptosis but DNA repair. Circulation 99:2757–2764
92. Kerr PM, Suleiman MS, Halestrap AP (1999) Reversal of permeability transition during recovery of hearts from ischemia and its enhancement by pyruvate. Am J Physiol 276:H496–H502

93. Keyse SM, Tyrrell RM (1989) Heme oxygenase is the major 32-kDa stress protein induced in human skin fibroblasts by UVA radiation, hydrogen peroxide, and sodium arsenite. Proc Natl Acad Sci 86:99–103
94. Kitada S, Krajewska M, Zhang X, Scudiero D, Zapata JM, Wang HG, Shabaik A, Tudor G, Krajewski S, Myers TG, Johnson GS, Sausville EA, Reed JC (1998) Expression and location of pro-apoptotic bcl-2 family protein BAD in normal human tissues and tumor cell lines. Am J Pathol 152:51–61
95. Kluck RM, Bossy-Wetzel E, Green DR, Newmeyer DD (1997) The release of cytochrome c from mitochondria: a primary site for bcl-2 regulation of apoptosis. Science 275:1132–1136
96. Kluck RM, Martin SJ, Hoffman BM, Zhou JS, Green DR, Newmeyer DD (1997) Cytochrome c activation of CPP32-like proteolysis plays a critical role in a Xenopus cell-free apoptosis system. Embo J 16:4639–4649
97. Knudsen CM, Tung CS, Tourtelotte WG, Brown GA, Korsmeyer SJ (1995) Bax-deficient mice with lymphoid hyperplasia and male germ cell death. Science 270:96–99
98. Kops GJPL, De Ruiter ND, De Vries-Smits AMM, Powell DR, Bos JL, Burgering BMT (1999) Direct control of the Forkhead transcription factor AFX by protein kinase B. Nature 398:630–634
99. Koseki T, Inohara N, Chen S, Nunez G (1998) ARC, an inhibitor of apoptosis expressed in skeletal muscle and heart that interacts selectively with caspases. Proc Natl Acad Sci 95:5156–5160
100. Kroemer G, Dallaporta B, Resche-Rigon M (1998) The mitochondrial death/life regulator in apoptosis and necrosis. Ann Rev Physiol 60:619–642
101. Krown KA, Page MT, Nguyen C, Zechner D, Gutierrez V, Comstock KL, Glembotski CC, Quintana PJE, Sabbadini RA (1996) Tumor necrosis factor alpha-induced apoptosis in cardiac myocytes - Involvement of the sphingolipid signaling cascade in cardiac cell death. J Clin Invest 98:2854–2865
102. Kubota T, McTiernan CF, Frye CS, Demetris AJ, Feldman AM (1997) Cardiac-specific overexpression of tumor necrosis factor-alpha causes lethal myocarditis in transgenic mice. J Card Fail 3:117–124
103. Kubota T, McTiernan CF, Frye CS, Slawson SE, Lemster BH, Koretsky AP, Demetris AJ, Feldman AM (1997) Dilated cardiomyopathy in transgenic mice with cardiac-specific overexpression of tumor necrosis factor-alpha. Circ Res 81:627–635
104. Kuwana T, Smith JJ, Muzio M, Dixit V, Newmeyer DD, Kornbluth S (1998) Apoptosis induction by caspase-8 is amplified through the mitochondrial release cytochrome c. J Biol Chem 273:16589–16594
105. Lavoie JN, Nguyen M, Marcellus RC, Branton BE, Shore GC (1998) E4orf4, a novel adenovirus death factor that induces p53-independent apoptosis by a pathway that is not inhibited by zVAD-fmk. J Cell Biol 140:637–645
106. Leri A, Claudio PP, Li Q, Wang X, Reiss K, Wang S, Malhotra A, Kajstura J, Anversa P (1998) Stretch-mediated release of angiotensin II induces myocyte apoptosis by activating p53 that enhances the local renin-angiotensin system and decreases the bcl-2-to-bax ratio in the cell. J Clin Invest 101:1326–1342
107. Leri A, Liu Y, Claudio PP, Kajstura J, Wang X, Wang S, Kang P, Malhotra A, Anversa P (1999) Insulin-like growth factor-1 induces Mdm2 and downregulates p53, attenuating the myocyte renin-angiotensin system and stretch-mediated apoptosis. Am J Pathol 154:567–580
108. Levine B, Kalman J, Mayer L, Fillit HM, Packer M (1990) Elevated circulation levels of tumor necrosis factor in severe chronic heart failure. N Engl J Med 323:236–241

109. Levkau B, Scatena M, Giachelli CM, Ross R, Raines EW (1999) Apoptosis overrides survival signals through a caspase-mediated dominant-negative NF-κB loop. Nature Cell Biol 1:227–233
110. Li H, Zhu H, Xu CJ, Yuan J (1998) Cleavage of BID by caspase 8 mediates the mitochondrial damage in the Fas pathway of apoptosis. Cell 94:491–501
111. Li J, Billiar TR, Talanian RV, Kim YM (1997) Nitric oxide reversibly inhibits seven members of the caspase family via S-nitrosylation. Biochem Biophys Res Comm 240:419–424
112. Li Q, Li B, Wang X, Levi A, Jana KP, Liu X, Kajstura J, Baserga R, Anversa P (1997) Overexpression of insulin growth factor-1 in mice protects from myocyte death after infarction, attenuating ventricular dilation, wall stress and cardiac hypertrophy. J Clin Invest 100:1991–1999
113. Li ZH, Bing OHL, Long XL, Robinson KG, Lakatta EG (1997) Increased cardiocyte apoptosis during the transition to heart failure in the spontaneously hypertensive rat. Am J Heart 272:H2313–H2319
114. Liao R, Gwathmey JK, Wang CK (1999) A possible mechanism for decreased myocardial contractility in idiopathic dilated cardiomyopathy: significance of spatial relationship between Helix A and $Ca2^+$-binding loop II in human cardiac troponin C (abstr). Circulation 100 (suppl):II–60
115. Lindenmayer GE, Harigaya S, Bajusz E, Schwartz A (1970) Oxidative phosphorylation and calcium transport of mitochondria isolated from cardiomyopathic hamster hearts. J Mol Cell Cardiol 9:249–259
116. Lindenmayer GE, Sordahl LA, Harigaya S, Allen JC, Besch HR, Schwartz A (1971) Some biochemical studies on subcellular systems isolated from fresh recipient human cardiac tissue obtained during transplantation. Am J Cardiol 27:277–283
117. Liu X, Kim CN, Yang J, Jemmerson R, Wang X (1996) Induction of apoptotic program in cell-free extracts: requirement for dATP and cytochrome c. Cell 86:147–157
118. Liu X, Li P, Widlack P, Zuo H, Luo X, Garrard WT, Wang X (1998) The 40-kDa subunit of DNA fragmentation factor induces DNA fragmentation and chromatin condensation during apoptosis. Proc Natl Acad Sci 95:8461–8466
119. Liu X, Zou H, Slaughter C, Wang X (1997) DFF, a heterodimeric protein that functions downstream of caspase 3 to trigger DNA fragmentation during apoptosis. Cell 89:175–184
120. Lorenzo HK, Susin SA, Penninger J, Kroemer G (1999) Apoptosis inducing factor (AIF): a phylogenetically old, caspase-independent effector of cell death. Cell Death Differ 6:516–524
121. Lotem J, Kama R, Sachs L (1999) Suppression or induction of apoptosis by opposing pathways downstream from calcium-activated calcineurin. Proc Natl Acad Sci USA 96:12016–12020
122. Luo X, Budihardjo I, Zou H, Slaughter C, Wang X (1998) Bid, a Bcl-2 interacting protein, mediates cytochrome c release from mitochondria in response to activation of cell surface death receptors. Cell 94:481–490
123. MacLellan WR, Schneider MD (1997) Death by design: programmed cell death in cardiovascular biology and disease. Circ Res 81:137–144
124. Maines MD (1997) The heme oxygenase system: a regulator of second messenger gases. Ann Rev Pharmacol Toxicol 37:517–554
125. Malhotra R, Brosius FC (1999) Glucose uptake and glycolysis reduce hypoxia-induced apoptosis in cultured neonatal rat cardiac myocytes. J Biol Chem 274:12567–12575
126. Mannick JB, Hausladen A, Liu LM, Hess DT, Zeng M, Miao QX, Kane LS, Gow AJ, Stamler JS (1999) Fas-induced caspase denitrosylation. Science 284:651–654

127. Mannick JB, Miao XQ, Stamler JS (1997) Nitric oxide inhibits Fas-induced apoptosis. J Biol Chem 272:24125–24128
128. Martinou I, Desagher S, Eskes R, Antonsson B, Andre E, Fakan S, Martinou JC (1999) The release of cytochrome c from mitochondria during apoptosis of NGF-deprived sympathetic neurons is a reversible event. J Cell Biol 144:883–889
129. Marzo I, Susin SA, Petit PX, Ravagnan L (1998) Caspases disrupt mitochondrial membrane barrier function. FEBS Lett 427:198–202
130. Maulik N, Engelman DT, Watanabe M, Engelman RM, Das DK (1996) Nitric oxide – a retrograde messenger for carbon monoxide signaling in ischemic heart. Mol Cell Biochem 157:75–86
131. Maulik N, Engelman DT, Watanabe M, Engelman RM, Rousou JA, Flack JE, Deaton DW, Gorbunov NV, Elsayed NM, Kagan VE, Das DK (1996) Nitric oxide/carbon monoxide: a molecular switch for myocardial preservation during ischemia. Circulation 94:II-398–II-406
132. Maulik N, Sharma HS, Das DK (1996) Induction of the haem oxygenase gene expression during the reperfusion of ischemic rat myocardium. J Mol Cell Cardiol 28:1261–1270
133. Maurer I, Zierz S (1993) Myocardial respiratory chain enzyme activities in idiopathic dilated cardiomyopathy, and comparison with those in atherosclerotic coronary artery disease and valvular aortic stenosis. Am J Cardiol 72:428–433
134. McCarthy NJ, Whyte MKB, Gilbert CS, Evan GI (1997) Inhibition of Ced-3/ICE-related proteases does not prevent cell death induced by oncogenes, DNA damage, or the Bcl-2 homologue Bak. J Cell Biol 136:215–227
135. McCord JM (1998) Iron, free radicals, and oxidative injury. Semin Hematol 35:5–12
136. Melkonyan HS, Chang WC, Shapiro JP, Mahadevappa M, Fitzpatrick PA, Kiefer MC, Tomei LD, Umansky SR (1997) SARPs: a family of secreted apoptosis-related proteins. Proc Natl Acad Sci 94:13636–13641
137. Mestril R, Dillmann WH (1991) Heat shock and adaptive response to ischemia. Trends Cardiovasc Med 1:240–244
138. Mestril R, Dillmann WH (1995) Heat shock proteins and protection against myocardial ischemia. J Mol Cell Cardiol 27:45–52
139. Molketin JD, Lu JR, Antos CL, Markham B, Richardson J, Robbins J, Grant SR, Olson EN (1998) A calcineurin-dependent transcriptional pathway for cardiac hypertrophy. Cell 93:215–228
140. Morawietz H, Rohrbach S, Darmer D, Hakim K, Zerkowski HR, Holtz J-B (1996) Angiotensin converting enzyme inhibitor treatment upregulates the expression of endothelial nitric oxide synthase in human atrial myocardium (abstr). Circulation 94 (suppl I):I-521
141. Mosser DD, Caron AW, Bourget L, Denis-Larose C, Massie B (1997) Role of the human heat shock protein hsp70 in protection against stress-induced apoptosis. Mol Cell Biol 17:5317–5327
142. Mukae N, Enari M, Sakahira H, Fukuda Y, Inazawa J, Toh H, Nagata S (1998) Molecular cloning and characterization of human caspase-activated DNase. Proc Natl Acad Sci 95:9123–9128
143. Müller SP, Pregla R, Holtz J (1998) Anti-apoptotic action of insulin-like growth factor I (IGF-I) in myocardium of rats with hypertension due to inhibition of nitric oxide synthase (abstr). Naunyn-Schmiedeberg's Arch Pharmacol 358 (suppl 3):94
144. Müller-Werdan U, Schumann H, Fuchs R, Reithmann C, Loppnow H, Koch S, Zimny-Arndt U, He C, Darmer D, Jungblut P, Stadler J, Holtz J, Werdan K (1997) Tumor-necrosis factor α (TNFα) is cardiodepressant in pathophysiologically relevant concentrations without inducing inducible nitric oxide-(NO)-synthase (iNOS) or triggering serious cytotoxity. J Mol Cell Cardiol 29:2915–2923

145. Müller-Werdan U, Schumann H, Loppnow H, Fuchs R, Darmer D, Stadler J, Holtz J, Werdan K (1998) Endotoxin and tumor necrosis factor α exert a similar proinflammatory effect in neonatal rat cardiomyocytes, but have different cardiodepressant profiles. J Mol Cell Cardiol 30:1027–1036
146. Musaro A, McCullagh KJ, Naya FJ, Olson EN, Rosenthal N (1999) IGF-1 induces skeletal myocyte hypertrophy through calcineurin in association with GATA-2 and NF-ATc1. Nature 400:581–585
147. Narula J, Haider N, Virmani R, DiSalvo T, Kolodgie FD, Hajjar RJ, Schmidt U, Semigran MJ, Dec W, Khaw BA (1996) Apoptosis in myocytes in end-stage heart failure. N Engl J Med 335:1182–1189
148. Narula J, Pandey P, Arbustini E, Haider N, Narula N, Kolodgie FD, Dal Bello B, Semigran MJ, Bielsa-Madeu A, Dec GW, Israels S, Ballester M, Virmani R, Saxena S, Kharbanda S (1999) Apoptosis in heart failure: release of cytochrome c from mitochondria and activation of caspase-3 in human cardiomyopathy. Proc Natl Acad Sci 96:8144–8149
149. Neubauer S, Horn M, Cramer M, Harre K, Newell JB, Peters W, Pabst T, Ertl G, Hahn D, Ingwall JS, Kochsiek K (1997) Myocardial phosphocreatine-to-ATP ratio is a predictor of mortality in patients with dilated cardiomyopathy. Circulation 96:2190–2196
150. Neubauer S, Remkes H, Spindler M, Horn M, Wiesmann F, Prestle J, Walzel B, Ertl G, Hasenfuss G, Wallimann T (1999) Downregulation of the Na(+)-creatine cotransporter in failing human myocardium and in experimental heart failure. Circulation 100:1847–1850
151. Nicholson DW, Thornberry NA (1997) Caspases: killer proteases. Trends Biochem Sci 22:299–306
152. Nicotera P, Leist P (1997) Energy supply and the shape of death in neurons and lymphoid cells. Cell Death Diff 4:435–442
153. Nishigaki K, Minatoguchi S, Seishima M, Asano K, Noda T, Yasuda N, Sano H, Kumada H, Takemura M, Noma A, Tanaka T, Watanabe S, Fujiwara H (1997) Plasma Fas ligand, an inducer of apoptosis, and plasma soluble Fas, an inhibitor of apoptosis, in patients with chronic congestive heart failure. JACC 29:1214–1220
154. Nunez G, Benedict MA, Hu Y, Inohara N (1998) Caspases: the proteases of the apoptotic pathway. Oncogene 17:3237–345
155. Nunez G, del Peso L (1998) Linking extracellular survival signals and the apoptotic machinery. Curr Opin Neurobiol 8:613–618
156. Okamura T, Miura T, Takemura G, Fujiwara H, Iwamoto H, Kawamura S, Kimura M, Ikeda Y, Iwatate M, Matsuzaki M (2000) Effect of caspase inhibitors on myocardial infarct size and myocyte DNA fragmentation on the ischemic-reperfused rat heart. Cardiovasc Res 45:642–650
157. Olivetti G, Abbi R, Quaini F, Kajstura J, Cheng W, Nitahara JA, Quaini E, DiLoreto C, Beltrami CA, Krajewski S, Reed JC, Anversa P (1997) Apoptosis in the failing human heart. N Engl J Med 336:1131–1141
158. Olivetti G, Quaini F, Sala R, Lagrasta C, Corradi D, Bonacina E, Gambert SR, Cigola E, Anversa P (1996) Acute myocardial infarction in humans is associated with activation of programmed myocyte cell death in the surviving portion of the heart. J Mol Cell Cardiol 28:2005–2016
159. Orkin SH, Weiss MJ (1999) Apoptosis: cutting red-cell production. Nature 401:433–436
160. O'Rourke B (1999) Apoptosis: rekindling the mitochondrial fire. Circ Res 85:880–883
161. Orth K, Chinnaiyan AM, Garg M, Froelich CJ, Dixit VM (1996) The CED-3/ICE-like protease Mch2 is activated during apoptosis and cleaves the death substrate lamin A. J Biol Chem 271:16443–16446

162. Oskarsson HJ, Coppey L, Weiss RM, Li WG (2000) Antioxidants attenuate myocyte apoptosis in the remote non-infarcted myocardium following large myocardial infarction. Cardiovasc Res 45:679–687
163. Ozes ON, Mayo LD, Gustin JA, Pfeffer SR, Pfeffer LM, Donner MB (1999) NF-κB activation by tumour necrosis factor requires the Akt serine-threonine kinase. Nature 401:82–85
164. Papoff G, Cascino I, Eramo A, Starace G, Lynch DH, Ruberti G (1996) An N-terminal domain shared by Fas/Apo-1 (CD95) soluble variants prevents cell death in vitro. J Immunol 156:4622–4630
165. Paradis P, Dali-Youcef N, Paradis FW, Thibault G, Nemer M (2000) Overexpression of angiotensin II type I receptor in cardiomyocytes induces cardiac hypertrophy and remodeling. Proc Natl Acad Sci 97:931–936
166. Patterson SD, Spahr CS, Daugas E, Susin SA, Irinopoulou T, Koehler C, Kroemer G (2000) Mass spectrometric identification of proteins released from mitochondria undergoing permeability transition. Cell Death Differ 7:137–144
167. Pawlowski J, Kraft AS (2000) Bax-induced apoptotic cell death. Proc Natl Acad Sci USA 97:529–531
168. Piot CA, Padmanaban D, Ursell PC, Sievers RE, Wolfe CL (1997) Ischaemic preconditioning decreases apoptosis in rat hearts in vivo. Circulation 96:1598–1604
169. Poss KD, Tonegawa S (1997) Heme oxygenase 1 is required for mammalian iron reutilization. Proc Natl Acad Sci 94:10919–10924
170. Poss KD, Tonegawa S (1997) Reduced stress defense in heme oxygenase 1-deficient cells. Proc Natl Acad Sci 94:10925–10930
171. Raczniak TJ, Chesney CF, Allen JR (1977) Oxidative phosphorylation and respiration by mitochondria from normal, hypertrophied and failing rat hearts. J Mol Cell Cardiol 9:215–223
172. Reed JC (1994) Mini-review: cellular mechanisms of disease series: bcl-2 and the regulation of programmed cell death. J Cell Biol 124:1–6
173. Reed JC (1997) Double identity for proteins of the Bcl-2 family. Nature 387:773–776
174. Reed JC, Paternostro G (1999) Postmitochondrial regulation of apoptosis during heart failure. Proc Natl Acad Sci 96:7614–7616
175. Rohrbach S, Yan X, Weinberg E, Hasan F, Bartunek J, Marchionni MA, Lorell BH (1999) Neuregulin in cardiac hypertrophy in rats with aortic stenosis: differential expression of erbB2 and erbB4 receptors. Circulation 100:407–412
176. Romashkova JA, Makarov SS (1999) NF-κB is a target of AKT in anti-apoptotic PDGF signalling. Nature 401:86–90
177. Roy N, Deveraux QL, Takahashi R, Salvesen GS, Reed JC (1997) The c-IAP-1 and c-IAP-2 proteins are direct inhibitors of specific caspases. Embo J 16:6914–6925
178. Sabbah HN, Sharov V, Riddle JM, Kono T, Lesch M, Goldstein S (1992) Mitochondrial abnormalities in myocardium of dogs with chronic heart failure. J Mol Cell Cardiol 24:1333–1347
179. Sahara S, Aoto M, Eguchi Y, Imamoto N, Yoneda Y, Tsujimoto Y (1999) Acinus is a caspase-3-activated protein required for apoptotic chromatin condensation. Nature 401:168–173
180. Sakahira H, Enari M, Nagata S (1998) Cleavage of CAD inhibitor in CAD activation and DNA degradation during apoptosis. Nature 391:96–99
181. Samali A, Zhivotovsky B, Jones DP, Orrenius S (1998) Detection of pro-caspase-3 in cytosol and mitochondria of various tissues. FEBS Lett 431:167–169
182. Saraste A, Pulkki K, Kallajoki M, Heikkilä P, Laine P, Mattila S, Nieminen MS, Parvinen M, Voipio-Pulkki LM (1999) Cardiomyocyte apoptosis and progression of heart failure to transplantation. Eur J Clin Invest 29:380–386

183. Saraste A, Pulkki K, Kallajoki M, Henriksen K, Parvinen M, Voipio-Pulkki LM (1997) Apoptosis in human acute myocardial infarction. Circulation 95:320–323
184. Scaffidi C, Fulda S, Srinivasan A, Friesen C, Li F, Tomaselli KJ, Debatin KM, Krammer PH, Peter ME (1998) Two CD95 (APO-1/Fas) signaling pathways. EMBO J 17:1675–1687
185. Schaper J, Froede R, Hein S, Buck A, Hashizume H, Speiser B, Briedl A, Bleese N (1991) Impairment of the myocardial ultrastructure and changes of the cytoskeleton in dilated cardiomyopathy. Circulation 83:504–514
186. Schaper J, Lorenz-Meyer S, Suzuki K (1999) The role of apoptosis in dilated cardiomyopathy. Herz 24:219–224
187. Scheid MP, Duronio V (1998) Dissociation of cytokine-induced phosphorylation of BAD and activation of PKB/akt: involvement of MEK upstream of BAD phosphorylation. Proc Natl Acad Sci 95:7439–7444
188. Schellenberger E, Szibor M, Holtz J (2000) In vivo imaging of apoptosis in overload-induced heart failure: potential approaches and application implications. Z Kardiol (in press)
189. Schumann H, Holtz J, Zerkowski HR, Hatzfeld M (2000) Expression of secreted frizzled related proteins 3 and 4 in human ventricular myocardium correlates with apoptosis related gene expression. Cardiovasc Res 45:720–728
190. Schumann H, Morawietz H, Hakim K, Zerkowski HR, Eschenhagen T, Holtz J, Darmer D (1997) Alternative splicing of the primary Fas transcript generating soluble Fas antagonists is suppressed in the failing human ventricular myocardium. Biochem Biophys Res Comm 239:794–798
191. Schwartz SM (1998) Cell death and the caspase cascade. Circulation 97:227–229
192. Schwarz F, Schaper J, Kittstein D, Flameng W, Walter P, Schaper W (1981) Reduced volume fraction of myofibrils in myocardium of patients with decompensated pressure overload. Circulation 63:1299–1304
193. Semsarian C, Wu MJ, Ju YK, Marciniec T, Yeoh T, Allen DG, Harvey RP, Graham RM (1999) Skeletal muscle hypertrophy is mediated by a $Ca2^{+}$-dependent calcineurin signalling pathway. Nature 400:576–581
194. Seta Y, Shan K, Bozkurt B, Oral H, Mann DL (1996) Basic mechanisms in heart failure: the cytokine hypothesis. J Cardiac Failure 2:243–249
195. Sharma HS, Maulik N, Gho BCG, Das DK, Verdouw PD (1996) Coordinated expression of heme oxygenase-1 and ubiquitin in the porcine heart subjected to ischemia and reperfusion. Mol Cell Biochem 157:111–116
196. Singh K, Communal C, Sawyer DB, Colucci WS (2000) Adrenergic regulation of myocardial apoptosis. Cardiovasc Res 45:713–719
197. Skulachev VP (1996) Role of uncoupled and non-coupled oxidations in maintenance of safely low levels of oxygen and its one-electron reductants. Quart Rev Biophys 29:169–202
198. Soares MP, Lin Y, Anrather J, Csizmadia E, Takigami K, Sato K, Grey ST, Colvin RB, Choi AM, Poss KD, Bach FH (1998) Expression of heme oxygenase-1 can determine cardiac xenograft survival. Nature Med 4:1073–1077
199. Srinivasula SM, Ahmad M, Fernandes-Alnemri T, Alnemri ES (1998) Autoactivation of procaspase-9 by Apaf-1-mediated oligomerization. Mol Cell 1:949–957
200. Stocker R, Yamamoto Y, McDonagh AF, Glazer AN, Ames BN (1987) Bilirubin is an antioxidant of physiological importance. Science 235:1043–1046
201. Stone JR, Marletta MA (1994) Soluble guanylate cyclase from bovine lung: activation by nitric oxide and carbon monoxide and spectral characterization of the ferrous and ferric states. Biochemistry 33:36–40
202. Stroh C, Schulze-Osthoff K (1998) Death by a thousand cuts: an ever increasing list of caspase substrates. Cell Death Diff 5:997–1000

203. Susin SA, Lorenzo HK, Zamzami N, Marzo I, Brenner C, Larochette N, Prévost MC, Alzari PM, Kroemer G (1999) Mitochondrial release of caspase-2 and -9 during the apoptotic process. J Exp Med 189:381–393
204. Susin SA, Lorenzo HK, Zamzami N, Marzo I, Snow BE, Brothers GM, Mangion J, Jacotot E, Costantini P, Loeffler M, Larochette N, Goodletti DR, Aebersold R, Siderovski DP, Penninger JM, Kroemer G (1999) Molecular characterization of mitochondrial apoptosis-inducing factor. Nature 397:441–446
205. Taigen T, De Windt LJ, Lim HW, Molketin JD (2000) Targeted inhibition of calcineurin prevents agonist-induced cardiomyocyte hypertrophy. Proc Natl Acad Sci 97:1196–1201
206. Takahashi A, Alnemri ES, Lazebnik YA, Fernandes-Alnemri T, Litwack G, Moir RD, Goldman RD, Poirier GG, Kaufmann SH, Earnshaw WC (1996) Cleavage of lamin A by Mch2α but not CPP32: multiple interleukin 1β-converting enzyme-related proteases with distinct substrate recognition properties are active in apoptosis. Proc Natl Acad Sci 93:8395–8400
207. Takemoto M, Egashira K, Usui M, Numaguchi K, Tomita H, Tsutsui H, Shimokawa H, Sueishi K, Takeshita A (1997) Important role of tissue angiotensin-converting enzyme activity in the pathogenesis of coronary vascular and myocardial structural changes induced by long-term blockade of nitric oxide synthesis in rats. J Clin Invest 99:278–287
208. Tanaka M, Ito H, Adachi S, Akimoto H, Nishikawa T, Kasajima T, Marumo F, Hiroe M (1994) Hypoxia induces apoptosis with enhanced expression of Fas antigen messenger RNA in cultured neonatal rat cardiomyocytes. Circ Res 75:426–433
209. Teiger E, Dam TV, Richard L, Wisnewsky C, Tea BS, Gaboury L, Tremblay J, Schwartz K, Hamet P (1996) Apoptosis in pressure overload-induced heart hypertrophy in the rat. J Clin Invest 97:2891–2897
210. Tewari M, Dixit VM (1995) Fas- and tumor necrosis factor-induced apoptosis is inhibited by the pox virus crmA gene product. J Biol Chem 270:3255–3260
211. Thornberry NA, Lazebnik Y (1998) Caspases: enemies within. Science 281:1313–1316
212. Torre-Amione G, Bozkurt B, Deswal A, Mann DL (1999) An overview of tumor necrosis factor α and the failing human heart. Curr Opin Cardiol 14:206–210
213. Torre-Amione G, Kapadia S, Benedict C, Oral H, Young JB, Mann DL (1996) Proinflammatory cytokine levels in patients with depressed left ventricular ejection fraction: a report from the Studies of Left Ventricular Dysfunction (SOLVD). J Am Coll Cardiol 27:1201–1206
214. Torre-Amione G, Kapadia S, Lee J, Bies RD, Lebovitz R, Mann DL (1995) Expression and functional significance of tumor necrosis factor receptors in human myocardium. Circulation 92:1487–1493
215. Torre-Amione G, Stetson SJ, Youker KA, Durand JB, Radovancevic B, Delgado RM, Frazier OH, Entman ML, Noon GP (1999) Decreased expression of tumor necrosis factor-alpha in failing human myocardium after mechanical circulatory support: a potential mechanism for cardiac recovery. Circulation 100:1189–1193
216. Torriglia A, Perani P, Brossas JY, Chaudun E, Treton J, Courtois Y, Counis MF (1998) L-DNase II, a molecule that links proteases and endonucleases in apoptosis, derives from the ubiquitous serpin leukocyte elastase inhibitor [published erratum appears in Mol Cell Biol 1998 Aug; 18(8):4947]. Mol Cell Biol 18:3612–3619
217. Trost SU, Omens JH, Karlon WJ, Meyer M, Mestril R, Covell JW, Dillmann WH (1998) Protection against myocardial dysfunction after a brief ischemic period in transgenic mice expressing inducible heat shock protein 70. J Clin Invest 101:855–862

218. Tsujimoto Y (1997) Apoptosis and necrosis: intracellular ATP levels as a determinant for cell death modes. Cell Death Diff 4:429–434
219. Tsujimoto Y (1998) Role of Bcl-2 family proteins in apoptosis: apoptosomes or mitochondria? Genes to Cells 3:697–707
220. Tsujimoto Y, Shimizu S (2000) Bcl-2 family: life-or-death switch. FEBS Lett 466:6–10
221. Vancompernolle K, Van Herreweghe F, Pynaert G, Van de Craen M, De Vos K, Totty N, Sterling A, Fiers W, Vandenbeele P, Grooten J (1998) Atractyloside-induced release of cathepsin B, a protease with caspase-processing activity. FEBS Lett 438:150–158
222. Van der Heiden MG, Chandel NS, Williamson EK, Schumacker PT, Thompson CB (1997) Bcl-x_L regulates the membrane potential and volume homeostasis of mitochondria. Cell 91:627–637
223. Van der Heiden MG, Thompson CB (1999) Bcl-2 proteins: regulators of apoptosis or of mitochondrial homeostasis? Nature Cell Biol 1:E209–E216
224. Villa P, Kaufmann SH, Earnshaw WC (1997) Caspases and caspases inhibitors. TIBS 22:388–393
225. Villani G, Greco M, Papa S, Attardi G (1998) Low reserve of cytochrome c oxidase capacity in vivo in the respiratory chain of a variety of human cell types. J Biol Chem 273:31829–31836
226. Wang CY, Mayo MW, Korneluk RG, Goeddel DV, Baldwin AS (1998) NF-kappaB antiapoptosis: induction of TRAF1 and TRAF2 and c-IAP1 and c-IAP2 to suppress caspase-8 activation. Science 281:1680–1683
227. Wang HG, Pathan N, Ethell IM, Krajewski S, Yamaguchi Y, Shibasaki F, McKeon F, Bobo T, Franke TF, Reed JC (1999) $Ca2^+$-induced apoptosis through calcineurin dephosphorylation of BAD. Science 284:339–343
228. Wang HG, Rapp UR, Reed JC (1996) Bcl-2 targets the protein kinase Raf-1 to mitochondria. Cell 87:629–638
229. Wickman A, Isgaard J, Adams MA, Friberg P (1997) Inhibition of nitric oxide in rats. Regulation of cardiovascular structure and expression of insulin-like growth factor I and its receptor messenger RNA. J Hypertens 15:751–759
230. Wolf V, Ke G, Dharmarajan AM, Bielke W, Artuso L, Saurer S, Friis R (1997) DDC-4, an apoptosis-associated gene, is a secreted frizzled relative. FEBS Lett 417:385–389
231. Wollert KC, Heineke J, Westermann J, Ludde M, Fiedler B, Zierhut W, Laurent D, Bauer MK, Schulze-Osthoff K, Drexler H (2000) The cardiac fas (APO-1/CD95) receptor/Fas ligand system: relation to diastolic wall stress in volume-overload hypertrophy in vivo and activation of the transcription factor AP-1 in cardiac myocytes. Circulation 101:1172–1178
232. Wu CF, Bishopric NH, Pratt RE (1997) Atrial natriuretic peptide induces apoptosis in neonatal rat cardiac myocytes. J Biol Chem 272:14860–14866
233. Wyllie AH, Kerr JFR, Currie AR (1980) Cell death: the significance of apoptosis. Int Rev Cytol 68:251–306
234. Yamaguchi S, Yamaoka M, Okuyama M, Nitoube J, Fukui A, Shirakabe M, Shirakawa K, Nakamura N, Tomoike H (1999) Elevated circulating levels and cardiac secretion of soluble Fas ligand in patients with congestive heart failure. Am J Cardiol 83:1500–1503
235. Yamamoto S, Sawada K, Shimomura H, Kawamura K, James TN (2000) On the nature of cell death during remodeling of hypertrophied human myocardium. J Mol Cell Cardiol 32:161–175
236. Yaoita H, Ogawa K, Maehara K, Maruyama Y (1998) Attenuation of ischemia/reperfusion injury in rats by a caspase inhibitor. Circulation 97:276–281

237. Zamzami N, Susin SA, Marchetti P, Hirsch T, I G-M, Castedo M, Kroemer G (1996) Mitochondrial control of nuclear apoptosis. J Exp Med 183:1533–1544
238. Zechner D, Craig R, Hanford DS, McDonough PM, Sabbadini RA, Glembotsky CC (1998) MKK6 activates myocardial cell NF-κB and inhibits apoptosis in a p38 mitogen-activated protein kinase dependent manner. J Biol Chem 273:8232–8239
239. Zha J, Harada H, Yang E, Jockel J, Korsmeyer SJ (1996) Serine phosphorylation of death agonist BAD in response to survival factor results in binding to 14-3-3 not BCL-X. Cell 87:619–628
240. Zhivotovsky B, Orrenius S, Brugustun OT, Doskeland SO (1998) Injected cytochrome c induces apoptosis. Nature 391:449–450
241. Zoratti M, Szabo I (1995) The mitochondrial permeability transition. Biochim Biophys Acta 1241:139–176
242. Zou H, Henzel WJ, Liu X, Lutschg A, Wang X (1997) Apaf-1, a human protein homologous to C. elegans CED-4, participates in cytochrome c-dependent activation of caspase-3. Cell 90:405–413
243. Zou H, Li Y, Liu X, Wang X (1999) An APAF-1 cytochrome c multimeric complex is a functional apoptosome that activates procaspase-9. J Biol Chem 274:11549–11556

Chapter 15

Strategies to prevent apoptosis

A. Haunstetter, S. Izumo [1]

Department of Cardiology, University of Heidelberg, Heidelberg, Germany, and

[1] Cardiovascular Division, Beth Israel Deaconess Medical Center, Harvard Medical School, Boston, MA, USA

Rationale

Cardiac myocytes are terminally differentiated cells with distinct electrical and mechanical characteristics that exhibit a high degree of functional specialization. Although some controversy exists, they are generally considered to be post-mitotic, having lost their regenerative capacity [4, 65]. On the other hand, loss of cardiac myocytes is a pathologic feature of several cardiac disease states among which massive necrosis of myocardial tissue is the one that comes to mind first. However, in recent years increasing evidence has accumulated that myocyte loss by apoptosis may also contribute to the pathophysiology of myocardial disease [25]. Among others apoptosis was detected in acute ischemia and reperfusion, chronic heart failure due to dilated cardiomyopathy and ischemic heart disease, and myocardial hypertrophy due to increased afterload. This, in conjunction with the fact that the number of cardiac myocytes is a critical determinant for cardiac function, has increased the interest of cardiovascular researchers in defining the mechanisms and potentials of a treatment strategy aimed at inhibiting apoptotic myocyte loss. Based on current knowledge about myocyte apoptosis, apoptotic mechanisms that may be targeted to prevent myocyte apoptosis will be delineated (Fig. 1). Both inhibition of pro-apoptotic pathways and promotion of anti-apoptotic mechanisms will be considered in more detail. In addition, potential problems inherent to an anti-apoptotic treatment approach are also discussed.

Disrupting the pro-apoptotic cascade

Elimination of the pro-apoptotic stimulus

Myocardial ischemia, hypertrophy, myocardial remodeling and neurohumoral factors such as catecholamines have been shown to induce apoptosis in experimental and pathologic studies [6, 13, 31, 55, 61, 71, 73]. Therefore, it could be assumed that therapy aimed at reducing the intensity of these pro-apoptotic stimuli will limit the loss of cardiac myocytes by apoptosis. Any therapy that improves myocardial perfusion (e.g., coronary by-

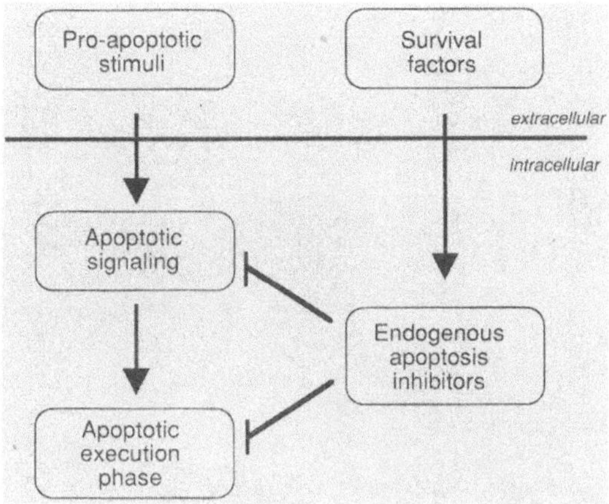

Fig. 1. Overview of potential strategies to interfere with apoptotic myocyte loss. Both pro-apoptotic and anti-apoptotic pathways may constitute targets for intervention.

pass grafting, angioplasty, and thrombolysis), reduces mechanical load [9, 73] (e.g., antihypertensive treatment, surgery for stenotic and regurgitant heart valves), and modulates neurohumoral derangement (e.g., ACE inhibition, β-blockade) [33, 89] is expected to limit pro-apoptotic stress on cardiac myocytes and, thus, should reduce the pace and extent of myocyte apoptosis. In addition, scavenging the ligand for the death receptors Fas and tumor necrosis factor receptor by soluble variants of these receptors may offer another possibility to prevent apoptosis by blocking the pro-apoptotic signal before it reaches the cell [21, 52].

Inhibition of intracellular pro-apoptotic signaling

Targeting the death receptor pathway. One major pathway that leads to the activation of caspases and finally to apoptotic myocyte death is through the activation of death receptors on the cell membrane (Fig. 2). At present, at least six different death receptor genes have been identified (Fas, TNF receptor 1, and the death receptors 3–6). All of these receptors show a high degree of homology and form a subgroup within the larger group of tumor necrosis factor receptors [5]. Their major distinctive feature is the presence of a death domain in the intracellular region of the protein. This domain is approximately 60–80 amino acids in length and is important in propagating the apoptosis signal within the cell [30, 72]. TNF receptor 1 and Fas are known to be expressed on cardiac myocytes. In fact, Fas seems to be upregulated during myocardial ischemia [32, 71, 76, 89].

Although the death domain is necessary for the induction of apoptosis by all death receptors, heterogeneity exists among death receptors regarding post-receptor signaling events [5]. Fas stimulation leads to the death domain-mediated recruitment of the adaptor protein FADD, which in turn binds the inactive caspase precursor procaspase-8 [11, 76]. It is believed

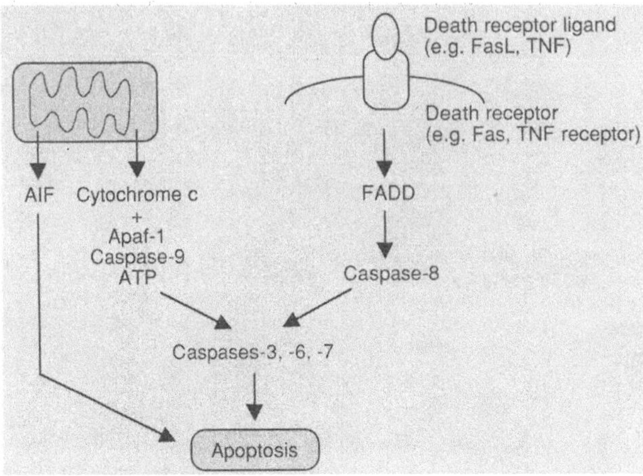

Fig. 2. Schematic diagram showing pro-apoptotic pathways that may be amenable to therapeutic intervention. *AIF* denotes apoptosis-inducing factor; *ATP,* adenosine triphosphate; *FasL,* Fas ligand; *TNF,* tumor necrosis factor; *FADD,* Fas-associated death domain protein.

that clustering of procaspase-8 at the Fas receptor complex is sufficient for its activation [49]. Activated caspase-8 is capable of activating downstream executioner caspases. Stimulation of TNF receptor 1 and death receptor 3 does not recruit FADD directly, but requires an intermediary adaptor protein called TRADD [12, 27]. In the future, pharmacologic inhibitors directed at the cell surface proteins Fas and TNF receptor 1 or membrane-permeant agents directed at the intracellular mediators FADD and caspase-8 may be developed. However, despite death receptor expression on cardiac myocytes being well documented, evidence for death receptor-mediated myocyte apoptosis in clinical cardiac disease is limited and relies mostly on correlational observations [32, 40, 89]. Therefore, further research is required to substantiate the role of death receptors in myocyte apoptosis and to estimate the potential benefit of any approach specifically targeted at the death receptor pathway in cardiac myocytes.

Mitochondrion-dependent pathway. Besides death receptors, mitochondria have been shown to be the second major mediator of apoptotic cell death (Fig. 2).

At present, two principal mechanisms are known whereby mitochondria can induce apoptosis

- caspase activation triggered by the release of cytochrome c from mitochondria and
- caspase-independent apoptosis induced by the release of apoptosis-inducing factor (AIF) from mitochondria [44, 67].

Release of the mature form of cytochrome c from the mitochondrial intermembrane space is the regulatory mechanism that initiates activation of caspase-3 [45]. Caspase-9, the scaffold protein apaf-1 and (deoxy)adenosine triphosphate were identified as essential co-factors for the activation of caspase-3. With regard to the mechanism of cytochrome c release, it was suggested that the voltage-dependent anion channel (VDAC), which is located in the outer mitochondrial membrane, may mediate cytochrome c release from mitochondria [64]. As shown in liposome particles, the pro-apoptotic regulators Bax seem to modulate pore size of the voltage-dependent anion channel (VDAC) such that cytochrome c can permeate through VDAC into the cytosol. Rupture of the outer mitochondrial membrane secondary to mitochondrial swelling has been proposed as an alternative mechanism to allow for the diffusion of cytochrome c into the cytosol [77].

Apoptosis mediated by apoptosis-inducing factor (AIF) also involves the translocation of the AIF protein from the mitochondrial intermembrane space into the cytosol and the cell nucleus. In contrast to the release of cytochrome c, translocation of AIF depends on the opening of the permeability transition pore, which is generated by the apposition of the VDAC of the outer mitochondrial membrane and the nucleotide transporter of the inner mitochondrial membrane [68, 90, 91]. In the open state the permeability transition pore induces the dissolution of the ion gradients across the inner mitochondrial membrane. To induce apoptotic cell death, AIF does not require caspase activity and AIF-induced cell death is therefore not inhibited by pharmacologic caspase inhibition [67].

Considering the role of mitochondria for apoptosis initiation, transformation of mitochondria into a pro-apoptotic state may provide targets for anti-apoptotic treatment. The pro-apoptotic Bax protein, the permeability transition pore and VDAC may be potential sites for intervention. However, at present suitable pharmacologic possibilities to test the efficacy of this strategy in the prevention of myocyte apoptosis *in vitro* or *in vivo* are limited.

Role of stress-activated protein kinases. Overexpression of constitutively active mutants of the stress-activated protein kinase p38α or its upstream activator MKK3 increases apoptotic cell loss in isolated cardiac myocytes, while dominant-negative p38α improves cell survival, suggesting a pro-apoptotic effect on the MKK3/p38α pathway in cardiac myocytes [81]. Likewise, overexpression of Gsα or Gqα induces myocyte apoptosis in transgenic mice and cultured cardiac myocytes, respectively [2, 23]. For these intracellular signal transduction pathways, the mechanisms of apoptosis regulation are not well understood. As downstream signaling of stress-activated protein kinases in general involves the regulation of transcription factors, transcriptional control of either pro-apoptotic or anti-apoptotic proteins may serve as the basis for survival control. Inhibitors of kinase activity and potentially transcriptional regulation may therefore provide additional anti-apoptotic targets. Considering the pleiotropic effect of these signaling proteins in both cardiac myocytes and other cell lineages side-effects may limit the applicability of this approach.

Inhibition of caspase activity. Caspases play a central role in the initiation and execution of apoptotic cell death [51, 74]. They constitute a unique class of intracellular proteases that characteristically cleave substrate proteins at aspartate residues within a tetrameric recognition motif specific for each caspase [75]. For example, caspase-3 efficiently recognizes and cleaves proteins at aspartate-glutamate-valine-aspartate (DEVD) peptide sequences. Based on functional and structural characteristics, caspases can be classified into three main functional groups: inflammatory (caspases-1, -3, -4, -5), upstream regulatory (caspases-2, -8, -9, -10), and downstream executioner caspases (caspases-3, -6, -7) [74]. Caspases within the latter group cleave a plethora of cellular target proteins, thus, inducing the morphologic alterations of apoptosis and finally cellular demise. Activation of all caspases involves the cleavage into a large (approx. 17–20 kD) and a small (approx. 10–12 kD) catalytic subunit that are held together by covalent cysteine bridges.

Induction of apoptosis through the death receptor pathway and the cytochrome c-dependent mitochondrial pathway converges at the level of the downstream executioner caspases. In addition, caspases-8 and -9 have been shown to be crucial upstream mediators in these two pathways. It therefore seems logical to inhibit caspase activity to prevent apoptotic cell death. In fact, potent pharmacologic agents (e.g., zVAD.fmk) have been developed that efficiently inhibit caspase activity *in vitro*. Some of these agents permeate the cell membrane and may therefore permit systemic administration of the inhibitor. Interestingly, initial attempts to use synthetic caspase inhibitors in an *in vivo* model of ischemia and reperfusion proved to be promising [85]. However, targeting a universal mechanism of apoptosis may be of concern as systemic toxicity due to inference with apoptosis in other cell lineages may become limiting for their use (see below). In addition, current evidence for efficacy is based on short-term observations and the long-term benefit of caspase inhibition in ischemic heart disease and other myocardial diseases requires further substantiation. Inhibition of caspases may not be effective when apoptosis is initiated by an AIF-dependent mechanism [67].

Promotion of anti-apoptotic pathways

Activation of endogenous anti-apoptotic mechanisms

Besides interfering with the pro-apoptotic sequence of events, promoting endogenous mechanisms that support myocyte survival will offer additional possibilities for intervention to increase net myocyte survival under pathophysiological conditions (Fig. 3).

Promoting anti-apoptotic signaling through Bcl-2 family proteins. Among the best-known protective mechanisms are the anti-apoptotic members of the Bcl-2 protein family (Bcl-2, Bcl-x, Bcl-w, Mcl-1, NR-13, Boo). Bcl-2 pre-

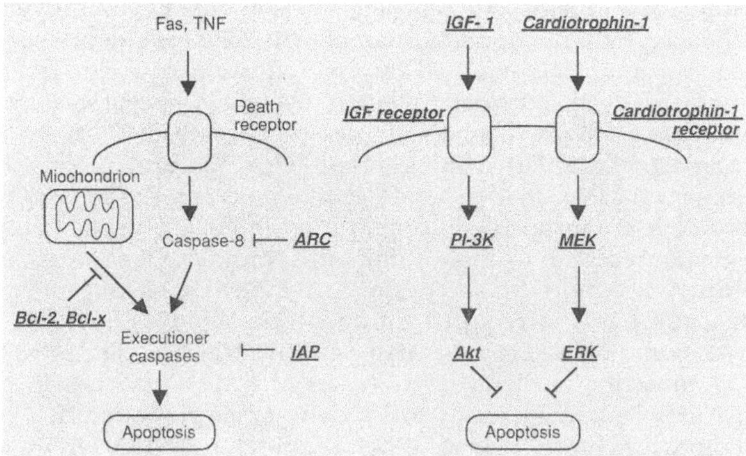

Fig. 3. Diagram showing endogenous anti-apoptotic pathways (underlined) and their presumed sites of interaction with pro-apoptotic signaling. *TNF* denotes tumor necrosis factor; *ARC*, apoptosis repressor with caspase recruitment domain; *IAP*, inhibitor of apoptosis protein; *IGF*, insulin-like growth factor; *PI-3K*, phosphatidylinositol 3-kinase; *ERK*, extracellular signal-regulated kinase; *MEK*, MAPK/ERK kinase.

vents the release of the pro-apoptotic factors cytochrome c and AIF from mitochondria [38, 67, 68, 86]. According to a recent model, pro-apoptotic Bax or Bak modulate the voltage-dependent anion channel (VDAC) of the outer mitochondrial membrane to permit the passage of proteins as large as cytochrome c [64]. In contrast, anti-apoptotic Bcl-2 family proteins prevent cytochrome c release by closing the VDAC channel even in the presence of Bax or Bak. In addition, Bcl-x was shown to interfere with the activation of caspase-3 by the complex formed by caspase-9, apaf-1, and cytochrome c released from mitochondria [10]. In conformity with mutant analysis in the model organism *C. elegans*, anti-apoptotic Bcl-2 family proteins regulate apoptosis upstream of caspases [10, 12, 83].

Although deficiency of Bcl-2, Bcl-x and Bcl-w does not induce a spontaneous cardiac phenotype in mice, this does not exclude a pathophysiologic significance of these apoptosis regulators in cardiac myocytes, as the role of anti-apoptotic Bcl-2 proteins may only become obvious under stress conditions [34, 47, 50, 60, 80]. In fact, in neonatal rat cardiac myocytes Bcl-2 inhibits apoptosis induced by overexpression of the nuclear transcription factor p53 [37]. Likewise, preliminary observations in mice indicate that overexpression of Bcl-2 reduces myocyte apoptosis after myocardial ischemia and reperfusion [7]. Although providing a powerful tool to assess the significance of apoptosis in myocardial disease states, it is currently not known how to efficiently activate anti-apoptotic members of the Bcl-2 protein family other than by gene overexpression. Interestingly, Bcl-2 can be activated by phosphorylation, and characterization of the enzymes involved would provide a target for pharmacologic modulation of regulatory kinases or phosphatases.

Regulation of apoptosis signaling through death receptors. As for apoptosis induced by mitochondria, mammalian cells have developed mechanisms to control apoptosis initiated by the activation of death receptors. Activation of the death receptor pathway involves consecutive steps of protein-protein interactions: ligand with receptor, receptor with the adaptor protein FADD, and FADD with caspase-8. One mechanism is based on the expression of genes that generate homologues of death receptors and caspase-8 that are incapable of propagating the death signal in the presence of the death receptor ligand. Within this group of apoptosis inhibitors are the decoy receptors for the death ligand TRAIL, lacking most of the intracellular part that is required for apoptotic signaling [57, 63], and the caspase-8 homolog CASH (also named FLIP, I-FLICE, FLAME-1) [24, 28, 29, 66]. A mutation in the catalytic center of CASH abolishes its caspase enzymatic activity. CASH seems to exert its anti-apoptotic effect by competing with the functional caspase-8 for binding to FADD within the activated death receptor complex.

In addition, ARC (apoptosis repressor with caspase recruitment domain) constitutes another type of inhibitor specifically interfering with death receptor-mediated apoptosis [39]. It contains two major domains: a CARD domain located at the carboxy-terminus which allows for its interaction with the upstream caspase and a domain which is rich in proline and glutamate residues. Functional analysis showed that ARC interacts with caspases-2 and -8, blocking their enzymatic activity. Interestingly, ARC is specifically expressed in skeletal and cardiac tissue, suggesting a special role of this inhibitor in cells of muscular lineage. To date, the role of endogenous inhibitors of death receptor-induced apoptosis in cardiac myocytes is largely unknown. In addition, mechanisms to promote the inhibitory potential of these proteins other than by overexpression remain to be elucidated. Strengthening these anti-apoptotic pathways therefore seems to be an attractive, although remote goal.

Promoting endogenous inhibitors of downstream caspases. Given the central role of caspases in the initiation and execution of apoptosis, it is not surprising that mammalian organisms developed potent inhibitors of caspases to prevent inadvertent apoptosis. So far, the inhibitor of apoptosis protein-1 (IAP-1), IAP-2, X-linked IAP, neuronal apoptosis inhibitor protein, and survivin have been shown to be potent inhibitors of the downstream caspases-3 and -7 [16]. Structurally, they are characterized by the presence of at least one baculoviral IAP repeat (BIR) domain. A single BIR domain as in survivin is sufficient to inhibit caspase activity, although not all BIR domains appear to have an equivalent anti-caspase activity as shown for the three BIR domains of X-linked IAP [3, 69]. As IAPs interfere with apoptotic signaling at a stage where most apoptotic initiation pathways converge into one common execution stage, they are expected to efficiently block apoptosis induced by a variety of pro-apoptotic stimuli. However, in contrast to Bcl-2, IAPs will not prevent apoptosis induced by AIF [67].

Promotion of survival by growth factor treatment

Several growth factors, such as nerve growth factor and interleukin-3, are essential to keep cells of the neuronal and hematopoietic lineages alive in culture. Withdrawal of growth factors induces extensive cellular apoptosis [18, 58, 84]. Interestingly, apoptosis of cultured cardiac myocytes induced by serum withdrawal or by treatment with the chemotherapeutic agent doxorubicin is inhibited by insulin-like growth factor I (IGF-1), suggesting a role for growth factors also for the survival of cardiac myocytes [62, 82]. Common to all of these growth factors is the intracellular activation of a signaling cascade involving phosphatidylinositol-3 kinase (PI-3K) and the serine/threonine kinase Akt [18, 22, 36, 58, 84]. The presumed anti-apoptotic mechanism of Akt involves phosphorylation and thus inactivation of Bad, a pro-apoptotic member of the Bcl-2 protein family [15].

Cardiotrophin-1 is a growth factor which induces a hypertrophic response in cultured cardiac myocytes [59]. In addition, cardiotrophin-1 promotes the survival of isolated cardiac myocytes kept under serum-free conditions [62]. Interestingly, in mice with cardiomyocytes deficient in gp130 (the common receptor subunit for cardiotrophin-1, interleukin-6, and leukemia inhibitory factor), pressure-overload induces myocyte apoptosis and ventricular dilation [26]. In contrast, in wild-type mice expressing gp130, pressure overload causes myocardial hypertrophy which is not followed by apoptosis and heart failure. This indicates that signaling through the gp130 receptor subunit can make cardiac myocytes resistant to apoptosis under cellular stress conditions *in vivo*. In contrast to IGF-1 and nerve growth factor, cardiotrophin-1 does not activate PI-3K, but the JAK/STAT and ERK kinase pathways [62]. However, only pharmacologic inhibition of the ERK pathway abolished the protective effect of cardiotrophin-1, suggesting a special role for ERK signaling in the survival signaling in cardiac myocytes.

Activation of growth factor receptors on cardiac receptors may represent a promising strategy to prevent myocyte apoptosis. The protein ligands for anti-apoptotic growth factor receptors are well characterized and are available for parenteral administration. Furthermore, cell surface receptors will be more easily amenable to the development of non-peptide pharmacologic agents. In fact, initial attempts have been made to treat chronic heart failure patients with human growth hormone, although it is currently not known whether this treatment reduces apoptotic myocyte loss in these patients [19, 56].

Limitations of anti-apoptosis as a new treatment approach

Uncertainties about the efficacy of anti-apoptotic strategy

The extent of a pathophysiologic phenomenon determines the potentials related to its inhibition. Therefore, detection of apoptotic myocytes in several cardiac diseases indicates a potential beneficial effect of anti-apoptotic treatment. Unfortunately, uncertainties exist with regard to the amount of myocardium that can be rescued by inhibition of apoptosis. In addition, implications of the preservation of myocyte number by anti-apoptotic treatment for cardiac function and survival of the organism have not been delineated. The reason for this is mostly related to shortcomings in methodology and experimental design of studies on myocyte apoptosis.

First, many studies have been performed in isolated cardiac myocytes to identify agents and conditions that either promote or inhibit apoptosis in cardiac cells. However, basal apoptotic rates in isolated myocytes are in the range of a few percent (ca. 1–10%) and thus by far exceed basal apoptotic cell loss in the myocardium which may be in the range of 0.001% [54]. This suggests that isolated cardiac myocytes are 'primed' to undergo apoptosis for reasons that are not exactly known, but which may be related to disrupted intercellular contact, altered electrical characteristics or deficiencies of extracellular survival factors. Therefore, quantitative data gained from isolated myocyte cultures have to be interpreted with caution.

Second, most *in vivo* studies of apoptosis in models of cardiac disease rely on TUNEL staining to estimate the extent of apoptosis in myocardial tissue. However, more recently concerns have been raised that TUNEL staining is not specific for apoptotic cell loss. In particular, in myocardial specimens from patients with dilated cardiomyopathy, positive-TUNEL staining was associated with markers for DNA repair [35]. Likewise, discrepancies have been noted between TUNEL staining and ultrastructural morphology with TUNEL-positive cells exhibiting characteristic features of necrotic myocytes [53]. Estimation of the potential benefit of apoptotic cell loss based on the extent of positive-TUNEL staining alone may therefore be misleading, as long as additional evidence for true apoptotic myocyte loss is not provided (e.g., evidence for caspase activation).

Third, some of the pro-apoptotic stimuli exert a pleiotropic effect on cardiac myocytes. For example, TNF was shown to induce apoptosis in cardiac myocytes and to have a negative inotropic effect [40, 41, 76]. Also other stimuli, such as activation of the death receptor Fas, myocyte stretch and ischemia, will affect myocyte function in several ways [20]. Salvage of myocytes from apoptotic cell death, therefore, cannot necessarily be equated with full functional recovery. In order to clarify these important issues, experimental studies using an interventional (in contrast to a descriptional) approach of apoptosis inhibition would be helpful to better delineate the potentials of anti-apoptotic treatment in myocardial disease.

Safety

Cell elimination by apoptosis is a physiologic process that helps to maintain tissue homeostasis. Ample evidence for the significance of apoptosis is provided by phenotype analysis in mice deficient in constituents of apoptotic pathways. For example, deficiency of caspase-3, caspase-9, and apaf-1, which are essential components of the mitochondrial pathway of apoptosis induction, causes embryonic lethality in mice associated with severe brain malformation [8, 42, 43, 47, 88]. Inhibition of Fas-induced apoptosis leads to a phenotype of lymphadenopathy, neoplastic disease and auto-immune disease in mice [1, 70] and mice deficient in FADD and caspase-8 die in utero due to impaired myocardial development and cardiac dilation [78, 87]. In man, hereditary mutations of the death receptor Fas result in a phenotype similar to the one seen in Fas-deficient mice, and Bcl-2 inactivation was shown to promote lymphoma development, indicating that concerns regarding side-effects and safety of anti-apoptotic treatment may actually apply to patients being treated with the anti-apoptotic approach [17, 46, 79]. These risks need to be kept in mind when defining the target for anti-apoptotic treatment of myocardial disease. While short-term inhibition of common downstream pathways of apoptosis in acute myocardial ischemia may be safe, chronic inhibition may be of concern. Unfortunately, apoptotic myocyte loss seems to be a continuously ongoing process in heart failure and during chronically increased load conditions, thus, necessitating chronic inhibition of apoptosis in order to be effective. One possible way to circumvent this problem is to identify upstream regulatory switches during apoptosis initiation which are unique to cardiac myocytes. At present, however, these mechanisms are ill-defined and should be an important focus of future research.

Acknowledgment. Armin Haunstetter was supported by the Deutsche Forschungsgemeinschaft (Ha 2606/1-1) and Seigo Izumo by the NIH (grant AG17008).

References

1. Adachi M, Suematsu S, Kondo T, Ogasawara J, Tanaka T, Yoshida N, Nagata S (1995) Targeted mutation in the Fas gene causes hyperplasia in peripheral lymphoid organs and liver. Nat Genet 11:294–300
2. Adams JW, Sakata Y, Davis MG, Sah VP, Wang Y, Liggett SB, Chien KR, Brown JH, Dorn GW (1998) Enhanced Galphaq signaling: a common pathway mediates cardiac hypertrophy and apoptotic heart failure. Proc Natl Acad Sci USA 95:10140–10145
3. Ambrosini G, Adida C, Altieri DC (1997) A novel anti-apoptosis gene, survivin, expressed in cancer and lymphoma. Nat Med 3:917–921
4. Anversa P, Kajstura J (1998) Ventricular myocytes are not terminally differentiated in the adult mammalian heart. Circ Res 83:1–14
5. Ashkenazi A, Dixit VM (1998) Death receptors: signaling and modulation. Science 281:1305–1308
6. Bardales RH, Hailey LS, Xie SS, Schaefer RF, Hsu SM (1996) In situ apoptosis assay for the detection of early acute myocardial infarction. Am J Pathol 149:821–829
7. Brocheriou V, Oubenaissa A, Hagege AA, Wassef M, Duriez M, Menasche P, Gilgenkrantz H (1999) Cardiac functional improvement by a Bcl2 transgene in a mouse model of ischemia/reperfusion injury. Circulation 100:1–774

8. Cecconi F, Alvarez-Bolado G, Meyer BI, Roth KA, Gruss P (1998) Apafl (CED-4 homolog) regulates programmed cell death in mammalian development. Cell 94:727–737
9. Cheng W, Li B, Kajstura J, Li P, Wolin MS, Sonnenblick EH, Hintze TH, Olivetti G, Anversa P (1995) Stretch-induced programmed myocyte cell death. J Clin Invest 96:2247–2259
10. Chinnaiyan AM, O'Rourke K, Lane BR, Dixit VM (1997) Interaction of CED-4 with CED-3 and CED-9: a molecular framework for cell death. Science 275:1122–1126
11. Chinnaiyan AM, O'Rourke K, Tewari M, Dixit VM (1995) FADD, a novel death domain-containing protein, interacts with the death domain of Fas and initiates apoptosis. Cell 81:505–512
12. Chinnaiyan AM, O'Rourke K, Yu GL, Lyons RH, Garg M, Duan DR, Xing L, Gentz R, Ni J, Dixit VM (1996) Signal transduction by DR3, a death domain-containing receptor related to TNFR-1 and CD95. Science 274:990–992
13. Communal C, Singh K, Pimentel DR, Colucci WS (1998) Norepinephrine stimulates apoptosis in adult rat ventricular myocytes by activation of the -adrenergic pathway. Circulation 98:1329–1334
14. Conradt B, Horvitz HB (1998) The *C. elegans* protein egl-1 is required for programmed cell death and interacts with the Bcl-2-like protein CED-9. Cell 93:519–529
15. Datta SR, Dudek H, Tao X, Masters S, Fu H, Gotoh Y, Greenberg ME (1997) Akt phosphorylation of BAD couples survival signals to the cell-intrinsic death machinery. Cell 91:231–241
16. Devereaux QL, Takahashi R, Salvesen GS, Reed JC (1997) X-linked IAP is a direct inhibitor of cell-death proteases. Nature 388:300–304
17. Drappa J, Vaishnaw AK, Sullivan KE, Chu JL, Elkon KB (1996) Fas gene mutations in the Canale-Smith syndrome, an inherited lymphoproliferative disorder associated with autoimmunity. N Engl J Med 335:1643–1649
18. Dudek H, Datta SR, Franke TF, Birnbaum MJ, Yao R, Cooper GM, Segal RA, Kaplan DR, Greenberg ME (1997) Regulation of neuronal survival by the serine-threonine protein kinase Akt. Science 275:661–665
19. Fazio S, Sabatini D, Capaldo B, Vigorito C, Giordano A, Guida R, Pardo F, Biondi B, Sacca L (1996) A preliminary study of growth hormone in the treatment of dilated cardiomyopathy. New Engl J Med 334:809–814
20. Felzen B, Shilkrut M, Less H, Sarapov I, Maor G, Coleman R, Robinson RB, Berke G, Binah O (1998) Fas (CD95/Apo-1)-mediated damage to ventricular myocytes induced by cytotoxic T lymphocytes from perforin-deficient mice. Circ Res 82:438–450
21. Ferrari R, Bachetti T, Confortini R, Opasich C, Febo O, Corti A, Cassani G, Visioli O (1995) Tumor necrosis factor soluble receptors in patients with various degrees of congestive heart failure. Circulation 92:1479–1486
22. Franke TF, Kaplan DR, Cantley LC (1997) PI3K: downstream AKTion blocks apoptosis. Cell 88:435–437
23. Geng Y, Ishikawa Y, Vatner DE, Wagner TE, Bishop SP, Vatner SF, Homcy CJ (1998) Apoptosis of cardiac myocytes in Gsα transgenic mice. Circ Res 84:34–42
24. Goltsev YV, Kovalenko AV, Arnold E, Varfolomeev EE, Brodianskii VM, Wallach D (1997) CASH, a novel caspase homologue with death effector domains. J Biol Chem 272:19641–19644
25. Haunstetter A, Izumo S (1998) Apoptosis. Circ Res 82:1111–1129
26. Hirota H, Chen J, Betz UAK, Rajewski K, Gu Y, Ross J, Muller W, Chien KR (1999) Loss of gp130 cardiac muscle cell survival pathway is a critical event in the onset of heart failure during biomechanical stress. Cell 97:189–198

27. Hsu H, Xiong J, Goeddel DV (1995) The TNF receptor 1-associated protein TRADD signals cell death and NF-kappa B activation. Cell 81:495–504
28. Hu S, Vincenz C, Buller M, Dixit VM (1997) A novel family of viral death effector domain-containing molecules that inhibit both CD-95- and tumor necrosis factor receptor-1-induced apoptosis. J Biol Chem 272:9621–9624
29. Irmler M, Thome M, Hahne M, Schneider P, Hofmann K, Steiner V, Bodmer JL, Schroter M, Burns K, Mattmann C, Rimoldi D, French LE, Tschopp J (1997) Inhibition of death receptor signals by cellular FLIP. Nature 388:190–195
30. Itoh N, Nagata S (1993) A novel protein domain required for apoptosis. Mutational analysis of human Fas antigen. J Biol Chem 268:10932–10937
31. Itoh G, Tamura J, Suzuki M, Suzuki Y, Ikeda H, Koike M, Nomura M, Jie T, Ito K (1995) DNA fragmentation of human infarcted myocardial cells demonstrated by the nick end labeling method and DNA agarose gel electrophoresis. Am J Pathol 146:1325–1331
32. Kajstura J, Cheng W, Reiss K, Clark WA, Sonnenblick EH, Krajewski S, Reed JC, Olivetti G, Anversa P (1996) Apoptotic and necrotic myocyte cell deaths are independent contributing variables of infarct size in rats. Lab Invest 74:86–107
33. Kajstura J, Cigola E, Malhotra A, Li P, Cheng W, Meggs LG, Anversa P (1997) Angiotensin II induces apoptosis of adult ventricular myocytes in vitro. J Mol Cell Cardiol 29:859–870
34. Kamada S, Shimono A, Shinto Y, Tsujimura T, Takahashi T, Noda T, Kitamura Y, Kondoh H, Tsujimoto Y (1995) bcl-2 deficiency in mice leads to pleiotropic abnormalities: accelerated lymphoid cell death in thymus and spleen, polycystic kidney, hair hypopigmentation, and distorted small intestine. Cancer Res 55:354–359
35. Kanoh M, Takemura G, Misao J, Hayakawa Y, Aoyama T, Nishigaki K, Noda T, Fujiwara T, Fukuda K, Minatoguchi S, Fujiwara H (1999) Significance of myocytes with positive DNA in situ nick end-labeling (TUNEL) in hearts with dilated cardiomyopathy. Circulation 99:2757–2764
36. Kauffmann-Zeh A, Rodriguez-Viciana P, Ulrich E, Gilbert C, Coffer P, Downward J, Evan G (1997) Suppression of c-Myc-induced apoptosis by Ras signalling through PI(3)K and PKB. Nature 385:544–548
37. Kirshenbaum LA, de Moissac D (1997) The bcl-2 gene product prevents programmed cell death of ventricular myocytes. Circulation 96:1580–1585
38. Kluck RM, Bossy-Wetzel E, Green DR, Newmeyer DD (1997) The release of cytochrome c from mitochondria: a primary site for Bcl-2 regulation of apoptosis. Science 275:1132–1136
39. Koseki T, Inohara N, Chen S, Nunez G (1998) ARC, an inhibitor of apoptosis expressed in skeletal muscle and heart that interacts selectively with caspases. Proc Natl Acad Sci USA 95:5156–5160
40. Krown KA, Page MT, Nguyen C, Zechner D, Gutierrez V, Comstock KL, Glembotski CC, Quintana PJ, Sabbadini RA (1996) Tumor necrosis factor alpha-induced apoptosis in cardiac myocytes. Involvement of the sphingolipid signaling cascade in cardiac cell death. J Clin Invest 98:2854–2865
41. Kubota T, McTiernan CF, Frye CS, Slawson SE, Lemster BH, Koretsky AP, Demetris AJ, Feldman AM (1997) Dilated cardiomyopathy in transgenic mice with cardiac-specific overexpression of tumor necrosis factor-alpha [In Process Citation]. Circ Res 81:627–635
42. Kuida K, Haydar TF, Kuan CY, Gu Y, Taya C, Karasuyama H, Su MS, Rakic P, Flavell RA (1998) Reduced apoptosis and cytochrome c-mediated caspase activation in mice lacking caspase 9. Cell 94:325–337
43. Kuida K, Zheng TS, Na S, Kuan C, Yang D, Karasuyama H, Rakic P, Flavell RA (1996) Decreased apoptosis in the brain and premature lethality in CPP32-deficient mice. Nature 384:368–372

44. Liu X, Kim CN, Yang J, Jemmerson R, Wang X (1996) Induction of apoptotic program in cell-free extracts: requirement for dATP and cytochrome c. Cell 86:147–157
45. Li P, Nijhawan D, Budihardjo I, Srinivasula SM, Ahmad M, Alnemri ES, Wang X (1997) Cytochrome c and ATP-dependent formation of Apaf-1/Caspase-9 complex initiates an apoptotic protease cascade. Cell 91:479–489
46. Martin DA, Zheng L, Siegel RM, Huang B, Fisher GH, Wang J, Jackson CE, Puck JM, Dale J, Straus SE, Peter ME, Krammer PH, Fesik S, Lenardo MJ (1999) Defective CD95/APO-1/Fas signal complex formation in the human autoimmune lymphoproliferative syndrome, type Ia. Proc Natl Acad Sci USA 96:4552–4557
47. Motoyama N, Wang F, Roth KA, Sawa H, Nakayama K, Nakayama K, Negishi I, Senju S, Zhang Q, Fujii S et al (1995) Massive cell death of immature hematopoietic cells and neurons in Bcl-x-deficient mice. Science 267:1506–1510
48. Muzio M, Chinnaiyan AM, Kischkel FC, O'Rourke K, Shevchenko A, Ni J, Scaffidi C, Bretz JD, Zhang M, Gentz R, Mann M, Krammer PH, Peter ME, Dixit VM (1996) FLICE, a novel FADD-homologous ICE/CED-3-like protease, is recruited to the CD95 (Fas/APO-1) death-inducing signaling complex. Cell 85:817–827
49. Muzio M, Stockwell BR, Stennicke HR, Salvesen GS, Dixit VM (1998) An induced proximity model of caspase-8 activation. J Biol Chem 273:2926–2930
50. Nakayama K, Negishi I, Kuida K, Sawa H, Loh DY (1994) Targeted disruption of Bcl-2 alpha beta in mice: occurrence of gray hair, polycystic kidney disease, and lymphocytopenia. Proc Natl Acad Sci USA 91:3700–3704
51. Nicholson DW, Thornberry NA (1997) Caspases: killer proteases. Trends Biochem Sci 22:299–306
52. Nishigaki K, Minatoguchi S, Seishima M, Asano K, Noda T, Yasuda N, Sano H, Kumada H, Takemura M, Noma A, Tanaka T, Watanabe S, Fujiwara H (1997) Plasma Fas ligand, an inducer of apoptosis, and plasma soluble Fas, an inhibitor of apoptosis, in patients with chronic congestive heart failure. J Am Coll Cardiol 29:1214–1220
53. Ohno M, Takemura G, Ohno A, Misao J, Hayakawa Y, Minatoguchi S, Fujiwara T, Fujiwara H (1998) "Apoptotic" myocytes in infarct area in rabbit hearts may be oncotic myocytes with DNA fragmentation. Circulation 98:1422–1430
54. Olivetti G, Abbi R, Quaini F, Kajstura J, Cheng W, Nitahara JA, Quaini E, Di Loreto C, Beltrami CA, Krajewski S, Reed JC, Anversa P (1997) Apoptosis in the failing human heart. N Engl J Med 336:1131–1141
55. Olivetti G, Quaini F, Sala R, Lagrasta C, Corradi D, Bonacina E, Gambert SR, Cigola E, Anversa P (1996) Acute myocardial infarction in humans is associated with activation of programmed myocyte cell death in the surviving portion of the heart. J Mol Cell Cardiol 28:2005–2016
56. Osterziel KJ, Strohm O, Schuler J, Friedrich M, Hänlein D, Willenbrock R, Anker SD, Poole-Wilson PA, Ranke MB, Dietz R (1998) Randomised, double-blind, placebo-controlled trial of human recombinant growth hormone in patients with chronic heart failure due to dilated cardiomyopathy. Lancet 351:1233–1237
57. Pan G, Ni J, Wei YF, Yu G, Gentz R, Dixit VM (1997) An antagonist decoy receptor and a death domain-containing receptor for TRAIL. Science 277:815–818
58. Parrizas M, Saltiel AR, LeRoith D (1997) Insulin-like growth factor 1 inhibits apoptosis using the phosphatidylinositol 3′-kinase and mitogen-activated protein kinase pathways. J Biol Chem 272:154–161
59. Pennica D, King KL, Shaw KJ, Luis E, Rullamas J, Luoh SM, Darbonne WC, Knutzon DS, Yen R, Chien KR (1995) Expression cloning of cardiotrophin-1, a cytokine that induces cardiac myocyte hypertrophy. Proc Natl Acad Sci USA 92:1142–1146
60. Ross AJ, Waymire KG, Moss JE, Parlow AF, Skinner MK, Russell LD, MacGregor GR (1998) Testicular degeneration in Bclw-deficient mice. Nat Gen 18:251–256

61. Saraste A, Pulkki K, Kallajoki M, Henriksen K, Parvinen M, Voipio-Pulkki LM (1997) Apoptosis in human acute myocardial infarction. Circulation 95:320–323
62. Sheng Z, Knowlton K, Chen J, Hoshijima M, Brown JH, Chien KR (1997) Cardiotrophin 1 (CT-1) inhibition of cardiac myocyte apoptosis via a mitogen-activated protein kinase-dependent pathway. Divergence from downstream CT-1 signals for myocardial cell hypertrophy. J Biol Chem 272:5783–5791
63. Sheridan JP, Marsters SA, Pitti RM, Gurney A, Skubatch M, Baldwin D, Ramakrishnan L, Gray CL, Baker K, Wood WI, Goddard AD, Godowski P, Ashkenazi A (1997) Control of TRAIL-induced apoptosis by a family of signaling and decoy receptors. Science 277:818–821
64. Shimizu S, Narita M, Tsujimoto Y (1999) Bcl-2 family proteins regulate the release of apoptogenic cytochrome c by the mitochondrial channel VDAC. Nature 399:483–487
65. Soonpaa MH, Field LJ (1998) Survey of studies examining mammalian cardiomyocyte DNA synthesis. Circ Res 83:15–26
66. Srinivasula SM, Ahmad M, Ottilie S, Bullrich F, Banks S, Wang Y, Fernandes-Alnemri T, Croce CM, Litwack G, Tomaselli KJ, Armstrong RC, Alnemri ES (1997) FLAME-1, a novel FADD-like anti-apoptotic molecule that regulates Fas/TNFR1-induced apoptosis. J Biol Chem 272:18542–18545
67. Susin SA, Lorenzo HK, Zamzami N, Marzo I, Snow BE, Brothers GM, Mangion J, Jacotot E, Costantini P, Loeffler M, Larochette N, Goodlett DR, Aebersold R, Siderovski DP, Penninger JM, Kroemer G (1999) Molecular characterization of mitochondrial apoptosis-inducing factor. Nature 397:441–446
68. Susin SA, Zamzami N, Castedo M, Hirsch T, Marchetti P, Macho A, Daugas E, Geuskens M, Kroemer G (1996) Bcl-2 inhibits the mitochondrial release of an apoptogenic protease. J Exp Med 184:1331–1341
69. Takahashi R, Deveraux Q, Tamm I, Welsh K, Assa-Munt N, Salvesen G, Reed J (1998) A single BIR domain of XIAP sufficient for inhibiting apoptosis. J Biol Chem 273:7787–7790
70. Takahashi T, Tanaka M, Brannan CI, Jenkins NA, Copeland NG, Suda T, Nagata S (1994) Generalized lymphoproliferative disease in mice, caused by a point mutation in the Fas ligand. Cell 76:969–976
71. Tanaka M, Ito H, Adachi S, Akimoto H, Nishikawa T, Kasajima T, Marumo F, Hiroe M (1994) Hypoxia induces apoptosis with enhanced expression of Fas antigen messenger RNA in cultured neonatal rat cardiomyocytes. Circ Res 75:426–433
72. Tartaglia LA, Ayres TM, Wong GH, Goeddel DV (1993) A novel domain within the 55 kd TNF receptor signals cell death. Cell 74:845–853
73. Teiger E, Than VD, Richard L, Wisnewsky C, Tea BS, Gaboury L, Tremblay J, Schwartz K, Hamet P (1996) Apoptosis in pressure overload-induced heart hypertrophy in the rat. J Clin Invest 97:2891–2897
74. Thornberry NA, Lazebnik Y (1998) Caspases: enemies within. Science 281:1312–1316
75. Thornberry NA, Rano TA, Peterson EP, Rasper DM, Timkey T, Garcia-Calvo M, Houtzager VM, Nordstrom PA, Roy S, Vaillancourt JP, Chapman KT, Nicholson DW (1997) A combinatorial approach defines specificities of members of the caspase family and granzyme B. Functional relationships established for key mediators of apoptosis. J Biol Chem 272:17907–17911
76. Torre-Amione G, Kapadia S, Lee J, Bies RD, Lebovitz R, Mann DL (1995) Expression and functional significance of tumor necrosis factor receptors in human myocardium. Circulation 92:1487–1493
77. Van der Heiden MG, Chandel NS, Williamson EK, Schumacker PT, Thompson CB (1997) Bcl-xL regulates the membrane potential and volume homeostasis of mitochondria. Cell 91:627–637

78. Varfolomeev EE, Schuchmann M, Luria V, Chiannilkulchai N, Beckmann JS, Mett IL, Rebrikov D, Brodianski VM, Kemper OC, Kollet O, Lapidot T, Soffer D, Sobe T, Avraham KB, Goncharov T, Holtmann H, Lonai P, Wallach D (1998) Targeted disruption of the mouse caspase 8 gene ablates cell death induction by the TNF receptors, Fas/Apo1, and DR3 and is lethal prenatally. Immunity 9:267–276
79. Vaux DL, Cory S, Adams JM (1988) Bcl-2 gene promotes haemopoietic cell survival and cooperates with c-myc to immortalize pre-B cells. Nature 335:440–442
80. Veis DJ, Sorenson CM, Shutter JR, Korsmeyer SJ (1993) Bcl-2-deficient mice demonstrate fulminant lymphoid apoptosis, polycystic kidneys, and hypopigmented hair. Cell 75:229–240
81. Wang Y, Huang S, Sah VP, Ross J Jr, Brown JH, Han J, Chien KR (1998) Cardiac muscle cell hypertrophy and apoptosis induced by distinct members of the p38 mitogen-activated protein kinase family. J Biol Chem 273:2161–2168
82. Wang L, Ma W, Markovich R, Chen J, Wang PH (1998) Regulation of cardiomyocyte apoptotic signaling by insulin-like growth factor I. Circ Res 83:516–522
83. Wu D, Wallen HD, Inohara N, Nunez G (1997) Interaction and regulation of the Caenorhabditis elegans death protease CED-3 by CED-4 and CED-9. J Biol Chem 272:21449–21454
84. Yao R, Cooper GM (1995) Requirement for phosphatidylinositol-3 kinase in the prevention of apoptosis by nerve growth factor. Science 267:2003-2006
85. Yaoita H, Ogawa K, Maehara K, Maruyama Y (1998) Attenuation of ischemia/reperfusion injury in rats by a caspase inhibitor. Circulation 97:276–281
86. Yang J, Liu X, Bhalla K, Kim CN, Ibrado AM, Cai J, Peng TI, Jones DP, Wang X (1997) Prevention of apoptosis by Bcl-2: release of cytochrome c from mitochondria blocked. Science 275:1129–1132
87. Yeh WC, Pompa JL, McCurrach ME, Shu HB, Elia AJ, Shahinian A, Ng M, Wakeham A, Khoo W, Mitchell K, El-Deiry WS, Lowe SW, Goeddel DV, Mak TW (1998) FADD: essential for embryo development and signaling from some, but not all, inducers of apoptosis. Science 279:1954–1958
88. Yoshida H, Kong Y, Yoshida R, Elia AJ, Hakem A, Hakem R, Penninger JM, Mak TW (1998) Apaf1 is required for mitochondrial pathways of apoptosis and brain development. Cell 94:739–750
89. Yue TL, Ma XL, Wang X, Romanic AM, Liu GL, Louden C, Gu JL, Kumar S, Poste G, Ruffolo RR Jr, Feuerstein GZ (1998) Possible involvement of stress-activated protein kinase signaling pathway and Fas receptor expression in prevention of ischemia/reperfusion-induced cardiomyocyte apoptosis by carvedilol. Circ Res 82:166–174
90. Zamzami N, Marchetti P, Castedo M, Zanin C, Vayssiere JL, Petit PX, Kroemer G (1995) Reduction in mitochondrial potential constitutes an early irreversible step of programmed lymphocyte death in vivo. J Exp Med 181:1661–1672
91. Zoratti M, Szabo I (1995) The mitochondrial permeability transition. Biochim Biophys Acta 1241:139–176

Chapter 16

Neurohumoral modulation of metalloproteinases in cardiac failure: *impact on remodeling*

D.A. Kass, H. Senzaki, N. Paolocci
Division of Cardiology, Department of Medicine, and Department of Biomedical Engineering, The Johns Hopkins Medical Institutions, Baltimore, MD, USA

Introduction

A dominant hallmark of cardiac failure is progressive chamber dilation and structural remodeling. This process is thought to play a major contributory role to the later stages of chamber dysfunction and is linked to increased morbidity and mortality in various clinical studies [9, 16, 28]. The magnitude of dilation far exceeds anything achievable with acute loading stress, but rather involves structural rearrangement within the myocardial wall notably of the fibrillar collagen matrix surrounding myocytes and blood vessels. This process of collagen degradation and remodeling is principally mediated by matrix metalloproteinases (MMPs), a large family of enzymes synthesized by several myocardial cell types, and secreted and activated within the cardiac interstitium [3, 5, 38, 39, 41]. Recent studies have reported elevation of MMP expression in failing experimental and human heart failure [21, 36, 38]. Furthermore, inhibition of this enzyme system has been shown to limit progressive chamber dilation both in a rodent infarct model [26], and in cardiac failure induced by rapid ventricular pacing in the pig [35], supporting a role in chamber remodeling.

In addition to demonstrating the presence and activation of MMPs during cardiac dilation and remodeling, recent studies suggest these enzymes may mediate exacerbation of diastolic dysfunction induced by the interaction of neurohormones within the failing heart. In particular, angiotensin II is an important late-stage contributor to the evolution of failure [22], and inhibition of angiotensin-converting enzyme reduces chronic chamber dilation [8, 25], as well as mortality in heart failure patients [34]. Over the past several years, our laboratory has studied the mechanisms by which angiotensin modulates evolving cardiac failure, focusing notably on its interactions with MMP activity [29]. These studies have raised the novel hypothesis that MMP activation is an important feature of neurohumoral modulation in the failing heart and that this pathway in particular contributes to elevated diastolic chamber pressures and stiffness. The present review discusses recent advances in our understanding of the role of MMPs and the influence of neurohumoral modulation of these enzymes.

Metalloproteinases

The field of matrix metalloproteinases is relatively recent, stemming from a study by Gross and Lapiere [10] in 1962, in which a vertebrate enzyme that was able to attack the triple helix of native type I collagen was first reported. Since then, interest in MMPs has exploded with a current rate of nearly 1000 new studies per year. MMPs play broad normal physiologic roles, including development (e.g., embryonic development, bone growth, tooth resorption), reproduction (e.g., endometrial cycling, postpartum mammary gland involution), and maintenance (e.g., hair folicle cycle, angiogenesis, wound healing, neutrophil function). They also play important roles in pathophysiologic states involving tissue destruction (e.g., rheumatoid arthritis, cancer invasion and metastasis, ulcerative syndromes), fibrosis (hepatic, pulmonary, atherosclerosis), and structural weakening (e.g., aortic aneurysms and dilated cardiomyopathy). Their contributions to these various processes have been recently summarized in several excellent reviews [1, 24].

MMPs form a subfamily (matrixin family) of proteinases, which primarily depend upon zinc for their catalytic action. There are nearly 20 enzymes in this class. Those that have been particularly prominent in the myocardium include interstitial collagenase (MMP-1), type IV collagenase (MMP-2), stromelysin-1 (MMP-3), and membrane-type MT1-MMP [2, 5, 29, 36, 38]. There is also an important class of tissue inhibitors of the MMPs (TIMPs-1, -2, -3, and -4) which play a major role in regulating the activities of the matrixins in tissue.

MMPs displays considerable redundancy in their activity. For example, MMP-1, -2, -8, and -13 all have activity against gelatins and collagen type I; many act on collagen II and III, on elastin, fibronectin, laminin, etc. [1]. Stromolysin-1 (MMP-3) can activate other members of the MMP family in addition to collagen II and IV, gelatin, and many other enzymes. In this respect, attempts at removing a specific MMP in genetically engineered mice can offer insight into specific roles in disease processes [14], but may also reveal this redundancy [32]. The redundancy may be less problematic in the myocardium for several reasons: MMP expression is normally quite low in healthy hearts [29], and the number of species that appear active in the heart appears to be more circumscribed. Recent reports regarding the MMP-9 –/– mouse have found significant effects in inhibiting post-infarction dilation [26], supporting this suspicion.

MMPs are synthesized in an inactive pro-form, secreted into the interstitium and then activated typically by cleavage to reveal the active site [23]. Activation can occur by an extensive number of factors, including cytokines such as interleukins and tumor necrosis factor, growth factors, cell surface-active agents such as fibronectin fragments and EMMPRIN, chemical agents such as lipopolysaccharide or phorbol ester, heat shock, mechanical injury, oxidative stress, etc. [1, 24]. In myocardium, synthesis by fibroblasts has been presumed to be the dominant source of these enzymes. However, recent evidence suggests that MMP-2 can be synthesized within left ventricular myocytes [4], displaying activity against collagen IV and fibronectin. This suggests that myocytes themselves may participate in the synthesis and activation of these enzymes and thus to the chamber-remodeling process. The relative role of MMP synthesis by matrix versus myocyte sources remains to be elucidated.

MMPs and dilated cardiomyopathy

While the number of studies reporting on MMP involvement in tumor pathophysiology, uterine function, or bone and tooth extends well into the thousands, there are remarkably few studies examining their role in dilated heart failure. These studies have consistently reported increased expression of MMPs, most commonly gelatinases A and B (MMP-2 and -9), and in some instances interstitial collagenase (MMP-1) and stromolysin (MMP-3). In an experimental study, Spinale et al. [36] reported a gradual decline in myocardial collagen content with progressive tachycardia-induced dilated heart failure which was preceded by increases in MMP-1, -2, and -3 (Fig. 1a). Selective upregulation of these enzymes were similarly reported in human myocardial tissue from DCM patients, particularly in MMP-9 and -3 which were found to rise by 422 and 563%, respectively [38].

While several investigators have demonstrated increases in MMPs with late stage cardiomyopathy, there is more controversy over the co-expression of the tissue inhibitors of MMPs (TIMPs). For example, Thomas et al. [38] reported substantial increases in TIMP-1 and -2 as measured by immunoblotting. In contrast, Li et al. [21] recently reported a reduction in TIMP-1 and -3 expression at both mRNA and protein levels, with no change in TIMP-2 and -4 mRNA, but a decline in TIMP-4 protein. These authors confirmed the rise

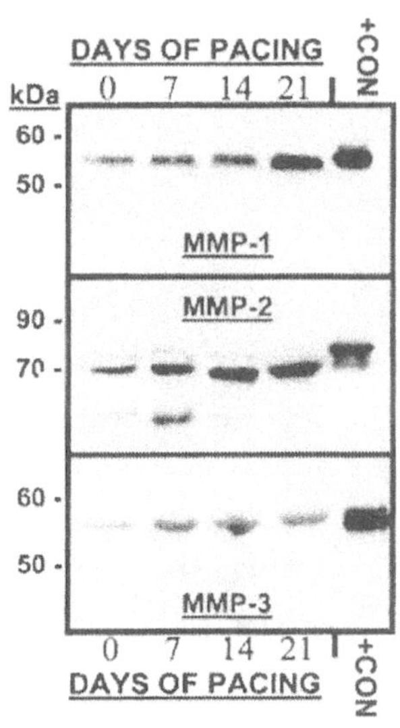

Fig. 1. Immunoblot of left ventricular myocardial extracts in a canine model of heart failure induced by tachycardia pacing (reprinted from [36] with permission). There was a time-dependent increase in MMP-1 and -2 which were maximal after 21 days of pacing. MMP-3 was also increased in this model, with a rise in expression observed after 7 days of pacing. Thus, multiple MMP species consistent with collagenase, gelatinase, and stromolysin are also activated in the pacing-tachycardia failure model.

in MMP-9, as well as net gelatinolytic activity of human failing myocardium supporting a balance-favoring matrix degradation and turnover.

In addition to studies demonstrating elevation of MMPs in failing hearts, recent reports have shown that inhibition of MMPs in models of failure can substantially dampen the extent of ongoing chamber dilation. Lee and colleagues [26] used a novel synthetic MMP inhibitor (CP-471,474) in mice exposed to a myocardial infarction. Animals receiving the inhibitor displayed significantly smaller increases in end-systolic and -diastolic dimensions, and had no significant net decline in fractional shortening as compared with controls. This effect [13] was most marked in animals with the greatest extent of initial chamber dilation (Fig. 2 a).

In another recent study, Spinale et al. [35] applied another inhibitor (PD166793) in pigs undergoing cardiac failure and dilation induced by rap-

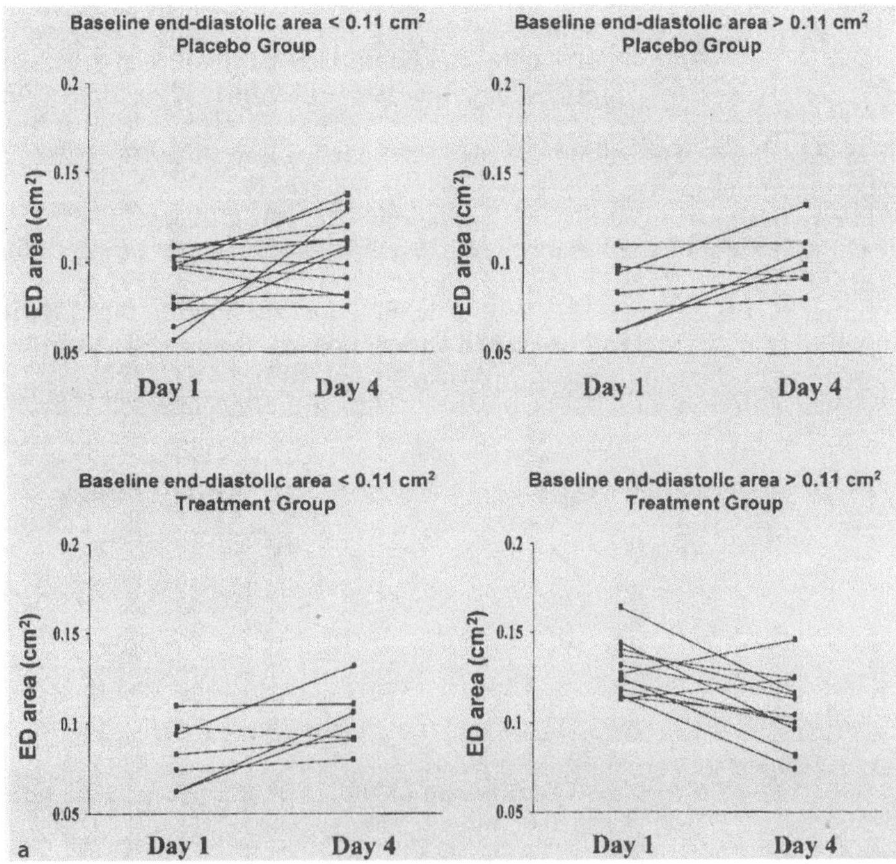

Fig. 2. a Reduction of post-infarct chamber dilation in rats by co-treatment with an MMP inhibitor. Animals with the largest rise in diastolic area after infarction demonstrated a reduction in chamber size with treatment. There was less influence of MMP inhibition in animals with little dilation post-MI (from [26] with permission).

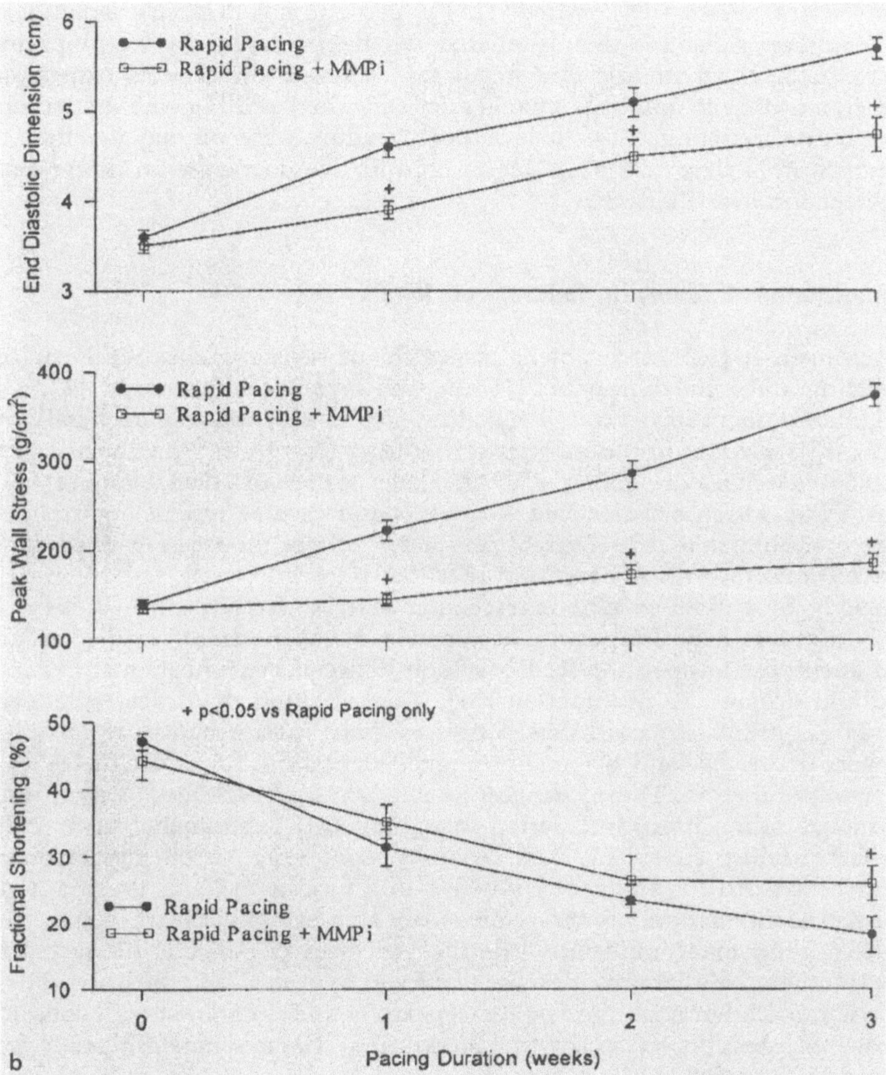

Fig. 2b. Similar effects on limiting chamber dilation in the rapid pacing failure model in animals treated with an MMP inhibitor (from [35] with permission).

id pacing. Treated animals displayed reduced end-diastolic dimension and peak wall stress, but greater endocardial shortening (Fig. 2b). These changes were accompanied by an increase in relative collagen fraction (from 2.3% in pacing only hearts to 10.6% in the treated, paced hearts). Myocyte elongation that is typically observed with pacing was diminished, yet myocyte-shortening velocity was not altered by MMP inhibition, suggesting that, while remodeling could be diminished, myocyte function itself was not necessarily restored. This is perhaps not that surprising given the complex signaling that is altered in the myocytes by rapid pacing which involves adrenergic downregulation, altered ion channel expression and function, and multiple changes in calcium handling and excitation-contraction coupling. Nonetheless, both studies were among the first to demonstrate a clear role of MMPs in chronic chamber dilation in two very different models of failure.

Angiotensin-II, evolving failure, and MMPs

Angiotensin-II (A-II) is a potent stimulator of myocardial extracellular remodeling and cellular necrosis [18, 39, 40], myocyte hypertrophy [27, 33], and alterations of myocyte cell signaling [7]. In addition to peripheral synthesis, it is directly produced within the heart [6, 19], and myocardial peptide levels reportedly increase in the later stages of dilated failure [17]. This juxtaposition of late-rising A-II levels and cardiac remodeling first led us to hypothesize that A-II might play a key role in modulating the decompensation of the failing heart and that this interaction was at least in part related to by its influence on extracellular matrix metabolism/catabolism.

To test this hypothesis, we developed a novel model of cardiac failure that attempted to open the feedback loop between neurohormonal stimulation and progressive dysfunction [29]. The evolution of cardiac failure involves an initial stimulus that depresses heart performance, which then triggers acute mechanical and hormonal adaptations to offset the decline in systolic function. These changes notably involve both catecholamine and hormonal stimulation (the latter including A-II, endothelin, AVP, BNP, adrenomedullin, etc.). The stimulation is itself toxic to the myocardium, further exacerbating the primary defect in a vicious cycle. If the goal is to study the interaction of neurohormones and evolving heart failure, the problem with many models is that the processes continually interact with one another. We therefore designed a novel approach in which neurohormonal stimulation could be applied separately and combined with subacute cardiac depression to study the interaction. Hormonal stimulation was provided by exogenously delivered i.v. A-II (at 10 or 17 ng/kg/min) for 4 days, and then continued as 48 hours of rapid pacing was superimposed (40/min).

The effect of superimposing A-II infusion and 48-h pacing is shown by the pressure-LV dimension loop analysis in Fig. 3. Each stimulus alone had little net effect on diastolic chamber function – as measured in conscious dogs. A-II infusion augmented systolic function, whereas 48-h pacing resulted in contractile depression and prolongation of chamber relaxation. However, their interaction proved synergistic, in that diastolic chamber stiffness and end-diastolic pressures rose markedly to levels that were otherwise only observed following 4–5 week exposure to rapid pacing with full evolution of cardiac failure. Systolic function was not synergistically af-

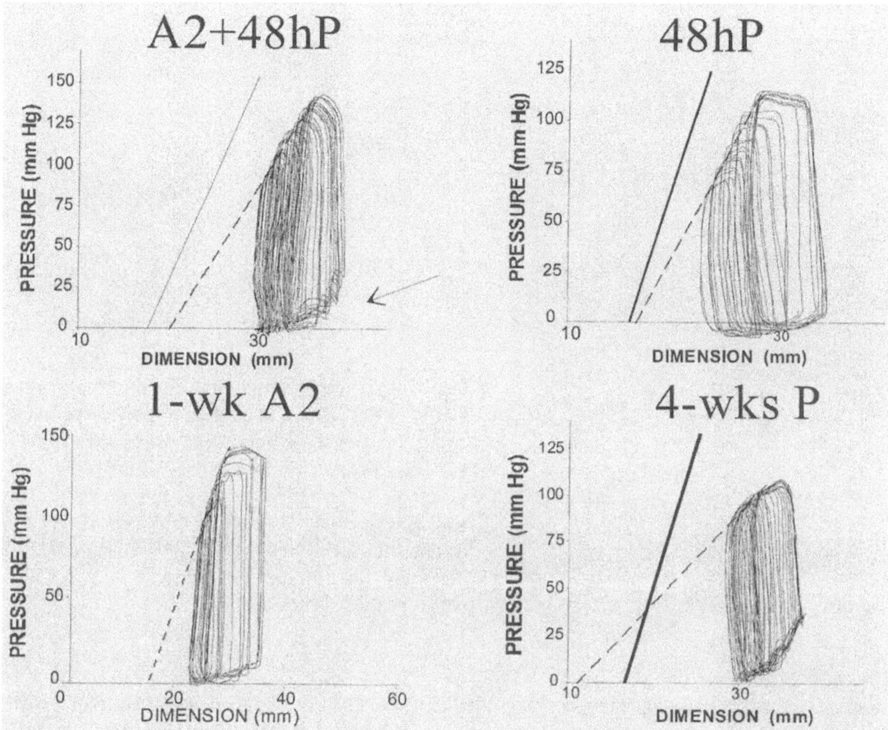

Fig. 3. Pressure-dimension relations demonstrating synergistic interaction of angiotensin-II infusion with evolving cardiac depression due to 48-h tachycardia pacing in the dog (A2+48hP). The result was a marked rise in diastolic pressures and stiffness (arrow), and contractile depression (downward rightward shift of ESPDV relation) (dashed line). Comparison data are also shown. 48hP – is the result with rapid pacing for two days only. The contractile depression is similar to A2+48hP, but there is no diastolic stiffening. 1-wk-A2 shows results with A-II infusion for 7 days only. There is no effect on systolic or diastolic function. The lower right panel shows data after 4 weeks of rapid pacing. The severity of diastolic changes is similar to that observed with the A2+48hP condition.

fected by the combination of A-II stimulation and 48-h-induced cardiodepression, – i.e., the level of depression observed with A-II plus pacing was similar to that with pacing alone. Interestingly, analogous findings were observed with active chamber relaxation, suggesting that the A-II/pacing synergy did not adversely influence active calcium handling – either in systole or diastole. Studies were also performed at lower doses of A-II that had no systemic vascular effect, and the results were virtually identical to those with the higher (vasoconstricting) dose, demonstrating that the interaction was independent of ventricular loading.

The specificity of the A-II-pacing interaction on diastolic chamber stiffening suggested a potential role for changes in the extracellular matrix. Figure 4 shows example zymograms [15] from endomyocardial biopsies taken from dogs during the progression of the A-II and A-II+pacing protocols. A-II

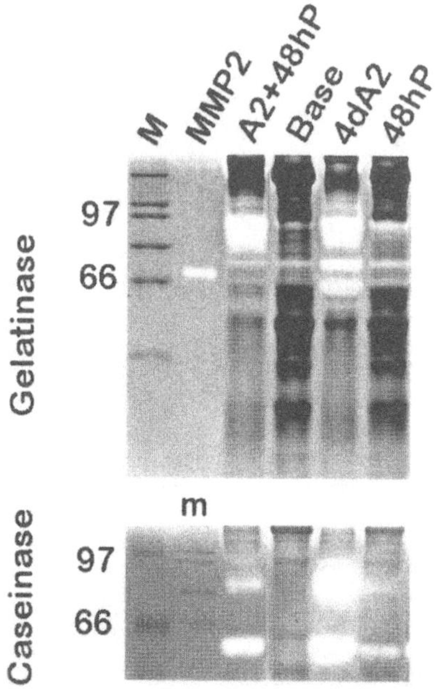

Fig. 4. *In vitro* zymography demonstrating increase in MMP species with A-II exposure alone for 4 days (4dA2) and with the superimposition with 48 h rapid pacing (A2+r8hP). Comparison control tissue (base) and 2-day rapid pacing only (48hP) are also shown. There is a strong lytic region in both the 92 and 72 kD territories consistent with gelatinases MMP-9 and MMP-2. The caseinase gel (bottom) shows lysis in a 52 kD region which is most likely MMP-1.

alone resulted in a marked increase in gel lysis (SDS gels containing gelatin or casein reveal enzyme abundance by local lytic bands), frequently with doublets in the bands (suggesting enzyme activation). This was not observed under basal conditions nor with 48-h rapid pacing alone. The increased MMP abundance persisted during the superimposition of A-II pacing. The molecular weights of these lytic bands were 72 kD (consistent with MMP-2), and 92 kD (consistent with MMP-9). Casein zymography further revealed lysis at a 52 kD location consistent with interstitial collagenase (MMP-1). The increase in MMPs was associated with inflammatory infiltrates and cellular necrosis, similar to that observed in rodents receiving A-II [12, 13, 37], but there was minimal collagen deposition.

One of the recognized limitations of *in vitro* zymography is that the isolation and processing of proteins and their separation by molecular weight on an SDS gel detaches MMPs from their *in situ* inhibitors (TIMPs). Since both are frequently co-expressed, MMP abundance on the gel may not indicate actual net tissue activity. Furthermore, protein activation is only indirectly reflected by a lower molecular weight of the active zymogen, often appearing as band doublets in the *in vitro* assay. This is not particularly sensitive, however. To further test if the changes in MMPs were reflecting tissue activity, we performed an *in situ* assay developed by Dr. Merry Lindsey [30]. In this assay, myocardial tissue is exposed to a solution containing a gelatin-linked fluorescent dye, and fluorescence can be observed microscopically when the gelatin is cleaved by MMPs. Figure 5 displays examples of this assay. Control tissue displayed minimal lysis *in situ*, with dark-

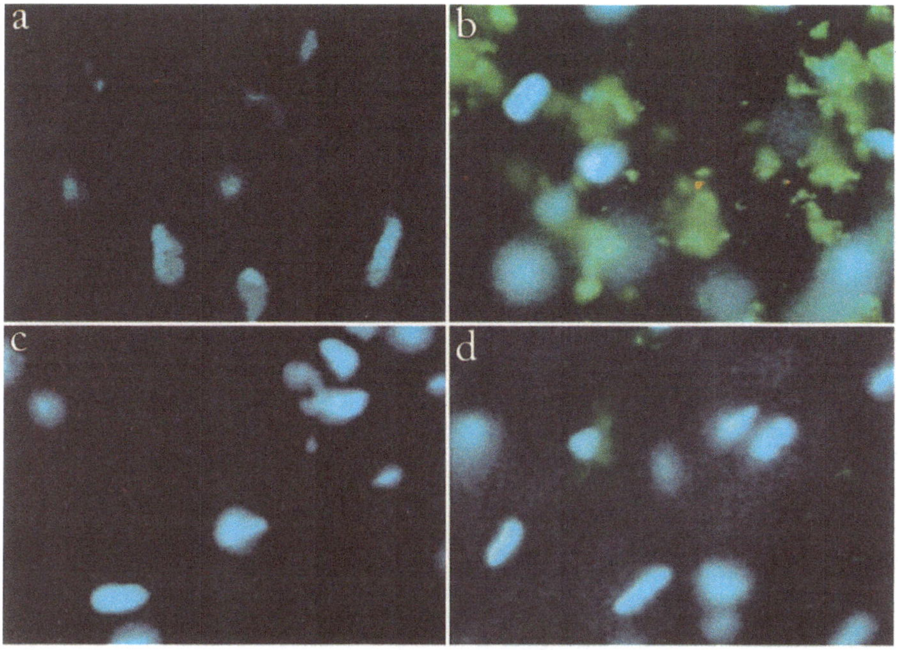

Fig. 5. *In situ* zymography demonstrating tissue activity of MMPs in the A-II+48 h pacing model. **a** is control tissue, with negligible MMP activity (dark background). The cell nuclei appear blue. **b** shows results with A2+48hP, revealing a green stain consistent with gelatin lysis by the myocardial tissue. This is inhibited by co-incubation with EDTA **c**, consistent with MMP inhibition by heavy metal chelation. Lastly, the gelatinase activity is largely inhibited by co-incubation with a blocking antibody for MMP-9 **d**, indicating that this species is playing an important role to total MMP activity.

blue nuclei co-stained separately (DAP1 nuclear stain) (panel a). However, the A-II-pacing tissue demonstrated marked fluorescence (green staining) (panel b). This was inhibited by co-incubation with the calcium chelator EDTA (panel c), which will broadly inhibit MMP activation. Also shown in this figure is the results of co-incubation with a blocking antibody to MMP-9 (panel d). This also markedly reduced the levels of *in situ* fluorescence, indicating that MMP-9 tissue activity was playing an important role in the overall MMP activation observed with this assay system.

To test whether continued exposure of myocardium to A-II was required to observe MMP activation and diastolic dysfunction, or if there was a *ghost* effect that remained after A-II exposure, we performed the following experiment. In a subset of animals, A-II was first infused for 1 week, then discontinued, and after 24 hours without A-II, 48-h rapid pacing was initiated. In these animals, diastolic pressure and chamber stiffness also rose substantially after pacing unlike that observed with pacing alone. MMP activation had declined after the A-II exposure, but was again reactivated upon removal of A-II in association with a fall in interstitial collagen.

Thus, in this setting where collagen content was reduced yet MMPs elevated, chamber diastolic stiffness paradoxically increased. This suggested that chamber stiffening may not simply be a function of the collagen content within the myocardium, but more its secondary structure and the activity of the enzymes involved with its turnover in the extracellular matrix.

Sympathomimetic effects of A-II

In previous studies performed in the rat, Janicki and colleagues reported that exogenously administered A-II induced direct toxic myocardial effects characterized by cellular damage, inflammatory infiltrates, and myocyte necrosis [37]. This was subsequently shown due to local release of catecholamines within the heart [13], and was inhibited by high dose propranolol [12, 13]. Based on these observations, we hypothesized that the accelerated diastolic dysfunction observed in the A-II combined with the 48-h pacing model might also be related to sympathomimetic effects from A-II [30, 31]. Animals were pretreated with atenolol at one of two doses for one week prior to exposure to A-II, and subsequent rapid pacing. The lower atenolol dose (200 mg/day) blocked maximal isoproterenol stimulated contractility by 30%, while the higher dose (nearly 2–3 g/day) fully inhibited this response. Interestingly, neither dose was associated with much change in baseline cardiac function or heart rate.

Figure 6 summarizes the results of this study. Treatment with high dose beta blockade prevented the diastolic stiffening observed with A-II+pacing alone, where this was not inhibited at the lower dose. Figure 6c summarizes the diastolic data for chamber stiffness and end-diastolic pressure. Figure 7 displays *in vitro* zymograms for low and high dose experiments. This reveals that the lytic bands observed with A-II+pacing (i.e., Fig. 4) were prevented by co-treatment with high dose but not low dose atenolol. Analogous results were obtained using the *in situ* zymography assay.

These data reveal a novel mechanism for ventricular diastolic dysfunction associated with A-II stimulation and evolving cardiac failure, based on sympathomimetic toxicity and sustained activation of MMP activation. They suggest an explanation for the favorable influence of beta blockade on chronic chamber remodeling [20] beyond those attributable to reduced cardiac work load and energy consumption.

Recent studies employing an A-II-type 1a receptor knock-out mouse have added further support to the link between A-II and chamber remodeling. In this study, Harada et al. [11] reported that the mutant animals developed less chamber dilation and had improved survival after suffering a myocardial infarction compared to wild-type animals. Diastolic pressures were nearly twice as great in wild-type versus knock-out animals after infarction, with much more interstitial fibrosis observed in the former. Yet despite what would seem to have been greater stiffness, chamber dilation was also greater in the control animals. This study did not report on the

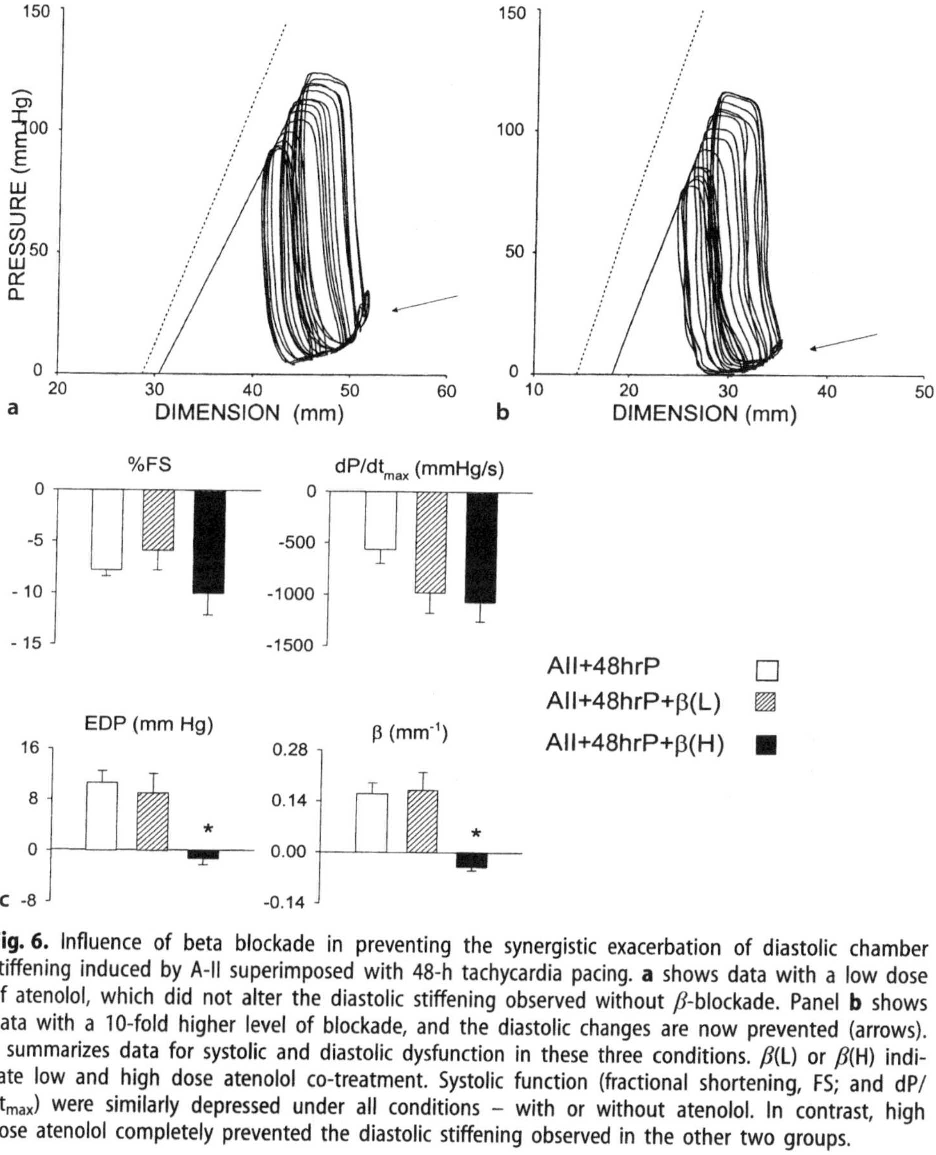

Fig. 6. Influence of beta blockade in preventing the synergistic exacerbation of diastolic chamber stiffening induced by A-II superimposed with 48-h tachycardia pacing. **a** shows data with a low dose of atenolol, which did not alter the diastolic stiffening observed without β-blockade. Panel **b** shows data with a 10-fold higher level of blockade, and the diastolic changes are now prevented (arrows). **c** summarizes data for systolic and diastolic dysfunction in these three conditions. β(L) or β(H) indicate low and high dose atenolol co-treatment. Systolic function (fractional shortening, FS; and dP/dt_{max}) were similarly depressed under all conditions – with or without atenolol. In contrast, high dose atenolol completely prevented the diastolic stiffening observed in the other two groups.

potential influence of MMP activation in this process, but it is quite possible that it played an important role. One might speculate that the AT_1 receptor knock-out animal had less MMP activation as well as less cellular sympathomimetic toxicity and reactive necrosis/fibrosis. The result was less collagen deposition and less dilation. Confirmation of this hypothesis awaits further studies.

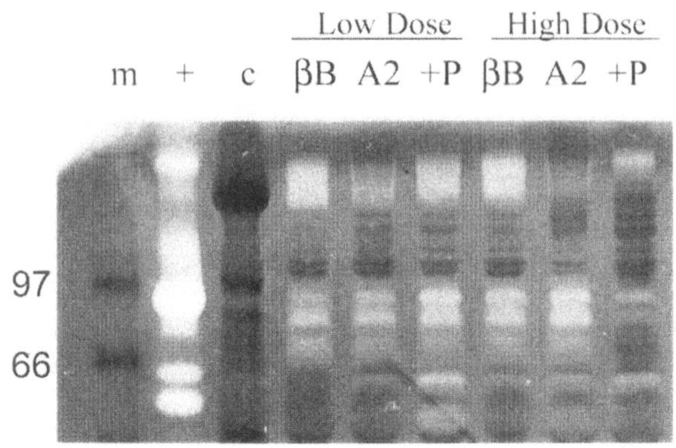

Fig. 7. *In vitro* zymography for β-blockade studies; m shows the marker lane, + is the positive control lane (MMP-9 and activated MMP-2), and c is the control tissue. βB is from animals treated with 1-week atenolol only, A2 is 4 days of A2 exposure with continued atenolol, and +P is final superimposition of 48-h rapid pacing with both other drugs continued. Low and high dose refer to the atenolol dose. Gel lysis in the region consistent with MMP-9 are observed with βB only, and A2. However, when pacing is superimposed and the diastolic dysfunction synergy observed, the low dose atenolol band shows persistent lysis, whereas this was markedly inhibited with high dose β-blockade.

Conclusion

The recognition that chamber remodeling itself plays an important contributory role in exacerbating progressive cardiac failure has led to focused efforts towards its inhibition. To date, successful therapies for cardiac failure, including ACE inhibitors and beta receptor blockade, share this feature. The growing appreciation of the role of MMP activation and related enzyme cascades in the cardiac remodeling process has opened up a new avenue for therapeutic intervention. Recognition and understanding of the mechanisms by which neurohormonal activation can influence MMP stimulation and thus remodeling is just beginning, but promises to forward this effort.

References

1. Parks WC, Mecham RP (eds) (1998) Matrix Metalloproteinases. Academic Press, San Diego
2. Armstrong PW, Moe GW, Howard RJ et al. (1994) Structural remodeling in heart failure: gelatinase induction. Can J Cardiol 10:214–220
3. Birkedal-Hansen H, Moore W, Bodden M, Windsor L, Birkedal-Hanse B, DeCarlo A, Engler J (1992) Matrix metalloproteinases: a review. Chir Rev Oral Biol Med 4:197–250
4. Coker ML, Doscher MA, Thomas CV, Galis ZS, Spinale FG (1999) Matrix metalloproteinase synthesis and expression in isolated LV myocyte preparations. Am J Physiol 277:H777–H787
5. Coker ML, Thomas CV, Clair MJ, Hendrick JW, Krombach RS, Galis ZS, Spinale FG (1998) Myocardial matrix metalloproteinase activity and abundance with congestive heart failure. Am J Physiol 274:H1516–H1523

6. Dostal DE, Baker KM (1999) The cardiac renin-angiotensin system. Conceptual, or a regulator of cardiac function. Circ Res 85:643–650
7. Dostal DE, Hunt RA, Kule CE, Bhat GJ, Karoor V, McWhinney CD, Baker KM (1997) Molecular mechanisms of angiotensin II in modulating cardiac function: intracardiac effect sand signal transduction pathways. J Mol Cell Cardiol 29:2893–2902
8. Goldstein S, Sabbah H (1994) Ventricular remodeling and angiotensin-converting enzyme inhibitors. J Cardiovasc Pharm 24 (Suppl 3):S27–S31
9. Goldstein S, Sharov VG, Cook JM, Sabbah HN (1995) Ventricular remodeling: insights from pharmacologic interventions with angiotensin-converting enzyme inhibitors. Mol Cell Biochem 147:51–55
10. Gross J, Lapiere CM (1962) Collagenolytic activity in amphibian tissues – A tissue culture assay. Proc Natl Acad Sci 48:1014–1022
11. Harada K, Sugaya T, Murakami K, Yazaki Y, Komuro I (1999) Angiotensin II type 1A receptor knockout mice display less left ventricular remodeling and improved survival after myocardial infarction. Circulation 100:2093–2099
12. Henegar JR, Brower GL, Kabour A, Janicki JS (1995) Catecholamine response to chronic ANG II infusion and its role in myocyte and coronary vascular damage. Am J Physiol 269:H1564–H1569
13. Henegar JR, Schwartz DD, Janicki JS (1998) Ang II-related myocardial damage: role of cardiac sympathetic catecholamines and β-receptor regulation. Am J Physiol 275:H534–H541
14. Itoh T, Tanioka M, Matsuda H, Nichimoto HYT, Suzuki R, Uehira M (1999) Experimental metastasis is suppressed in MMP-9-deficient mice. Clin Exp Metastasis 17:177–181
15. Kleiner DE, Stetler-Stevenson WG (1994) Quantitative zymography: detection of picogram quantities of gelatinases. Anal Biochem 218:325–329
16. Koilpillai C, Guinones MA, Greenberg B, Limacher MC, Shindler D, Pratt CM, Benedict CR, Kopelen H, Shelton B for the SOLVD Investigators (1996) Relation of ventricular size and function to heart failure status and ventricular dysrhythmia in patients with severe left ventricular dysfunction. Am J Cardiol 77:606–611
17. Lee YA, Liang CS, Lee MA, Lindpaintner K (1996) Local stress, not systemic factors, regulate gene expression of the cardiac renin-angiotensin system in vivo: a comprehensive study of all its components in the dog. Proc Natl Acad Sci 93:11035–11040
18. Leri A, Claudio PP, Li Q, Wang X, Reiss K, Wang S, Malhotra A, Kajstura J, Anversa P (1998) Stretch-mediated release of angiotensin II induces myocyte apoptosis by activating p53 that enhances the local renin-angiotensin system and decreases the Bcl-2-to-Bax protein ratio in the cell. J Clin Invest 101:1326–1342
19. Leri A, Dostal D, Liu Y, Wang X, Meggs LG, Anversa P (1998) Local renin-angiotensin system (RAS) is upregulated in myocytes following pacing-induced heart failure in dogs. Circulation 98:I 405 (abstr)
20. Lenarda A, Sabbadini G, Salvatore L, Sinagra G, Pinamonti B, Gregori D, Ciani F, Muzzi A, Klugmann S, Camerini F (1999) Long-term effects of carvedilol in idiopathic dilated cardiomyopathy with persistent left ventricular dysfunction despite chronic metoprolol. The Heart-Muscle Disease Study Group. J Am Coll Cardiol 33:1926–1934
21. Li YY, Feldman AM, Sun Y, McTiernan CF (1998) Differential expression of tissue inhibitors of metalloproteinases in the failing human heart. Circulation 98:1728–1734
22. Luchner A, Stevens TL, Borgeson DD, Redfield MM, Bailey JE, Sandberg SM, Heublein DM, Burnett JC Jr (1996) Angiotensin II in the evolution of experimental heart failure. Hypertension 28:472–477

23. Murphy G, Stanton H, Cowell S, Butler G, Knauper V, Atkinson S, Gavrilovic J (1999) Mechanisms for pro matrix metalloproteinase activation. APMIS 107:38–44
24. Nagase H, Woessner JF Jr (1999) Matrix metalloproteinases. J Biol Chem 274:21491–21494
25. Pitt B, Segal R, Martinez FA, Meurers G, Cowley AJ, Thomas I, Deedwania PC, Ney DE, Snavely DB, Chang PI (1997) Randomized trial of losartan versus captopril in patients over 65 with heart failure. Lancet 349:747–752
26. Rohde LE, Ducharme A, Arroyo LH, Aikawa M, Sukhova GH, Lopez-Anaya A, McClure KF, Mitchell PG, Libby P, Lee RT (1999) Matrix metalloproteinase inhibition attenuates early left ventricular enlargement after experimental myocardial infarction in mice. Circulation 99:3063–3070
27. Sadoshima J, Yuhui X, Slayter HS, Izumo S (1993) Autocrine release of angiotensin II mediates stretch-induced hypertrophy of cardiac myocytes *in vitro*. Cell 75:977–984
28. St John Sutton M, Pfeffer MA, Moye L, Plappert T, Rouleau JL, Lamas G, Rouleau J, Parker JO, Arnold MO, Sussex B, Braunwald E (1997) Cardiovascular death and left ventricular remodeling two years after myocardial infarction: baseline predictors and impact of long-term use of captopril: information from the Survival and Ventricular Enlargement (SAVE) trial. Circulation 96:3294–3299
29. Senzaki H, Gluzband YA, Pak PH, Crow MT, Janiki JS, Kass DA (1998) Synergistic exacerbation of diastolic stiffness from short-term tachycardial-induced cardiodepression and angiotensin II. Circ Res 82:503–512
30. Senzaki H, Paolocci N, Gluzband YA, Lindsey ML, Janicki JS, Crow MT, Kass DA (2000) β-blockade prevents sustained metalloproteinase activation and diastolic stiffening induced by angiotensin II combined with evolving cardiac dysfunction. Circ Res 86:807–815
31. Senzaki H, Paolocci N, Kass DA (1998) β-adrenergic blockade prevents angiotensin-mediated exacerbation of diastolic stiffness in conscious dogs with tachycardia-induced cardiodepression. Circulation 98:1–554 (abstr)
32. Shapiro SD (1997) Mighty mice: transgenic technology "knocks out" questions of matrix metalloproteinase function. Matrix Biol 15:527–533
33. Sodoshima J, Izumo S (1993) Molecular characterization of angiotensin II-induced hypertrophy of cardiac myocytes and hyperplasia of cardiac fibroblasts: critical role of the AT_1 receptor subtype. Circ Res 73:413–423
34. SOLVD Investigators (1991) Effect of enalapril on survival in patients with reduced left ventricular ejection fractions and congestive heart failure. N Engl J Med 325:293-302
35. Spinale FG, Coker ML, Krombach SR, Mukherjee R, Hallak H, Houck WV, Clair MJ, Kribbs SB, Johnson LL, Peterson JT, Zile MR (1999) Matrix metalloproteinase inhibition during the development of congestive heart failure. Circ Res 85:364–376
36. Spinale FG, Coker ML, Thomas CV, Walker JD, Mukherjee R, Hebbar L (1998) Time-dependent changes in matrix metalloproteinase activity and expression during the progression of congestive heart failure. Circ Res 82:482–495
37. Tan LB, Jalil JS, Janicki JE, Weber KT (1991) Cardiac myocyte necrosis induced by angiotensin II. Circ Res 69:1185–1195
38. Thomas CV, Coker ML, Zellner JL, Handy JR, Crumbley AJ 3rd, Spinale FG (1998) Increased matrix metalloproteinase activity and selective upregulation in LV myocardium from patients with end-stage dilated cardiomyopathy. Circulation 97:1708–1715
39. Weber KT, Anversa P, Armstrong PW, Brilla CG, Burnett JC Jr, Cruickshank JM, Devereux RB, Giles TD, Kordgaard N, Leier CV, Mendelsohn FAO, Motz WH, Mulvany MJ, Stuer BE (1992) Remodeling and reparation of the cardiovascular system. J Am Coll Cardiol 20:3–16

40. Weber KT, Brilla CG (1991) Pathological hypertrophy and cardiac interstitium: fibrosis and renin-angiotensin-aldosterone system. Circulation 83:1849–1865
41. Woessner J (1991) Matrix metalloproteinases and their inhibitors in connective tissue remodeling. FASEB J 5:2145–2154

Chapter 17

Oxidative stress in heart failure

D. B. Sawyer, W. S. Colucci

Myocardial Biology Unit, Boston University School of Medicine and the Cardiovascular Division, Boston University Medical Center, Boston, MA, USA

Introduction

There is growing evidence that oxidative stress is increased in heart failure, and may contribute to the structural and functional changes leading to disease progression. Our understanding of the role of oxidative stress in myocardial dysfunction remains incomplete. In this review, we will discuss the evidence for increased oxidative stress in heart failure, *in vivo* evidence suggesting a role for oxidative stress in the pathogenesis of heart failure, and recent *in vitro* studies that suggest potential mechanisms by which ROS might mediate myocardial remodeling and contractile dysfunction. Collectively, these studies suggest possible genetic and pharmacologic strategies both to approach the role of oxidative stress in the pathogenesis of heart failure as well as to develop novel therapeutics.

Reactive oxygen species, antioxidant systems, and oxidative stress

The myocardium is highly metabolically active and rich in reactive oxygen species (ROS). ROS are a byproduct of aerobic metabolism, and are handled in the myocardium by soluble and enzymatic antioxidant systems. When the production of ROS exceeds the capacity of antioxidant defense systems, there is 'oxidative stress'. ROS cascades classically begin with the formation of superoxide anion (O_2^-) by either enzymatic or non-enzymatic transfer of a single electron to molecular oxygen (Fig. 1). O_2^- is a free radical and reacts quickly with itself and other oxygen-containing species, and directly or indirectly with lipids, nucleic acids, and proteins to disrupt cellular function. Thus all aerobic organisms, from E. coli to man, have evolved a complex system of enzymatic and non-enzymatic antioxidant systems to defend against the obligate oxidative stress [64]. Interestingly, organisms have also evolved ways to exploit the toxicity of ROS as in the immune system, where powerful oxidase and nitric oxide synthase enzymes join forces to generate high localized concentrations of ROS on demand to wipe out invading microbes [52].

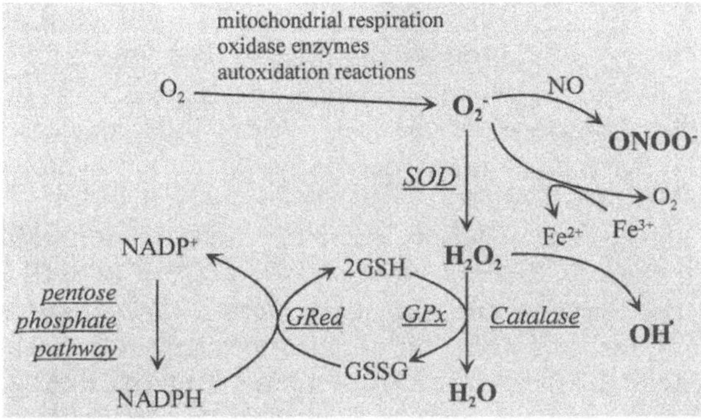

Fig. 1. Reactive oxygen species (ROS) and antioxidant enzyme systems: enzymatic or non-enzymatic formation of superoxide anion leads to the formation of other ROS, shown in bold. Potentially toxic ROS are removed by the enzymes superoxide dismutase (SOD), glutathione peroxidase (GPx), and catalase. The presence of Fe^{2+}, or nitric oxide (NO), can allow the formation of hydroxyl radical (OH) and peroxynitrate ($ONOO^-$), respectively. These latter reactions are favored when the activity of SOD is decreased. O_2^- can increase the formation of OH by reducing Fe^{3+} to Fe^{2+}. Glutathione plays a central role in cellular antioxidant defenses not only as a reducing agent for the action of GPx, but also through direct reactions with ROS. Glutathione is recycled by the enzyme glutathione reductase, which requires NADPH. Thus indirectly, the pentose phosphate pathway, by supplying NADPH, also plays an important role in antioxidant defenses.

Endogenous antioxidant enzymes include superoxide dismutases (SOD), catalase, and peroxidases. Of these, the mitochondrial enzymes manganese superoxide dismutase (MnSOD) and glutathione peroxidase (GPx) appear to be the most important in controlling myocardial levels of O_2^- and H_2O_2. MnSOD makes up approximately 70% of the SOD activity in the heart, and approximately 90% of the activity in cardiac myocytes [5]. The remaining fraction consists primarily of Cu/ZnSOD, with less than 1% extracellular SOD (ECSOD) [13]. This is in contrast to other organs, where MnSOD plays a lesser role. The importance of MnSOD in the regulation of ambient O_2^- levels in the myocardium is highlighted by the demonstration that homozygous knockout mice deficient in MnSOD develop normally *in utero*, but die soon after birth with dilated cardiomyopathy [55]. In contrast, mice deficient in CuZnSOD or ECSOD have no overt cardiovascular phenotype [13]. As the only SOD located in the mitochondria, MnSOD plays a critical role in the control of mitochondrial O_2^- generation during normal oxidative phosphorylation. The phenotype of the MnSOD knockout mouse underscores the importance of the mitochondria as a source of O_2^- in the myocardium.

Like MnSOD, GPx is localized to the mitochondria. Unlike MnSOD, mice deficient in GPx have no overt abnormality in myocardial function. GPx requires selenium for its activity [84], and it is interesting that dietary deficiency of selenium, as occurs in some areas of China, is associated with dilated cardiomyopathy [104]. Although there is evidence of increased oxidative stress in humans and animals with selenium deficiency, it appears that the pathogenesis of the dilated cardiomyopathy is not due to direct effects of this oxidative stress, but perhaps due to increased susceptibility to cardiotrophic viral infections [7, 8]. This may also apply to patients with AIDS, where selenium deficiency is a risk factor for the development of heart failure [49].

Glutathione plays an important role in maintaining cellular redox state (Fig. 1) both through the actions of GPx, as well as direct reactions with reactive oxygen and nitrogen species. Cells replenish reduced glutathione through the action of glutathione reductase. Thus, increased oxidative stress will lower the ratio of reduced to oxidized glutathione (GSH/GSSG), and this has been used as a measure of myocardial oxidative stress in models of heart failure [38]. Unlike the level of lipid peroxidation products, an indicator of oxidative stress both within and outside the cell, the GSH/GSSG ratio is a measure of intracellular oxidative stress. As the activity of glutathione reductase requires NADPH, the pentose phosphate pathway is also an important part of the cellular antioxidant defense system.

Vitamin antioxidants play a major role in the control of ROS cascades and the prevention of free radical chain reactions. In particular α-tocopherol and ascorbic acid, vitamins E and C, act synergistically to prevent runaway lipid peroxidation and membrane breakdown. α-Tocopherol is a fat-soluble molecule that concentrates in cellular membranes. α-Tocopherol has an aromatic ring headgroup attached to its hydrocarbon chain, and is able to form a 'stable' tocopheryl radical when it reacts with ROS and lipid peroxy radicals. Through reactions with ascorbic acid, the tocopheryl radical is converted back to tocopherol. α-Tocopherol has been used both as a measure of antioxidant capacity and oxidative stress [38], as well as a therapeutic intervention in animal models of heart failure [23].

Oxidative stress in human heart failure

Oxidation products of lipids, proteins, and nucleic acids have been used as markers of relative oxidative stress in heart failure (Table 1). While several of the methods employed can be criticized for their relative non-specificity, collectively these data suggest that systemic and myocardial oxidative stress are increased in CHF. Several investigators have reported elevations of malonyldialdehyde (MDA) as well as decreased thiol levels in patients with ischemic and non-ischemic cardiomyopathy compared to subjects without heart failure [10, 25, 64, 65]. More recently, Keith et al. used a similar approach to show that circulating markers of oxidative stress are increased with worsening NYHA functional class [50]. In addition they were able to show increased levels of oxidative stress that correlated with circulating levels of soluble receptors to tumor necrosis factor, a marker of prognosis in heart failure [28]. One group was able to show increased levels of exhaled pentane, a volatile lipid peroxidation product, in patients

Table 1. Studies of oxidative stress markers in human heart failure

Study	Markers	Findings
McMurray et al., 1990 [65]	MDA/Thiol	Increased plasma MDA, decreased plasma thiols in patients with CAD and LV dysfunction
Belch et al., 1991 [10]	MDA/Thiol	Increased plasma MDA, decreased plasma thiols in patients with CHF. Weak correlation between decreasing thiols and worsening LV function
McMurray 1993 [64]	MDA/Thiol	Increased MDA, decreased plasma thiols in both CAD and non-CAD patients with CHF
Sobotka et al., 1993 [94]	Breath pentane	Increased exhaled pentane in CHF compared to controls. Pentane levels reduced by captopril therapy
Ghatak et al., 1996 [31]	MDA, SOD, GPx	Increased MDA, and reduced erythrocyte SOD and GPx activities in patients with heart failure. Weak correlation with LV function. Improved by vitamin E administration
Diaz-Velez et al., 1996 [26]	MDA	Increased MDA in CHF No correlation with LV function. Some correlation between MDA and chronicity of illness
Keith et al., 1998 [50]	MDA, Lipid peroxides, GPx, Vit. C+E	Correlated oxidative stress with NYHA clinical class, as well as levels of soluble TNF receptor levels as marker of prognosis
Mallat et al., 1998 [61]	8-isoprostanes	Pericardial 8-isoprostanes in patients undergoing open-heart surgery correlated with pre-operative NYHA functional class

with CHF [91]. Interestingly, pentane normalized in patients taking captopril, but not angiotensin converting enzyme inhibitors without a thiol moiety. Ghatak et al. showed that circulating markers of oxidative stress normalized in patients with heart failure after 4 weeks of vitamin E therapy [31].

Perhaps the most direct evidence of increased myocardial oxidative stress in heart failure comes from measurements of 8-iso-prostaglandin $F_{2\alpha}$ (8-isoprostanes) in pericardial fluid of patients at time of open heart surgery. 8-Isoprostanes are a family of prostaglandin F2α isomers that are formed by the peroxidation of arachidonic acid mainly through a noncyclooxygenase-mediated reaction catalyzed by free radicals [57]. In contrast to reactive aldehydes, lipid hydroperoxides and conjugated dienes, 8-isoprostanes are more stable products of lipid peroxidation and thus are a more accurate indicator of oxidative stress *in vivo* [68]. 8-Isoprostanes are elevated in tissue subjected to increased oxidative stress, and can be extracted and measured quantitatively using an enzyme-linked immunoassay [22]. Mallat et al. measured 8-isoprostanes in fluid taken from the pericardial space of patients with NYHA functional class I–III HF undergoing open heart surgery for ischemic or valvular disease [60]. They found that the level of 8-isoprostanes increased with increasing NYHA functional class in patients pre-operatively, consistent with the concept that worsening heart failure is associated with increased myocardial oxidative stress.

Animal models of heart failure: oxidative stress and antioxidant therapy

While there are studies showing increased levels of systemic circulating markers of oxidative stress in heart failure patients, support for a role of myocardial oxidative stress in the progression of heart failure comes from work with animal models of heart failure. Singal and colleagues have worked with several animal models of heart failure to characterize changes in myocardial oxidative stress and antioxidant capacity in both myocardial hypertrophy and transition to failure. In a model of stable hypertrophy in response to abdominal aortic banding they found an increase in the activity of SOD and GPx [35]. However, in a model of pressure-overload leading to failure in the guinea pig, there was a fall in SOD and GPx activity during the failure stage with a decreased ratio of GSH/GSSG, consistent with an increase in myocardial oxidative stress [24].

Singal and colleagues have found similar changes in antioxidant capacity and oxidative stress in the rat late after myocardial infarction (MI) [38]. In that model there was a small increase in antioxidant enzyme activity early after MI. However, late after MI they found evidence for increased oxidative stress. During the period from 4 to 16 weeks after MI, there was a progressive decrease in systolic function and an increase in end-diastolic pressure.

These changes were accompanied by
- a progressive decline in GPx and catalase activity,
- an increase in lipid peroxidation,
- a decrease in GSH/GSSG ratio, and
- depletion of vitamin E. SOD activity decreased at the latest time point examined.

Thus, in both the pressure overload and post-MI models of myocardial remodeling leading to heart failure, there is evidence for increased oxidative stress and a maladaptive decrease in antioxidant enzyme capacity that correlate in time with declining ventricular function.

In a canine model of volume overload-induced heart failure secondary to mitral regurgitation, there is also evidence of increased myocardial levels of lipid peroxidation, decreased antioxidant enzyme capacity, and depletion of vitamin E [78]. Administration of vitamin E to dogs with surgically induced mitral regurgitation in part prevented the decline in ventricular function over a 4 month study. Interestingly, while the administration of vitamin E prevented in part the down-regulation of GPx and catalase activity as well as the increase in MDA, the decrease in SOD activity was not prevented by vitamin E.

Singal and colleagues also examined the effect of vitamin E administration on ventricular remodeling and transition to heart failure in their guinea pig aortic banding model of pressure overload [23]. In animals treated with implanted tablets of α-tocopherol, there was a measurable increase in myocardial α-tocopherol levels. There was no difference in the compensatory hypertrophy that occurs at early time points after banding. However at late time points, α-tocopherol administration prevented clinical signs of heart failure, and prevented in part the decline in cardiovascular function, as evidenced by improved left ventricular peak-developed pressure compared to the untreated banded animals. Collectively these data suggest that deficits in antioxidant capacity in the remodeling myocardium contribute to increased oxidative stress and the progression to heart failure. Moreover, the beneficial effects seen with α-tocopherol administration suggest that antioxidant strategies may be of use both for the prevention and treatment of heart failure.

Sources of oxidative stress in heart failure

There are many potential sources of O_2^- and other ROS in all eukaryotic cells, and several of these may be important sources of ROS in the failing myocardium. Several enzyme systems generate O_2^-, and some may produce pathophysiological amounts of O_2^-. Xanthine oxidase, derived from xanthine dehydrogenase during purification, may be activated in myocardial cells in response to ischemia and reperfusion [95]. It is yet unclear if there is any appreciable xanthine oxidase activity in the chronically failing heart, though a beneficial effect of a xanthine oxidase inhibitor in the rapid pacing model of heart failure suggests that this may be the case [27]. NADPH oxidase, originally described as a potent ROS generator important for the phagocytic antimicrobial activity of macrophages [50], appears to mediate some of the hypertrophic and proliferative effects of angiotensin II in vascular tissue [97].

Non-enzymatic autoxidation reactions may also contribute to the formation of ROS in vivo. Oxidation of norepinephrine and epinephrine occurs in aqueous solution forming adrenochrome and O_2^-, and this has been proposed as a mechanism for myocardial injury in the presence of chronic adrenergic stimulation [88]. As this reaction can be inhibited by small amounts of ascorbic acid, and there are clearly direct adrenergic receptor-mediated deleterious effects of adrenergic stimulation [21], it is unclear whether adrenochrome-mediated injury contributes to heart failure. Thiol compounds including cysteine and GSH can autoxidize to form O_2^-, particularly in the presence of transition metals. This and catalysis via the Fenton reaction to form hydroxyl radicals may in part account for the cardiotoxicity of iron overload. Given the myoglobin stores in cardiac myocytes, another potentially important source of ROS is the autoxidation of oxymyoglobin to metmyoglobin with the release of O_2^- [34]. The pH dependence of this reaction would favor O_2^- formation during cellular acidification, as occurs during hypoxia.

Growing evidence supports the mitochondria as a principle source of pathophysiologically significant levels of myocardial ROS. The majority of electrons entering the mitochondrial electron transport chain reduce molecular oxygen to water. However, there is 'leakage' of single electrons, particularly at the NADH-coenzyme Q reductase complex, to molecular oxygen to form O_2^- (Fig. 2). Given the density of mitochondria in cardiac myocytes and the high rate of oxidative phosphorylation, this can result in a high flux of O_2^-. Ide et al. have found convincing evidence that mitochondria from the myocardium of dogs with rapid pacing-induced heart failure are a source of ROS [40]. Similar to other models of heart failure, there were increased lipid peroxidation products in the myocardium of the failing animals compared to controls. They isolated the mitochondrial fraction from the hearts of these animals and examined the formation of O_2^- using electroparamagnetic resonance (EPR) with the O_2^- spin-trap 5,5′-dimethyl-

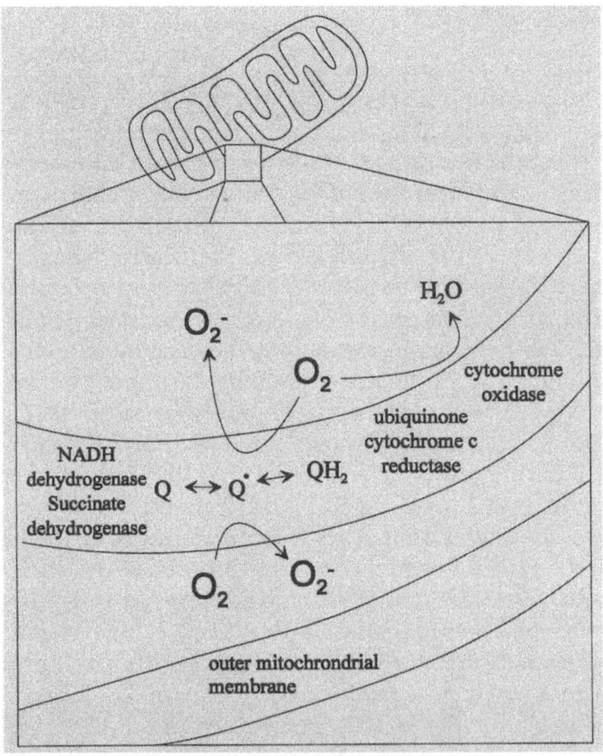

Fig. 2. The mitochondria as a source of ROS. The mitochondrial electron transport chain creates a proton-motive force through the transfer of electrons from NADH dehydrogenase (complex I) and succinate dehydrogenase (complex II) to ubiquinone (Q) to form reduced ubiquinone (QH_2). Partially reduced ubiquinone ($Q^•$) is a radical that can reduce O_2 to O_2^-. This oxygen 'leakage' is a potentially large source of ROS and has been implicated in the increased oxidative stress in heart failure (see text).

1-pyrroline-N-oxide (DMPO). Using EPR, these authors found a 2.8-fold higher DMPO spin signal in mitochondria from failing hearts compared to non-failing controls. They were able to determine that there was a functional blockade of complex I with an ~50% decrease in the enzymatic activity of mitochondria from the failing heart. Thus, in this model there is increased oxidative stress and increased mitochondrial formation of O_2^-. The exact mechanism by which this occurs in the failing hearts, and whether these results apply to other models of heart failure remains to be seen.

Effects of oxidative stress on myocardial structure and function

Role of ROS in myocardial remodeling

Following a myocardial injury such as myocardial infarction there is progressive "remodeling" of the remaining, viable myocardium, a process characterized by chamber enlargement, myocardial thinning, and pump dysfunction [19]. Progressive LV remodeling results in clinical heart failure [20], and therapeutic strategies that alter myocardial remodeling improve long-term survival in patients with myocardial dysfunction [75]. Multiple mechanisms contribute to myocardial remodeling. Chamber enlargement may reflect myocyte hypertrophy [30], myocyte slippage [74], myocyte apoptosis [58], and/or alterations in the turnover and properties of the extracellular matrix [103]. Pump dysfunction may reflect loss of functional myocytes, a shift in the contractile phenotype of surviving cells [56] or the consequences of abnormal LV geometry.

The stimuli for chronic remodeling include increased wall stress [2], inflammatory cytokines [87], and neurohormones including catecholamines [61] and angiotensin II [73]. *In vitro* and *in vivo* experimental studies have shown that oxidative stress can mimic many of the effects of remodeling stimuli, raising the possibility that ROS may mediate the effects of remodeling stimuli on myocardial structure and function (Fig. 3).

ROS play a role in growth pathways in many cell types, including the cardiovascular system. For example, as mentioned above, the hypertrophic effect of angiotensin II on vascular smooth muscle cells depends on increased production of O_2^- via NADPH oxidase [07]. Likewise, the growth effects of diverse stimuli acting via *ras* appear to be mediated by increases in O_2^- [42]. These growth effects of ROS also appear to occur in the myocardium. We have found that small alterations in cellular oxidative stress in cardiac myocytes *in vitro* lead to dose-dependent changes in myocyte hypertrophy. We used the copper chelator diethyldithiocarbamic acid (DDC) to inhibit the activity of CuZnSOD. DDC caused a dose-dependent decrease in SOD activity and thereby increases in cellular O_2^- levels as assessed by lucigenin chemiluminescence or NBT reduction [90]. The increase in O_2^- levels was prevented by the antioxidant tiron or the SOD-mimetic Euk-8. Exposure to a low concentration of DDC (1 μM) for 24 h caused myocyte growth, with increased protein

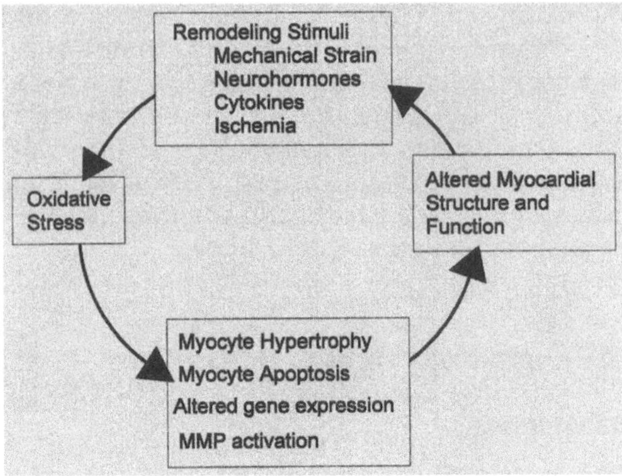

Fig. 3. The cycle of myocardial remodeling. Oxidative stress may be a primary stimulus for changes in cellular structure or function, or may mediate the effects of inflammatory cytokines, chronic neurohormonal stimulation, or mechanical strain. *MMP* matrix metalloproteinase; *TIMP* tissue inhibitor of matrix metalloproteinase.

synthesis and cell size. There was also increased myocyte expression of ANF mRNA, and decreased expression of SERCA2 mRNA [90]. These effects of DDC were prevented by antioxidants. Thus, small decreases in SOD activity lead to ROS-dependent activation of myocyte hypertrophy.

In contrast to these growth effects, we found that high concentrations of DDC (1 mM) cause myocyte apoptosis [90]. High concentrations of DDC resulted in an approximately 50% inhibition of SOD activity, with a greater increase in the formation of ROS. After 24 hours there was an increase in myocyte apoptosis as assessed by nuclear morphology and TUNEL staining for DNA fragmentation. The cytotoxic concentration, but not the hypertrophic concentration, DDC caused an increase in myocyte expression of bax, a pro-apoptotic member of the bcl-2 family. Like the growth stimulatory effect of low concentrations of DDC, the cytotoxic effect of higher concentrations of DDC were prevented by the antioxidant tiron or the SOD-mimetic Euk-8. Thus, larger decreases in SOD activity result in ROS-dependent activation of myocyte apoptosis.

Direct addition of ROS, or ROS-generating systems, to cardiac myocytes in culture also causes apoptosis. Aikawa et al. found that treatment of cardiac myocytes with H_2O_2 induced myocyte death through what appeared to be apoptosis [1]. We have found that the cardiotoxic anthracyclines, well known to generate intracellular ROS [79], induced both myocyte apoptosis and necrosis in a dose-dependent manner [85]. The apoptosis, but not necrosis, could be inhibited by the addition of dexrazoxane, an iron chelator used clinically in the prevention of anthracycline cardiotoxicity [92]. Iron chelation with dexrazoxane does not prevent anthracycline-induced O_2^- formation in cardiac myocytes (author's unpublished observation). Thus, together with inhibition of apoptosis by a SOD mimetic, these results implicate hydroxyl radicals formed via the Fenton reaction in anthracycline-induced apoptosis. A similar role for hydroxyl radicals could apply to the results of Aikawa et al. [1] discussed above, or von Harsdorf et al. who showed similar effects of high levels of extracellular ROS in isolated ventricular myocytes [99]. In those experiments, either a source of extracellular O_2^- or H_2O_2 caused myocyte apoptosis. Thus, multiple studies have shown that oxidative stress can cause myocyte apoptosis *in vitro*.

Work from several labs, including our own, has implicated ROS in mediating the effects of remodeling stimuli on myocyte growth and apoptosis. Cheng et al. implicated oxidative stress in myocyte apoptosis *in vitro* using an isolated papillary muscle preparation [16]. Application of a static mechanical load ($\sim$6-fold estimated normal end-diastolic wall stress) for 4 hours caused both increased production of O_2^- and apoptosis. We found similar effects of cyclic mechanical stretch in isolated cardiac myocytes [76]. Neonatal rat ventricular myocytes were subjected to cyclic mechanical strain at a frequency of 1 Hz for 24 h. Cyclic strain caused an increase in the production of O_2^- as measured by SOD-inhibitable cytochrome c reduction. When cells were stretched at a high amplitude (25%), there was an increase in the number of apoptotic myocytes. Treatment of myocytes with an SOD-mimetic prevented stretch-induced apoptosis.

Mechanical strain is a well-known stimulus for myocyte hypertrophy, and we have found that ROS mediate the hypertrophic effect of mechanical strain as well [76]. Low (5%) and high (25%) amplitude strain of cardiac myocytes cause dose-dependent increases in ROS formation as well as myocyte hypertrophy as assessed by protein synthesis and ANF expression. The increase in protein synthesis as well as the increase in ANF expression were inhibited by a SOD mimetic. Unlike high amplitude strain, there was no effect of low amplitude strain on the frequency of apoptosis as measured by TUNEL or DNA laddering. Thus, mechanical strain causes a graded increase in ROS that mediates myocyte hypertrophy, fetal gene expression, and apoptosis. As we found with inhibition of SOD (above) the smaller increase in ROS caused by low amplitude strain was associated with hypertrophy and fetal gene expression, whereas the larger increase in ROS caused by high amplitude strain also caused apoptosis.

Nakamura et al. have reported that myocyte hypertrophy stimulated by angiotensin II or TNF-α is also mediated by ROS [69]. Using a ROS-reactive fluorescent probe, these investigators were able to demonstrate an increase in the formation of ROS in myocytes after treatment with TNF-α or angiotensin II. The increase in protein synthesis as well as cell size induced by these stimuli was inhibited by concomitant treatment with soluble antioxidants including vitamin E. As formation of both angiotensin II and TNF-α has been demonstrated in myocytes subjected to mechanical strain [48, 54], these observations may be related to our own observations in mechanically-stimulated myocytes. In any case, ROS appear to play a critical role in mediating the phenotypic response of cardiac myocytes to remodeling stimuli, such as mechanical strain, angiotensin, and TNF-α. Furthermore, these observations suggest that the type and/or magnitude of ROS may be a determinant of myocyte phenotype.

Mechanisms of ROS-induced phenotype in cardiac myocytes

Mitochondria appear to be involved at an early step in the regulation of apoptosis through the release of cytochrome c from the intermembrane space (Fig. 4). Cytochrome c release activates caspase-3 and is also associated with mitochondrial generation of ROS, probably through effects on electron transport [51, 81]. This process is modulated by the bcl-2 family of proteins [47, 82]. Pro-apoptotic members of the bcl-2 family, bax, Bad, and bak, interact with components of the mitochondrial permeability transition pore thereby promoting cytochrome c release and dissipation of the membrane potential [47, 70, 83]. Anti-apoptotic members, bcl-2 and bcl-xL, inhibit bax-mediated cyochrome c release, caspase-3 activation, and the generation of ROS [70, 98].

In myocytes treated with apoptotic concentrations of DDC, we found an increase in bax expression, consistent with an increase in p53 activity, that can be inhibited with antioxidants [90]. In myocytes treated with ROS, von Harsdorf et al. saw an increase in p53 activity, but not in bax protein expression [99]. They did find, however, translocation of bax and Bad from the cytosol to the mitochondrial fraction, with associated release of cytochrome c. Interestingly, they found evidence that apoptosis induced by exogenous O_2^- occurs by a pathway distinct from H_2O_2. While treatment with H_2O_2 induced mitochondrial release of cytochrome c and activation of caspase 3, treatment with xanthine and xanthine oxidase (in the presence of catalase) as a source of O_2^- induced apoptosis without evidence of cytochrome c release or activation of caspase 3. O_2^--induced apoptosis did involve activation of the laminase Mch2α and was inhibited by the pan-caspase inhibitor Z-VAD-fmk. Together with the effects of DDC, these data suggest that exogenous O_2^- may trigger apoptosis via a different mechanism than intracellular O_2^-. This would not be surprising, as exogenous O_2^-

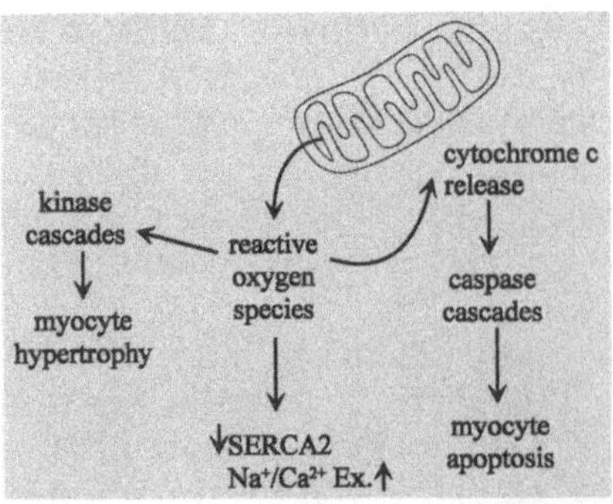

Fig. 4. Schematic of effects of ROS on myocyte phenotype. Through activation of kinase cascades such as MAPK, ROS can induce myocyte hypertrophy. ROS can also alter activity and expression of Ca^{2+} handling proteins including SERCA2 and Na^+/Ca^{2+} exchanger to alter myocardial contractility. Mitochondrial ROS may be particularly prone to induce apoptosis through induction of the mitochrondrial release of cytochrome c necessary for the activation of caspase cascades.

should enter the cell minimally given its negative charge and the negative resting membrane potential. Exogenous O_2^- might trigger apoptosis via changes in matrix/integrin interactions. We found that treatment of myocytes with xanthine/xanthine oxidase causes many myocytes to become detached [90], which itself may can be a trigger for apoptosis.

The effects of ROS on myocyte hypertrophy and apoptosis may involve activation of the stress-responsive protein kinases of the MAPK superfamily [94] which includes extracellularly-responsive kinases (ERKs) [89] and two stress-responsive MAPK subfamilies (SR-MAPKs), the p38-kinases and the c-Jun N-terminal kinases (JNKs). The JNKs consist of 46 or 54 kDa proteins [94]. The p38-kinases consist of at least 6 isoforms (α_1, α_2, β_1, β_2, γ and δ) of which the α and β isoforms appear to predominate in cardiac myocytes [44, 94]. In neonatal rat ventricular myocytes, constitutive activation of p38 kinase(β) or JNKs causes a hypertrophic response, whereas expression of a constitutively-active p38-kinase(α) causes apoptosis [101, 102]. There is also evidence that SR-MAPKs could participate in determining the phenotypic response to remodeling stimuli including hemodynamic overload [29].

ROS activate both SR-MAPKs and ERKs in the cardiovascular system [17, 18, 42, 53, 94]. In neonatal rat ventricular myocytes, H_2O_2 activates p38-kinase, JNKs, and ERKs [18]. In perfused rat hearts, H_2O_2 activated SR-MAPKs, but there was minimal activation of ERKs. Both ischemia and ischemia/reperfusion activated p38-kinase, whereas only ischemia/reperfusion activated JNKs, and neither ischemia nor ischemia/reperfusion activated ERKs [17]. The O_2^- scavenger spin-trap (N-tert-butyl-α-phenyl nitrone) inhibited p38-kinase activation, whereas the $OH^\bullet$ scavenger DMSO prevented activation of both p38-kinases and JNKs during ischemia/reperfusion, raising the possibility that specific ROS differentially activate specific SR-MAPKs. Wei and colleagues found that oxidative stress-induced apoptosis in the H9C2 cardiac cell line was associated with activation of JNKs and that transfection of a dominant negative JNK markedly diminished the extent of DNA fragmentation [96]. Feuerstein and colleagues were able to show in an ischemia/reperfusion model of myocardial injury that treatment with antioxidant/beta-blocker carvedilol blocked activation of JNK and decreased the number of apoptotic myocytes [110], again supporting a role for JNK in ROS-induced myocyte injury.

Aikawa et al. found that treatment with H_2O_2 activated ERKs in cardiac myocytes [1]. Inhibition of activation of ERKs increased the apoptotic response to ROS, suggesting that ERKs activate a survival pathway. While the authors did not look for evidence of myocyte hypertrophy in response to H_2O_2, the ERK pathway has been shown to play an important role in signaling myocyte hypertrophy by various hypertrophic stimuli [6, 109]. We have found that increased oxidative stress (by inhibition of SOD) leading to myocyte hypertrophy is accompanied by activation of ERKs. Collectively these data suggest that ROS act through redox-sensitive signaling cascades to activate distinct hypertrophic, apoptotic, and survival phenotypes in cardiac myocytes.

ROS-induced changes in calcium handling

The contribution of the Ca^{2+} handling proteins to contractile dysfunction in the failing heart are discussed in detail by other authors in this compilation. Myocytes isolated from the failing heart show markedly abnormal intracellular Ca^{2+} transients that appear to result from alterations in expression and/or activity of Ca^{2+} handling proteins [3]. Of note, the downregulation of sarcoplasmic reticulum Ca^{2+} ATPase (SERCA2) expression and activity appears to contribute to contractile dysfunction in both animal models of heart failure [11, 111] and human heart failure [86]. We have found that oxidative stress can decrease SERCA2 expression in primary cultures of cardiac myocytes [90]. Thus oxidative stress may be a proximal stimulus to alterations of Ca^{2+} handling proteins and dysregulation of intracellular [Ca^{2+}].

There are other direct and indirect effects of ROS on myocyte Ca^{2+} handling that can result in changes in contractile function. ROS alter Ca^{2+} transients and excitation-contraction coupling in isolated myocytes [34] in part by increasing the activity of the Na^{+}/Ca^{2+} exchanger, which in some situations may lead to Ca^{2+} overload [32]. A similar alteration in Na^{+}/Ca^{2+} exchanger activity can be seen in some models of heart failure. Investigations of Ca^{+2} transients and force-frequency behavior of myocytes isolated from the myocardium late after MI show increased Na^{+}/Ca^{2+} exchanger activity together with a depressed force-frequency relationship [56]. Electrophysiological studies in isolated myocytes have also shown direct effects of O_2^-, NO, and $ONOO^-$ on the voltage-dependent Ca^{2+} channel and the calcium release channel [12, 107]. Thus, there are direct effects of ROS on Ca^{2+} handling proteins *in vitro*, and some of these may be active *in vivo* in the chronically failing heart.

Nitric oxide and its interaction with ROS

Nitric oxide (NO) can modify the myocardial response to oxidative stress both directly and indirectly. NO is a ubiquitous molecule synthesized in the conversion of L-arginine to L-citrulline by a family of nitric oxide synthases [71]. NO is a free radical gas and is buffered in the cell by reactions with glutathione. NO reacts reversibly with sulfhydryl groups of proteins forming S-nitrosothiols which may alter protein function [93]. Through chemical reactions with ROS, NO can *decrease* or *increase* the oxidative stress in a cell or tissue.

Under normal circumstances, myocardial NO is produced primarily by the calcium-sensitive nitric oxide synthase NOS_3. The activity of this enzyme, present constitutively in virtually all cell types in the myocardium including myocytes, fibroblasts and endothelial cells, is regulated by a calcium-sensitive interaction with calmodulin [66]. Inducible nitric oxide synthase (NOS_2) is not regulated by Ca^{2+}, and when expressed is capable of producing high levels of cellular NO. Though NOS_2 is not normally expressed in the myocardium, after exposure to cytokines, hypoxia, and perhaps other stimuli, NOS_2 is induced in both myocytes and nonmyocytes within the myocardium due to activation of specific transcription factors, leading to a marked increase in the production of NO [89]. Of note, there is evidence for increased expression and activity of the inducible isoform of nitric oxide synthase (NOS_2) in the myocardium of patients with both idiopathic and ischemic dilated cardiomyopathies [36, 37].

Low levels of NO may reduce the level of oxidative stress by decreasing the production of O_2^- through inhibition of oxidative enzymes [106]. Indirectly, low levels of NO may also exert beneficial effects on myocardial remodeling. NO through the activation of guanylate cyclase can inhibit the hypertrophic effect of adrenergic stimulation [11]. NO may also be able to promote cell survival by inactivating proteases involved in the apoptotic cascade [62].

Higher levels of NO may increase oxidative stress by reacting with O_2^- to generate peroxynitrite ($ONOO^-$), a free radical which may be more toxic and long-lived than either NO or O_2^- [9]. $ONOO^-$ can react with tyrosine residues of susceptible proteins, including MnSOD, causing irreversible inactivation [43]. Based on the relative rate constants of O_2^- with superoxide dismutase (SOD) and NO, the formation of $ONOO^-$ is favored when the levels of O_2^- or NO are high, or the level of SOD is low [9]. Interestingly, Wang and Zweier have shown that NOS_2 is also capable of catalyzing the formation of O_2^- [105] particularly when there is depletion of arginine. Thus expression of NOS_2 may contribute directly to the formation of ROS.

High concentrations of NO can have direct toxic effects on cardiac myocytes *in vitro*. Pinsky et al. demonstrated that adult rat ventricular myocytes in culture died in response to stimulation with cytokines known to induce the expression of NOS_2 [77]. This myocytotoxic effect of the cytokines could be prevented by inhibition of NOS with L-NMMA, suggesting that NOS_2- derived NO is required for myocyte death. Bishopric and colleagues went on to show that in neonatal rat ventricular myocytes cytokines induce cell death via NO-dependent apoptosis [41]. We have found that cytokine-induced apoptosis can be prevented by either an inhibitor of NOS_2 or an SOD-mimetic implicating $ONOO^-$ [4].

Animal models of autoimmune and viral myocarditis have implicated a direct toxic effect of NO and $ONOO^-$ *in vivo*. In these models there is massive inflammation in the heart that results in overt myocyte necrosis [45]. Ishiyama et al. were able to reduce the amount of necrotic myocardium as well as the elevation of serum CK in rats with experimental autoimmune myocarditis using aminoguanidine, an inhibitor of NOS_2 [44]. Interestingly, in that system treatment with aminoguanidine also decreased the amount of superoxide anion formed. While it is possible that superoxide anion was formed by NOS_2 in this system, it is also possible that an increase in superoxide anion resulted from the inactivation of MnSOD by $ONOO^-$ [59].

Mikama et al. were able to reveal both good and bad aspects of NO when they examined the effect of inhibition of NO synthesis with L-NAME on mortality and the extent of myocardial injury in a murine model of viral myocarditis [67]. Mice were infected with coxsackievirus B3 in the presence of increasing doses of L-NAME. At the highest dose of L-NAME, there was decreased survival. At a low dose, however, L-NAME improved survival and reduced the severity of heart failure and extent of myocardial necrosis.

The exact mechanisms at play in determining the "optimal" NO concentration remains to be determined. Interestingly, in a papillary muscle preparation, stretch-induced myocyte apoptosis was inhibited by the addition of an NO donor [16]. Coincident with the decrease in apoptosis was a decrease in the level of O_2^-, leading the authors to conclude that NO might exert a beneficial action by scavenging O_2^- generated by mechanical stretch. However, as discussed above, the addition of NO could lead to formation of $ONOO^-$, which would exert deleterious effects of its own. In other cell types it appears that NO can reduce apoptosis by inhibiting specific enzymes in the programmed cell death pathway [62], and this may have been the mechanism for the beneficial effect of NO seen in the papillary muscle preparation. Another possibility is that the NO donor decreased production of ROS through its actions on mitochondria. NO is known to decrease mitochondrial respiration and myocardial oxygen consumption [72, 106], and this may indirectly control the rate of ROS production.

Potential therapeutic antioxidant strategies for the treatment of heart failure

If indeed oxidative stress is a therapeutic target in heart failure, there are many strategies to consider. Pharmacologic antioxidants are attractive in that many are food-derived compounds and readily available, easy to administer, with little to no toxic potential. Moreover, as discussed above, α-tocopherol has already been proven effective in some models of heart failure. There has been no definitive clinical trial of α-tocopherol in heart failure, though the ability of α-tocopherol therapy to lower oxidative stress in patients with heart failure has been shown [31], providing the basis for an antioxidant therapeutic trial. Many other plant-derived compounds contain antioxidant properties similar to α-tocopherol, and may also be important dietary and pharmacologic antioxidants [39].

Antioxidant enzyme expression is also an attractive target for therapeutic intervention. The myocardium regulates the expression and activity of antioxidant enzymes in response to ROS, thereby controlling oxidative stress. For example, after ischemia and reoxygenation, neonatal cardiac myocytes *in vitro* rapidly increase the expression of MnSOD [108]. This regulation appears to be part of the hypoxic preconditioning response, as inhibition of MnSOD upregulation with antisense oligonucleotides to MnSOD inhibits the protective effect of ischemic preconditioning to subsequent prolonged hypoxia. Thus the decrease in antioxidant activity that occurs in the failing myocardium in the face of increased oxidative stress is clearly maladaptive. At present we understand very little about the regulation of antioxidant expression and activity, and by what mechanism dysregulation occurs.

Even in the absence of strategies to prevent the maladaptive down-regulation of antioxidant enzymes, gene therapy approaches to effect targeted overexpression of antioxidant enzymes may be of use if vectors achieve stable long-term myocardial expression. The use of transgenic mice with stable overexpression of antioxidant enzymes may be able to guide overexpression strategies. To date these genetically altered animals have only been studied in models of ischemia/reperfusion. Transgenic mice that overexpress each of the three forms of SOD have improved recovery after ischemia/reperfusion. Wang et al. reported that in transgenic mice overexpressing Cu/ZnSOD the burst of O_2^- upon reperfusion is markedly diminished, with concomitant decreases in the extent of myocardial injury [100]. Chen et al. showed improved functional recovery in mice overexpressing EC-SOD after ischemia/reperfusion [14], while Chen et al. showed similar beneficial effects of mice overexpressing MnSOD [15]. As ischemia/reperfusion injury occurs in the setting of large fluxes of ROS, these results may not apply to chronic myocardial dysfunction where the elevations of oxidative stress are more subtle.

Conclusions

There is evidence that oxidative and nitrositive stress is elevated systemically and in the myocardium of patients with chronic systolic LV failure. The cause of increased ROS in the setting of chronic heart failure is not known, but may relate to increased production due to increased metabolic activity, stimulated production by mechanical strain, neurohormonal activation, inflammatory cytokines, and/or decreased antioxidant activity. Based on *in vitro* studies, these increases in oxidative and nitrositive stress may be contributing to the ventricular remodeling and contractile dysfunction in patients with heart failure.

Oxidative stress has many effects on myocardial structure and function *in vitro*. As in other tissues, oxidative stress can stimulate growth or lead to myocyte death by apoptosis or necrosis. The mechanism by which various ROS activate cell signaling pathways remains an area of active investigation and promises to offer new therapeutic targets for pharmacologic antioxidants. It is clear that oxidative stress can trigger many responses in myocytes *in vitro*, and these changes occur *in vivo* in many situations leading to myocardial dysfunction.

There remain many unanswered questions. In developing therapeutic strategies, we will need to understand in more detail

- what the relative contributions of decreased antioxidant activity vs. increased formation of ROS are to myocardial oxidative stress in heart failure,

- in what situations oxidative and nitrositive stress contribute to the pathogenesis of myocardial dysfunction *in vivo*; and
- where the optimal place in ROS cascades to intervene is to prevent adverse effects on myocardial structure and function.

Advances in our understanding of antioxidant enzymes and technology for manipulation of these genes, as well as the development of animal models for acute and chronic myocardial injury, are likely to provide new insight into the potential therapeutic value of antioxidants in the treatment and prevention of myocardial dysfunction.

References

1. Aikawa R, Komuro I, Yamazaki T, Zou Y, Kudoh S, Tanaka M, Shiojima I, Hiroi Y, Yazaki Y (1997) Oxidative stress activates extracellular signal-regulated kinases through Src and Ras in cultured cardiac myocytes of neonatal rats. J Clin Invest 100(7):1813–1821
2. Anversa P, Olivetti G, Capasso JM (1991) Cellular basis of ventricular remodeling after myocardial infarction. Am J Cardiol 68:7D–16D
3. Arai M, Alpert NR, MacLennan DH, Barton P, Periasamy M (1993) Alterations in sarcoplasmic reticulum gene expression in human heart failure. A possible mechanism for alterations in systolic and diastolic properties of the failing myocardium. Circ Res 72:463–469
4. Arstall MA, Sawyer DB, Fukazawa R, Kelly RA (1999) Cytokine-mediated apoptosis in cardiac myocytes: the role of inducible nitric oxide synthase induction and peroxynitrite generation [see comments]. Circ Res 85:829–840
5. Assem M, Teyssier JR, Benderitter M, Terrand J, Laubriet A, Javouhey A, David M, Rochette L (1997) Pattern of superoxide dismutase enzymatic activity and RNA changes in rat heart ventricles after myocardial infarction. Am J 151:549–555
6. Baliga RR, Pimental DR, Zhao YY, Simmons WW, Marchionni MA, Sawyer DB, Kelly RA (1999) NRG-1-induced cardiomyocyte hypertrophy. Role of PI-3-kinase, p70(S6K), and MEK-MAPK-RSK. Am J Physiol 277:H2026–H2037
7. Beck MA, Kolbeck PC, Rohr LH, Shi Q, Morris VC, Levander OA (1994) Benign human enterovirus becomes virulent in selenium-deficient mice. J Med Virol 43(2):166–170
8. Beck MA, Shi Q, Morris VC, Levander OA (1995) Rapid genomic evolution of a non-virulent coxsackievirus B3 in selenium-deficient mice results in selection of identical virulent isolates [see comments]. Nat Med 1(5):433–436
9. Beckman JS, Koppenol WH (1996) Nitric oxide, superoxide, and peroxynitrite: the good, the bad, and ugly. Am J Physiol 271(5 Pt 1):C1424–1437
10. Belch JJ, Bridges AB, Scott N, Chopra M (1991) Oxygen free radicals and congestive heart failure. Br Heart J 65:245–248
11. Calderone A, Takahashi N, Izzo NJ Jr, Thaik CM, Colucci WS (1995) Pressure- and volume-induced left ventricular hypertrophies are associated with distinct myocyte phenotypes and differential induction of peptide growth factor mRNAs. Circulation 92:2385–2390
12. Campbell DL, Stamler JS, Strauss HC (1996) Redox modulation of L-type calcium channels in ferret ventricular myocytes. Dual mechanism regulation by nitric oxide and S-nitrosothiols. J Gen Physiol 108:277–293

13. Carlsson LM, Jonsson J, Edlund T, Marklund SL (1995) Mice lacking extracellular superoxide dismutase are more sensitive to hyperoxia. Proc Natl Acad Sci USA 92(14):6264–6268
14. Chen EP, Bittner HB, Davis RD, Van Trigt P, Folz RJ (1998) Physiologic effects of extracellular superoxide dismutase transgene overexpression on myocardial function after ischemia and reperfusion injury. J Thorac Cardiovasc Surg 115(2):450–458; discussion 458–459
15. Chen Z, Siu B, Ho YS, Vincent R, Chua CC, Hamdy RC, Chua BH (1998) Overexpression of MnSOD protects against myocardial ischemia/reperfusion injury in transgenic mice. J Mol Cell Cardiol 30(11):2281–2289
16. Cheng W, Li B, Kajstura J, Li P, Wolin MS, Sonnenblick EH, Hintze TH, Olivetti G, Anversa P (1995) Stretch-induced programmed myocyte cell death. J Clin Invest 96:2247–2259
17. Clerk A, Fuller SJ, Michael A, Sugden PH (1998) Stimulation of "stress-regulated" mitogen-activated protein kinases (stress-activated protein kinases/c-Jun N-terminal kinases and p38-mitogen-activated protein kinases) in perfused rat hearts by oxidative and other stresses. J Biol Chem 273:7228–7234
18. Clerk A, Michael A, Sugden PH (1998) Stimulation of multiple mitogen-activated protein kinase sub-families by oxidative stress and phosphorylation of the small heat shock protein, HSP25/27, in neonatal ventricular myocytes. Biochem J 333:581–589
19. Cohn JN (1995) New concepts regarding events that lead to end-stage heart disease. Cardiovasc Drugs Ther 9 (Suppl 3):489–492
20. Colucci WS, Braunwald E (1995) Pathophysiology of heart failure. In: Braunwald E (ed) Heart disease. WB Saunders Co, Philadelphia
21. Communal C, Singh K, Pimentel DR, Colucci ED (1998) Norepinephrine stimulates apoptosis in adult rat ventricular myocytes by activation of the β-adrenergic pathway. Circulation 98:1329–1334
22. Delanty N, Reilly MP, Pratico D, Lawson JA, McCarthy JF, Wood AE, Ohnishi ST, Fitzgerald DJ, FitzGerald GA (1997) 8-epi PGF2 alpha generation during coronary reperfusion. A potential quantitative marker of oxidant stress in vivo. Circulation 95(11):2492–2499
23. Dhalla AK, Hill MF, Singal PK (1996) Role of oxidative stress in transition of hypertrophy to heart failure. J Am Coll Cardiol 28(2):506–514
24. Dhalla AK, Singal PK (1994) Antioxidant changes in hypertrophied and failing guinea pig hearts. Am J Physiol 266:H1280–H1285
25. Diaz-Velez CR, Garcia-Castineiras S, Mendoza-Ramos E, Hernandez-Lopez E (1996) Increased malondialdehyde in peripheral blood of patients with congestive heart failure. Am Heart J 131(1):146–152
26. Diaz-Velez CR, Garcia-Castineiras S, Mendoza-Ramos E, Hernandez-Lopez E (1996) Increased malondialdehyde in peripheral blood of patients with congestive heart failure. Am Heart J 131(1):146–152
27. Ekelund UE, Harrison RW, Shokek O, Thakkar RN, Tunin RS, Senzaki H, Kass DA, Marban E, Hare JM (1999) Intravenous allopurinol decreases myocardial oxygen consumption and increases mechanical efficiency in dogs with pacing-induced heart failure. Circ Res 85:437–445
28. Ferrari R, Bachetti T, Confortini R, Opasich C, Febo O, Corti A, Cassani G, Visioli O (1995) Tumor necrosis factor soluble receptors in patients with various degrees of congestive heart failure [see comments]. Circulation 92:1479–1486
29. Fischer TA, Ludwig A, Singh K, Peter F, Gambaryan S, Kelly RA, Pfeffer MA, Pfeffer JM (1998) Mechanical load induces stress-regulated mitogen-activated protein kinases (JNK-1/p38) in acute pressure overload in rat heart. Circulation (Supp 1):1–119

30. Gerdes AM, Liu Z, Zimmer HG (1994) Changes in nuclear size of cardiac myocytes during the development and progression of hypertrophy in rats. Cardioscience 5:203–208
31. Ghatak A, Brar MJ, Agarwal A, Goel N, Rastogi AK, Vaish AK, Sircar AR, Chandra M (1996) Oxy free radical system in heart failure and therapeutic role of oral vitamin E. Int J Cardiol 57(2):119–127
32. Goldhaber JI (1996) Free radicals enhance Na^{+}/Ca^{2+} exchange in ventricular myocytes. Am J Physiol 271(3 Pt 2):H823–833
33. Goldhaber JI, Liu E (1994) Excitation-contraction coupling in single guinea-pig ventricular myocytes exposed to hydrogen peroxide. J Physiol (Lond) 477(Pt 1):135–147
34. Goto T, Shikama K (1974) Autoxidation of native oxymyoglobin from bovine heart muscle. Arch Biochem Biophys 163:476–481
35. Gupta M, Singal PK (1989) Higher antioxidative capacity during a chronic stable heart hypertrophy. Circ Res 64:398–406
36. Habib FM, Springall DR, Davies GJ, Oakley CM, Yacoub MH, Polak JM (1996) Tumour necrosis factor and inducible nitric oxide synthase in dilated cardiomyopathy [see comments]. Lancet 347(9009):1151–1155
37. Haywood GA, Tsao PS, von der Leyen HE, Mann MJ, Keeling PJ, Trindade PT, Lewis NP, Byrne CD, Rickenbacher PR, Bishopric NH, Cooke JP, McKenna WJ, Fowler MB (1996) Expression of inducible nitric oxide synthase in human heart failure [see comments]. Circulation 93(6):1087–1094
38. Hill MF, Singal PK (1996) Antioxidant and oxidative stress changes during heart failure subsequent to myocardial infarction in rats. Am J Cardiol 148(1):291–300
39. Hollman PC, Katan MB (1998) Bioavailability and health effects of dietary flavonols in man. Arch Toxicol Suppl 20:237–248
40. Ide T, Tsutsui H, Kinugawa S, Utsumi H, Kang D, Hattori N, Uchida K, Arimura K, Egashira K, Takeshita A (1999) Mitochondrial electron transport complex I is a potential source of oxygen free radicals in the failing myocardium. Circ Res 85:357–363
41. Ing DJ, Zang J, Dzau VJ, Webster KA, Bishopric NH (1999) Modulation of cytokine-induced cardiac myocyte apoptosis by nitric oxide, Bak, and Bcl-x. Circ Res 84(1):21–33
42. Irani K, Xia Y, Zweier JL, Sollott SJ, Der CJ, Fearon ER, Sundaresan M, Finkel T, Goldschmidt-Clermont PJ (1997) Mitogenic signaling mediated by oxidants in Ras-transformed fibroblasts. Science 275:1649–1652
43. Ischiropoulos H, Zhu L, Chen J, Tsai M, Martin JC, Smith CD, Beckman JS (1992) Peroxynitrite-mediated tyrosine nitration catalyzed by superoxide dismutase. Arch Biochem Biophys 298(2):431–437
44. Ishiyama S, Hiroe M, Nishikawa T, Abe S, Shimojo T, Ito H, Ozasa S, Yamakawa K, Matsuzaki M, Mohammed MU, Nakazawa H, Kasajima T, Marumo F (1997) Nitric oxide contributes to the progression of myocardial damage in experimental autoimmune myocarditis in rats. Circulation 95:489–496
45. Izumi T, Suzuki K, Saeki M, Ookura Y, Hirono S, Inomata T, Hanawa H, Kodama M (1995) An ultrastructural study on experimental autoimmune myocarditis with special reference to effector cells. Eur Heart J 16 (Suppl O):75–77
46. Jiang Y, Gram H, Zhao M, New L, Gu J, Feng L, Di Padova F, Ulevitch RJ, Han J (1997) Characterization of the structure and function of the fourth member of p38 group mitogen-activated protein kinases, p28δ J Biol Chem 272:30122–30128
47. Jurgensmeier JM, Xie Z, Deveraux Q, Ellerby L, Bredesen D, Reed JC (1998) Bax directly induces release of cytochrome c from isolated mitochondria. Proc Natl Acad Sci USA 95(9):4997–5002

48. Kapadia SR, Taffet GE, Mann DL (1995) Hemodynamic regulation of tumor necrosis factor-α gene and protein expression in adult mammalian myocardium. Circulation 92 (Suppl 1):1-12 (abstr)
49. Kavanaugh-McHugh AL, Ruff A, Perlman E, Hutton N, Modlin J, Rowe S (1991) Selenium deficiency and cardiomyopathy in acquired immunodeficiency syndrome. JPEN J Parenter Enteral Nutr 15(3):347–349
50. Keith M, Geranmayegan A, Sole MJ, Kurian R, Robinson A, Omran AS, Jeejeebhoy KN (1998) Increased oxidative stress in patients with congestive heart failure. J Am Coll Cardiol 31:1352–1356
51. Kojima H, Endo K, Moriyama H, Tanaka Y, Alnemri ES, Slapak CA, Teicher B, Kufe D, Datta R (1998) Abrogation of mitochondrial cytochrome c release and caspase-3 activation in acquired multidrug resistance. J Biol Chem 273(27):16647–16650
52. Krueger GG, Ogden BE, Weston WL (1976) In vitro quantitation of cell-mediated immunity in guinea-pigs by macrophage reduction of nitro-blue tetrazolium. Clin Exp Immunol 23:517–524
53. Lander HM, Ogiste JS, Teng KK, Novogrodsky A (1995) $p21^{ras}$ as a common signaling target of reactive free radicals and cellular redox stress. J Biol Chem 270:21195–21198
54. Leri A, Claudio PP, Li Q, Wang X, Reiss K, Wang S, Malhotra A, Kajstura J, Anversa P (1998) Stretch-mediated release of angiotensin II induces myocyte apoptosis by activating p53 that enhances the local renin-angiotensin system and decreases the Bcl-2-to-Bax protein ratio in the cell. J Clin Invest 101(7):1326–1342
55. Li Y, Huang T-T, Carlson EJ, Melov S, Ursell PC, Olson JL, Noble LJ, Yoshimura MP, Berger C, Chan PH, Wallace DC, Epstein CJ (1995) Dilated cardiomyopathy and neonatal lethality in mutant mice lacking manganese superoxide dismutase. Nature Genetics 11:376–381
56. Litwin SE, Bridge JH (1997) Enhanced $Na(^{+})$-Ca^{2+} exchange in the infarcted heart. Implications for excitation-contraction coupling. Circ Res 81(6):1083–1093
57. Liu TZ, Stern A, Morrow JD (1998) The isoprostanes: unique bioactive products of lipid peroxidation. An overview [in process citation]. J Biomed Sci 5(6):415–420
58. MacLellan WR, Schneider MD (1997) Death by design. Programmed cell death in cardiovascular biology and disease. Circ Res 81:137–144
59. MacMillan-Crow LA, Crow JP, Kerby JD, Beckman JS, Thompson JA (1996) Nitration and inactivation of manganese superoxide dismutase in chronic rejection of human renal allografts. Proc Natl Acad Sci USA 93:11853–11858
60. Mallat Z, Philip I, Lebret M, Chatel D, Maclouf J, Tedgui A (1998) Elevated levels of 8-iso-prostaglandin F2alpha in pericardial fluid of patients with heart failure: a potential role for in vivo oxidant stress in ventricular dilatation and progression to heart failure. Circulation 97(16):1536–1539
61. Mann DL, Kent RL, Parsons B, Cooper G (1992) Adrenergic effects of the biology of the adult mammalian cardiocyte. Circulation 85:790–804
62. Mannick JB, Miao XQ, Stamler JS (1997) Nitric oxide inhibits Fas-induced apoptosis. J Biol Chem 272:24125–24128
63. McCord JM, Fridovich I (1969) Superoxide dismutase. An enzymic function for erythrocuprein (hemocuprein). J Biol Chem 244:6049-6055
64. McMurray J, Chopra M, Abdullah I, Smith WE, Dargie HJ (1993) Evidence of oxidative stress in chronic heart failure in humans. Eur Heart J 14(11):1493–1498
65. McMurray J, McLay J, Chopra M, Bridges A, Belch JJ (1990) Evidence for enhanced free radical activity in chronic congestive heart failure secondary to coronary artery disease. Am J Cardiol 65:1261–1262

66. Michel JB, Feron O, Sacks D, Michel T (1997) Reciprocal regulation of endothelial nitric-oxide synthase by Ca^{2+}-calmodulin and caveolin. J Biol Chem 272(25):15583–15586
67. Mikami S, Kawashima S, Kanazawa K, Hirata K, Hotta H, Hayashi Y, Itoh H, Yokoyama M (1997) Low-dose N omega-nitro-L-arginine methyl ester treatment improves survival rate and decreases myocardial injury in a murine model of viral myocarditis induced by coxsackievirus B3. Circ Res 81(4):504–511
68. Moore K, Roberts LJ Jr (1998) Measurement of lipid peroxidation. Free Radic Res 28(6):659–671
69. Nakamura K, Fushimi K, Kouchi H, Mihara K, Miyazaki M, Ohe T, Namba M (1998) Inhibitory effects of antioxidants on neonatal rat cardiac myocyte hypertrophy induced by tumor necrosis factor-alpha and angiotensin II. Circulation 98(8):794–799
70. Narita M, Shimizu S, Ito T, Chittenden T, Lutz RJ, Matsuda H, Tsujimoto Y (1998) Bax interacts with the permeability transition pore to induce permeability transition and cytochrome c release in isolated mitochondria [in process citation]. Proc Natl Acad Sci USA 95(25):14681–14686
71. Nathan C (1995) Natural resistance and nitric oxide. Cell 82(6):873–876
72. Oddis CV, Finkel MS (1995) Cytokine-stimulated nitric oxide production inhibits mitochondrial activity in cardiac myocytes. Biochem Biophys Res Commun 213:1002–1009
73. Ohta K, Kim S, Wanibuchi H, Ganten D, Iwao H (1996) Contribution of local renin-angiotensin system to cardiac hypertrophy, phenotypic modulation, and remodeling in TGR (mRen2)27 transgenic rats. Circulation 94(4):785–791
74. Olivetti G, Capasso JM, Sonnenblick EH, Anversa P (1990) Side-to-side slippage of myocytes participates in ventricular wall remodeling acutely after myocardial infarction in rats. Circ Res 67:23–34
75. Pfeffer MA, Braunwald E, Moye LA, et al (1992) Effect of captopril on mortality and morbidity in patients with left ventricular dysfunction after myocardial infarction. Results of the Survival and Ventricular Enlargement Trial. N Engl J Med 327:669–677
76. Pimentel DR, Amin JK, Baliga RR, Siwik DA, Chang DL, Pagano PJ, Colucci WS, Sawyer DB (1998) Reactive oxygen species mediate hypertrophy and apoptosis in cyclically-stretched cardiac myocytes. Circulation Suppl:1–743 (abstr)
77. Pinsky DJ, Cai B, Yang X, Rodriguez C, Sciacca RR, Cannon PJ (1995) The lethal effects of cytokine-induced nitric oxide on cardiac myocytes are blocked by nitric oxide synthase antagonism or transforming growth factor β. J Clin Invest 95:677–685
78. Prasad K, Gupta JB, Kalra J, Lee P, Mantha SV, Bharadwaj B (1996) Oxidative stress as a mechanism of cardiac failure in chronic volume overload in canine model. J Mol Cell Cardiol 28:375–385
79. Rajagopalan S, Politi PM, Sinha BK, Myers CE (1988) Adriamycin-induced free radical formation in the perfused rat heart: implications for cardiotoxicity. Cancer Res 48(17):4766–4769
80. Rapaport E, Gheorghiade M (1996) Pharmacologic therapies after myocardial infarction. Am J Med 101:4A61S–4A69S
81. Reed JC (1997) Cytochrome c: can't live with it – can't live without it [comment]. Cell 91(5):559–562
82. Reed JC (1997) Double identity for proteins of the Bcl-2 family. Nature 387(6635): 773–776
83. Rosse T, Olivier R, Monney L, Rager M, Conus S, Fellay I, Jansen B, Borner C (1998) Bcl-2 prolongs cell survival after Bax-induced release of cytochrome c [see comments]. Nature 391(6666):496–499

84. Rotruck JT, Pope AL, Ganther HE, Swanson AB, Hafeman DG, Hoekstra WG (1973) Selenium: biochemical role as a component of glutathione peroxidase. Science 179(73):588–590
85. Sawyer DB, Fukazawa R, Arstall MA, Kelly RA (1999) Daunorubicin-induced apoptosis in rat cardiac myocytes is inhibited by dexrazoxane. Circ Res 84:257–265
86. Schmidt U, Hajjar RJ, Helm PA, Kim CS, Doye AA, Gwathmey JK (1998) Contribution of abnormal sarcoplasmic reticulum ATPase activity to systolic and diastolic dysfunction in human heart failure. J Mol Cell Cardiol 30:1929–1937
87. Shatrov VA, Ratter F, Gruber A, Droge W, Lehmann V (1996) HIV type 1 glycoprotein 120 amplifies tumor necrosis factor-induced NF-kappa B activation in Jurkat cells. AIDS Res Hum Retroviruses 12(13):1209–1216
88. Singal PK, Dhillon KS, Beamish RE, Kapur N, Dhalla NS (1982) Myocardial cell damage and cardiovascular changes due to i.v. infusion of adrenochrome in rats. Br J Exp Pathol 63:167–176
89. Singh K, Balligand JL, Fischer TA, Smith TW, Kelly RA (1996) Regulation of cytokine-inducible nitric oxide synthase in cardiac myocytes and microvascular endothelial cells. Role of extracellular signal-regulated kinases 1 and 2 (ERK1/ERK2) and STAT1 alpha. J Biol Chem 271:1111–1117
90. Siwik DA, Tzortzis JD, Pimental DR, Chang DL, Pagano PJ, Singh K, Sawyer DB, Colucci WS (1999) Inhibition of copper-zinc superoxide dismutase induces cell growth, hypertrophic phenotype, and apoptosis in neonatal rat cardiac myocytes in vitro. Circ Res 85:147–153
91. Sobotka PA, Brottman MD, Weitz Z, Birnbaum AJ, Skosey JL, Zarling EJ (1993) Elevated breath pentane in heart failure reduced by free radical scavenger [see comments]. Free Radic Biol Med 14:643–647
92. Speyer JL, Green MD, Kramer E, Rey M, Sanger J, Ward C, Dubin N, Ferrans V, Stecy P, Zeleniuch-Jacquotte A (1988) Protective effect of the bispiperazinedione ICRF-187 against doxorubicin-induced cardiac toxicity in women with advanced breast cancer. N Engl J Med 319:745–752
93. Stamler JS, Simon DI, Osborne JA, Mullins ME, Jaraki O, Michel T, Singel DJ, Loscalzo J (1992) S-nitrosylation of proteins with nitric oxide: synthesis and characterization of biologically active compounds. Proc Natl Acad Sci USA 89:444–448
94. Sugden PH, Clerk A (1998) "Stress-responsive" mitogen-activated protein kinases (c-Jun N-terminal kinases and p38 mitogen-activated protein kinases) in the myocardium. Circ Res 83:345–352
95. Thompson-Gorman SL, Zweier JL (1990) Evaluation of the role of xanthine oxidase in myocardial reperfusion injury. J Biol Chem 265(12):6656–6663
96. Turner NA, Xia F, Azhar G, Zhang X, Liu L, Wei JY (1998) Oxidative stress induces DNA fragmentation and caspase activation via the c-Jun NH_2-terminal kinase pathway in H9c2 cardiac muscle cells. J Mol Cell Cardiol 30(9):1789–1801
97. Ushio-Fukai M, Zafari AM, Fukui T, Ishizaka N, Griendling KK (1996) p22phox is a critical component of the superoxide-generating NADH/NADPH oxidase system and regulates angiotensin II-induced hypertrophy in vascular smooth muscle cells. J Biol Chem 271(38):23317–23321
98. Van der Heiden MG, Chandel NS, Williamson EK, Schumacker PT, Thompson CB (1997) Bcl-xL regulates the membrane potential and volume homeostasis of mitochondria [see comments]. Cell 91(5):627–637
99. von Harsdorf R, Li PF, Dietz R (1999) Signaling pathways in reactive oxygen species-induced cardiomyocyte apoptosis. Circulation 99(22):2934–2941
100. Wang P, Chen H, Qin H, Sankarapandi S, Becher MW, Wong PC, Zweier JL (1998) Overexpression of human copper, zinc-superoxide dismutase (SOD1) prevents postischemic injury. Proc Natl Acad Sci USA 95(8):4556–4560

101. Wang Y, Huang S, Sah VP, Ross J, Brown JH, Han J, Chien KR (1998) Cardiac muscle hypertrophy and apoptosis induced by distinct members of the p38 mitogen-activated protein kinase family. J Biol Chem 273:2161–2168
102. Wang Y, Su B, Sah VP, Brown JH, Han J, Chien KR (1998) Cardiac hypertrophy induced by mitogen-activated protein kinase 7, a specific activator for c-Jun NH_2-terminal kinase in ventricular muscle cells. J Biol Chem 273:5423–5426
103. Weber KT, Anversa P, Armstrong PW, Brilla CG, Burnett JC Jr, Cruickshank JM, Devereux RB, Giles TD, Korsgaard N, Leier CV (1992) Remodeling and reparation of the cardiovascular system. J Am Coll Cardiol 20:3–16
104. Wu J, Xu GL (1987) Plasma selenium content, platelet glutathione peroxidase and superoxide dismutase activity of residents in Kashin-Beck disease affected area in China. J Trace Elem Electrolytes Health Dis 1(1):39–43
105. Xia Y, Zweier JL (1997) Superoxide and peroxynitrite generation from inducible nitric oxide synthase in macrophages. Proc Natl Acad Sci USA 94(13):6954–6958
106. Xie YW, Shen W, Zhao G, Xu X, Wolin MS, Hintze TH (1996) Role of endothelium-derived nitric oxide in the modulation of canine myocardial mitochondrial respiration in vitro. Implications for the development of heart failure. Circ Res 79(3):381–387
107. Xu L, Eu JP, Meissner G, Stamler JS (1998) Activation of the cardiac calcium release channel (ryanodine receptor) by poly-S-nitrosylation [in process vitation]. Science 279:234–237
108. Yamashita N, Nishida M, Hoshida S, Kuzuya T, Hori M, Taniguchi N, Kamada T, Tada M (1994) Induction of manganese superoxide dismutase in rat cardiac myocytes increases tolerance to hypoxia 24 hours after preconditioning. J Clin Invest 94(6):2193–2199
109. Yamazaki T, Komuro I, Zou Y, Kudoh S, Shiojima I, Hiroi Y, Mizuno T, Aikawa R, Takano H, Yazaki Y (1997) Norepinephrine induces the raf-1 kinase/mitogen-activated protein kinase cascade through both alpha 1- and beta-adrenoceptors. Circulation 95(5):1260–1268
110. Yue TL, Ma XL, Gu JL, Ruffolo RR Jr, Feuerstein GZ (1998) Carvedilol inhibits activation of stress-activated protein kinase and reduces reperfusion injury in perfused rabbit heart. Eur J Pharmacol 345(1):61–65
111. Zarain-Herzberg A, Afzal N, Elimban V, Dhalla NS (1996) Decreased expression of cardiac sarcoplasmic reticulum $Ca^{(2+)}$-pump ATPase in congestive heart failure due to myocardial infarction. Mol Cell Biochem 163/164:285–290

CHAPTER 18

Modulation of cardiac function by essential myosin light chains in health and disease

I. MORANO

Max-Delbrück-Center for Molecular Medicine, Berlin-Buch and Humboldt-University, Medical Faculty (Charité), Institute of Physiology, Berlin, Germany

Summary

Cardiac contraction is performed by the ATP-consuming cyclic interaction of the "molecular motor" myosin with the actin filament. The myosin heavy chain (MHC) contains the actin and ATP binding sites. Two different MHC genes (α and β) with distinct biochemical features are expressed in the human atrium, but only the β-MHC is expressed in the ventricle. Mutations in genes coding for ventricular myosin subunits are associated with hypertrophic cardiomyopathy. Motor function could be tuned by essential myosin light chain (MLC-1) isoforms. Expression of the atrial MLC-1 isoform in the hypertrophied human ventricle increases cross-bridge cycling kinetics and contractility. It is suggested that MLC-1 acts as a MHC/actin tether. Weakening of this tether increased myosin function.

Myosin structure of striated muscle

The three-dimensional structure of the S1 domain of the myosin molecule of chicken skeletal muscle was elucidated by X-ray crystallographic analysis [46]. It consists of an alpha-helical heavy chain (MHC), which folds at the N-terminus into an asymmetric globular head domain (Fig. 1). This head has a length of 16.5 nm, a width of 6.5 nm, and a thickness of 4 nm, comprises a seven-stranded β-sheet connected by flanking α-helices and/or loops which constitute the catalytic domain. Limited proteolysis revealed three major segments, a 25 kDa N-terminal, a central 50 kDa, and a 20 kDa C-terminal domain [38]. The 50 kDa domain is split by a long narrow cleft with actin-binding sites located on both sites of the cleft. Also, the ATP-binding (active) site forms an open cleft and is located opposite from the actin-binding site at the 25 kDa/50 kDa junction. The apex of the long cleft through the 50 kDa domain is very close to the nucleotide-binding cleft, thus, mediating signal transduction between the actin- and nucleotide-binding clefts. Amino acids (aa) 771–843 at the C-terminus form a 8.5 nm α-helical structure – the neck region – which binds two types of light chains that join the catalytic domain. The essential myosin light chain binds between aa 783 and 806 and the regulatory light chains further downstream between aa 808 and 842. The catalytic and light chain binding domains are joined by a so-called converter domain (around aa 711–771). Further downstream, not represented by the three-dimensional structure, the 140 nm α-helical "rod" domain joins the light chain-binding domain which forms the myosin filament. Therefore, the basic structure of the myosin molecule is a trimer. *In vivo*, two trimers associate to the native double-headed myosin molecule with Mr around 470.

Function of the molecular motor

In the intact contractile structure, the ATP- or ADP-Pi-loaded MHC binds as the "cross-bridge" to the N-terminus of actin. During the cycle, myosin undergoes changes of actin affinity and structure, being strongly attached to actin (having high affinity) or weakly attached (having low affinity) [5, 11]. Force is generated upon the transition from the weakly to the strongly attached state. This transition is considered to be coupled to the Pi release step [10].

These structural changes of the cross-bridges are associated with the strain of an elastic component present in the cross-bridges which operates over a range of around 8–10 nm [22]. In a contemporary model, the α-helical neck domain is believed to function as a lever arm that swings relative to the catalytic domain: picometer changes in the active site of S1 are magnified into nanometers of motion by rotation of the converter domain [11, 19]. In fact, truncation and elongation of the light chain-binding domains showed that the sliding velocity of actin filaments is proportional to the length of the lever arm [59]. Furthermore, the light chain-binding domain, rather than the catalytic domain, revealed tilting motions during length perturbations of an isometrically contracting muscle [20, 23, 25] (Fig. 1). This is in contrast to textbook illustrations which show tilting S1 portions. The elastic element of the cross-bridge may, therefore, reside in the lever arm [21].

Myosin heavy chain expression in the human heart

In the human heart, two sarcomeric myosin II genes are expressed generating two isoenzymes of the myosin heavy chain (designated α- and β-MHC). They are located in tandem on the long arm of human chromosome 14q11.2-q13 [48]. In the normal adult human heart, both MHC isoenzymes are expressed in a tissue-specific manner: the α-MHC is preferentially expressed in the atrium and the β-MHC is almost exclusively expressed in the ventricle [4, 15]. In the rodent, β-MHC revealed a lower ATPase activity and was associated with a decreased maximal shortening velocity of the cardiac fibers compared to α-MHC. It is still not clear to what extent the different myosin light chain subunit isoforms present in atrium and ventricle (see below) contributed to the higher cycling kinetics of human atrial myosin compared to human ventricular myosin [33].

In the hypertrophied human atrium, considerable amounts of β-MHC were expressed [9, 15], which was associated with a decrease of maximal shortening velocity [19].

In small mammals, cardiac overload is associated with increased ventricular expression of the β-MHC gene. The same mechanism was also suggested for the human ventricle, based on the observation of α-MHC mRNA in the human ventricle and its downregulation in the hypertrophied and failung myocardium [26, 39]. However, it is not yet clear at all, whether the human ventricle expresses α-MHC. Immunohistochemistry and peptide map studies [4, 15, 18] demonstrated the predominant expression of β-MHC in the ventricle, but those studies did not contribute to a quantification of α- and β-MHC protein expression. Using monoclonal antibodies raised against chicken and rat β-MHC and α-MHC, respectively, some low α-MHC protein could be demonstrated in the normal human ventricle using purified myosin from autopsy samples [29]. In the same study, myosin preparations with α-MHC revealed similar ATPase activities as myosin without α-MHC. Furthermore, similar amounts of α-MHC were reported in fetal ventricles and ventricles of hypertrophied human hearts [29] suggesting that putative human ventricular α-MHC has no enzymatic property distinct from β-MHC and that its expression is neither developmentally regulated nor modulated during hypertrophy.

Recently, we applied a qualitative Western blot method using a monoclonal antibody raised against human α-MHC and SDS extracts of quickly frozen human ventricular tissue to describe the amount of α-MHC expression in the human ventricle [47]. We could not detect any α-MHC signal in normal, hypertrophied left (patients with hypertrophic cardiomyopathy) and right (patients with tetralogy of Fallot, Double-Outlet Right Ventricle) ventricles, nor in the left ventricle of terminally failing (dilative and ischemic cardiomyopathy) human hearts [47]. Since the detection level was found to be 0.10 μg α-MHC and since we analyzed 10 μg ventricular MHC in the Wester blot, the relative amount of α-MHC in the human ventricles must be below 1%, i.e., in functionally insignificant proportions. The reason for undetectable levels of α-MHC in the human ventricle may reside in the very low α-MHC mRNA levels which was more than 40-fold smaller than β-MHC mRNA expression in the normal human heart [47]. Thus, unlike rodents, human beings did not regulate ventricular contractility by MHC gene variation.

Myosin heavy chain mutations

Around 40 mutations – predominantly missense mutations – of the β-MHC gene, and an α-β-MHC chimeric gene have been described in some familiar forms of hypertrophic cardiomyopathy, an autosomal dominant inherited heart disease. Some of these mutations have already been characterized at the functional level using *in vitro* motility assays and demembranated fiber mechanics. Since it is not within the scope of this paper to review myosin mutations (excellent articles have already been published, cf. [44, 60]), only some will be considered. Thus, Arg403Gln [24] in the actin-binding site revealed a decreased function and coincided with a high incidence of sudden cardiac death and decreased life expectancy [12]. Normal myosin function and low incidence of sudden cardiac death was associated with Gly256Glu mutation [24].

Myosin light chain expression in the human heart

Two types of myosin light chains (MLC), essential and regulatory, are associated with the neck region of the MHC. The essential MLC is designated as the MLC-1 or alkali MLC. The regulatory MLC is designated as MLC-2 or phosphorylatable MLC or DTNB-MLC [46]. Together with calmodulin and troponin C, both types belong to the superfamily of EF-hand Ca^{2+}-binding proteins [31].

In the human heart, two different genes encode the essential myosin light chain isoforms, the ventricular specific (VLC-1) and an atrial specific (ALC-1). VLC-1 is located on chromosome 3p21 [14] coding for a 194aa protein, which is the same isoform as the MLC-1s present in the adult slow skeletal muscle. ALC-1 is located on chromosome 17q21 [50] coding a 196aa protein.

Several MLC-2 isoforms exist in the human, preferentially expressed in the atrium (ALC-2) or in the ventricle (VLC-2). VLC-2 has been mapped to chromosome 12q23-qz24 [27] in human encoding a 166 aa protein. ALC-2 is composed of 175 aa [16], but no data are available yet about the chromosomal localization of ALC-2. Biochemical experiments revealed that the human ALC-2 was slightly more acidic than the VLC-2 [42]. Furthermore, sequence analysis suggested the existence of two VLC-2 isoforms in chicken [28], cow and rabbit [61]. In addition, electrophoretic analysis suggested the existence of two different VLC-2 isoforms in the human heart having the same molecular weight but different isoelectric points (VLC-2a for the more acidic and VLC-2b for the more basic isoform) [42].

Expression regulation of essential MLC in the human heart

Expression of ALC-1 is tissue specific and developmentally regulated

Human embryos expressed large amounts of ALC-1 in the whole heart as well as in skeletal muscle [3]. ALC-1 protein levels decreased in the ventricle to undetectable levels during early postnatal development but persisted in the atrium throughout the whole life [9].

Expression of ALC-1 is increased in the compensated state of ventricular overload

The hypertrophied right ventricle of children with Tetralogy of Fallot (TOF) expressed large amounts ALC-1 in the ventricle, up to adulthood [2]. Similarly, the hypertrophied left ventricle of patients with hypertrophic cardiomyopathy as well as valvular heart diseases expressed ALC-1 [35, 43, 49, 55]. Surgical intervention and subsequent normalization of the hemodynamic state decreased ALC-1 expression in these patients [55]. ALC-1 expression in the hypertrophied human ventricle was very heterogenous and varied between 0% and 35% of total MLC-1. However, mean amount of ALC-1 appeared higher in hypertrophied ventricles of patients with HOCM compared to the failing ventricles of patients with dilated cardiomyopathy (DCM). Thus, patients with HOCM expressed mean ALC-1 levels of 13% (range 0–32%) [43] while DCM revealed much lower mean ALC-1 levels of 4% (range: 0–10%) [35] in their ventricles.

These data show an interesting phenomenon: there is a large variation in ALC-1 expression in the human ventricle and some patients did not express any ALC-1 in their ventricles. At present, we do not know the reasons for that.

Transcription factors involved in ALC-1 expression

Regulation of ALC-1 expression in the human heart is still not well understood. In the mouse, two E boxes that interact with muscle-specific basic helix-loop-helix (bHLH) regulatory proteins of the MyoD family and a diverged CArG box that binds the serum response factor exist within the first 630 bp of the ALC-1 promoter region [6]. E boxes have been shown to be sufficient for ALC-1 transcription regulation during skeletal muscle differentiation [6]. bHLH regulatory factors of the MyoD family regulate skeletal muscle differentiation by forming heterodimers with E12 bHLH factors that bind to E-box elements, thus, increasing the transcription rate of target genes (for review see [40]). Recently, two cardiac-specific bHLH proteins homologous to the MyoD family were detected in the heart, designated as eHAND and dHAND [8, 51]. They are important for early development and looping of the embryonic heart [52]. Since both HAND transcription factors bind to E-box as E12 heterodimers, the ALC-1 may be a target gene. In the human hypertrophied ventricle there was indeed an upregulation of HAND gene expression as well as a positive correlation between HAND and ALC-1 mRNA [43]. Beside an E-box element, the human ALC-1 promoter contains consensus-binding sequences for GATA and NF-AT3 transcription factors known to mediate the hypertrophic response of the heart. Recently, the molecular events which could explain increased GATA activity in the heart were presented [30]: upon increased intracellular Ca^{2+}, NF-AT3 becomes dephosphorylated by the Ca^{2+}-dependent protein phosphatase calcineurin, translocates to the nucleus, and interacts with GATA, thus, increasing its DNA-binding activity. In addition, NF-AT3 may have the capability to directly activate ALC-1 transcription of target genes.

ALC-1 expression is regulated by endogenous antisense mRNA

ALC-1 expression may be regulated by endogenous antisense ALC-1 mRNA present in the human ventricle [43]. In fact, there was a dependency of ALC-1 protein expression on the ratio between antisense/sense ALC-1 mRNA present in the hypertrophied human heart: the higher the antisense/sense ALC-1 mRNA, the lower the ALC-1 protein expression was. ALC-1 protein being almost zero at a antisense/sense ALC-1 mRNA ratio of 1 [43].

Modulation of cross-bridge function by essential myosin light chains

The functional role of the essential MLC in the heart has remained obscure for many years. Recently, we described for the first time that maximal shortening velocity (V_{max}; which equals the cross-bridge detachment rate), the rate of tension redevelopment (which equals the cross-bridge detachment+attachment rate), isometric force generation per cross-section, and Ca^{2+} sensitivity of isometric force generation increased upon partial replacement of VLC-1 by ALC-1 in the human ventricle [32, 37]. Furthermore, there was a significant positive correlation between ALC-1 expression and dP/dt_{max} of patients with HOCM in vivo [47]. Thus, cross-bridge cycling kinetics and perhaps force per cross-bridge is modulated by differential expression of MLC-1 genes. However, it is not yet clear which step in the cross-bridge cycle is modified by ALC-1. Since expression of ALC-1 increased force per cross-section at saturating Ca^{2+} [37], force generation per cross-bridge could be increased. Hence, ventricular cross-bridges with ALC-1 could then more easily overcome the high internal loads present in cardiac fibers leading to a higher shortening velocity at a given external load [37]. This would increase contractility without additional consumption of ATP and oxygen, i.e., increased economy of tension production. In fact, increased Ca^{2+} sensitivity and rate of isometric tension generation observed in the presence of ALC-1 [35, 37] is theoretically predicted using an increased attachment rate [5].

These results demonstrated that there is a molecular mechanism which allows the ventricular cardiomyocyte to adjust to enhanced work load through modification of the structure of the molecular motor: partial substitution of VLC-1 by ALC-1 increased power output of the sarcomeric motor macromolecules and improved cardiac contractility. These results could be supported in a transgenic mouse model which overexpressed atrial essential MLC in the ventricle: working heart function increased upon atrial essential MLC expression in the ventricle of transgenic rats overexpressing ALC-1 [13]. In the same mouse model, rise of cardiac beating frequency caused by running was significantly lower in the transgenic group, demonstrating a large contractile reserve in ventricles with ALC-1 [13].

Thus, ALC-1 expression could be considered as a molecular adaptation mechanism to compensate an increased work demand or impaired sarcomeric function. In DCM, expressed ALC-1 levels may be too low to adequately balance decreased contractile function. Hence, patients with DCM may be a target for therapeutical upregulation of ALC-1 expression either by genetic (viral) transfer of ALC-1 cDNA into the cardiomyocyte or by upregulation of ALC-1 gene transcription.

The essential MLC isoforms act as a MHC/actin tether

MLC-1 binds not only to the neck domain of the MHC [46], but also with its N-terminus to the C-terminus domain of actin [17, 34, 54, 57, 58]. Thus, MLC-1 tethers the MHC to the actin filament. It could be demonstrated that MHC and MLC-1 bind to different actin monomers [57]. Binding of MLC-1 to actin cannot be predicted from the crystal structure of myosin S1, due to the limited resolution of the three-dimensional structure of the N-terminus of MLC-1 [46]. In fact, aro- und 40 N-terminal amino acid residues of MLC-1 are not seen in the crystal structure. This missing part of MLC-1 contains 10 Pro and 10 Ala residues [14], which could form an antenna-like structure long enough to bridge the gap to the actin filament.

Experimental evidence for the functional importance of the MHC/actin tether could be obtained by weakening the tether on the MLC-1/actin interface and/or MLC-1/MHC interface and simultaneous registration of cross-bridge function. Inhibition of the MLC-1/actin interaction by peptide competition using synthetic N-terminal MLC-1 peptides increases force production and shortening velocity of both demembranated (skinned) and of intact electrically driven human ventricular fibers [36] as well as myofibrillar ATPase activity [45]. We proposed that tethering MHC to the actin filament via MLC-1 imposes a load on the myosin cross-bridge. Relieving or weakening the MHC/actin tether decreases this load and accelerates cross-bridge cycling kinetics and at the same time enhances tension output per cross-bridge, thus, increasing contractility [36].

To explain the effects on contractility by partial VLC-1/ALC-1 replacement in the hypertrophied human ventricle [35, 37], we suggested that binding of ALC-1 to actin is weaker than the binding of VLC-1 to actin, representing a weaker MHC/actin tether. Interestingly, the primary structure of the N-terminus of the ALC-1 and VLC-1 are different [14] (Table 1). Indeed, the affinity of actin to the N-terminal peptide 5–14 derived from ALC-1 is significantly lower than the actin affinity to the corresponding N-terminal peptide of VLC-1 [34]. These results supported the initial hypothesis [37]: because of its low actin affinity, ALC-1 is a weaker MHC/actin tether than VLC-1, and has increased cross-bridge cycling kinetics and force generation.

Table 1. Primary structures (three-letter symbols; bold: positively charged residues; italics: negatively charged residues) of the N-terminal domains of human ventricular (VLC-1) and atrial (ALC-1) essential myosin-light chain isoforms

Isoform	Primary structure	Ref.
Human VLC-1	Ala-Pro-**Lys-Lys**-Pro-*Glu*-Pro-**Lys-Lys**-*Asp-Asp*-Ala-**Lys**-Ala-Ala-Pro-Ala-Pro-**Lys**-Ala-Ala-	[14]
Human ALC-1	Ala-Pro-**Lys-Lys**-Pro-*Glu*-Pro-**Lys-Lys**-*Glu*-Ala-Ala-Lys-Pro-Ala-Pro-Ala-Pro-Ala-Pro-Ala-	[50]

There is more experimental evidence in favor of this hypothesis: reconstitution of demembranated skeletal muscle fibers with MLC-1, where charged residues were substituted by uncharged Ala at the N-terminus, increased shortening velocity [56]. The N-terminus of ALC-1 contained 7 charged aa while VLC-1 contained 9 [14]. From these data, it appears that cross-bridge kinetics can be regulated by charge interactions between the N-terminus of MLC-1 and the actin C-terminus. Decreasing the amount of charged amino acid aa – by Ala substitution or differential MLC-1 isoform expression – weakened the MHC/actin tether and increased cross-bridge function.

Interaction between the N-terminus of essential MLC and actin may depend on the ionic conditions. In the test tube, the N-terminus of essential MLC could be cleaved by proteases only in the presence of Ca^{2+} [53]. Thus, different conformational states of the N-terminus of essential MLC may exist: an extended state with Ca^{2+} and a bent state without Ca^{2+} [53]. In the cardiomyocyte this would require a fluctuation of the N-terminus from an extended antenna-like form which could bind to actin during systole (high Ca^{2+}), and a bent form during diastole (low Ca^{2+}) dissociated from actin.

The molecular mechanism proposed of force generation and essential MLC action are schematically represented in Fig. 1.

There is an additional interpretation of the functional effects of essential MLC isoforms. Maximal force production of the myosin cross-bridge may depend on the stiffness of the lever arm, i.e., the smaller the stiffness, the smaller the force that would be generated per cross-bridge [21]. Since the light chains are associated with the lever arm, different MLC isoforms may influence the cross-bridge stiffness. It could, therefore, be suggested that the β-MHC associated with the VLC-1 has a higher stiffness than β-MHC with the ALC-1, thus, generating more force per motor molecule.

Another important feature of the regulation of the contractile cardiac system by essential MLC is the sensitivity. Relative small changes of the VLC-1/ALC-1 ratio were required to produce strong effects in the human heart [35, 37]. This is in contrast to the transgenic mouse model, where VLC-1 became almost completely replaced by ALC-1 with moderate in-

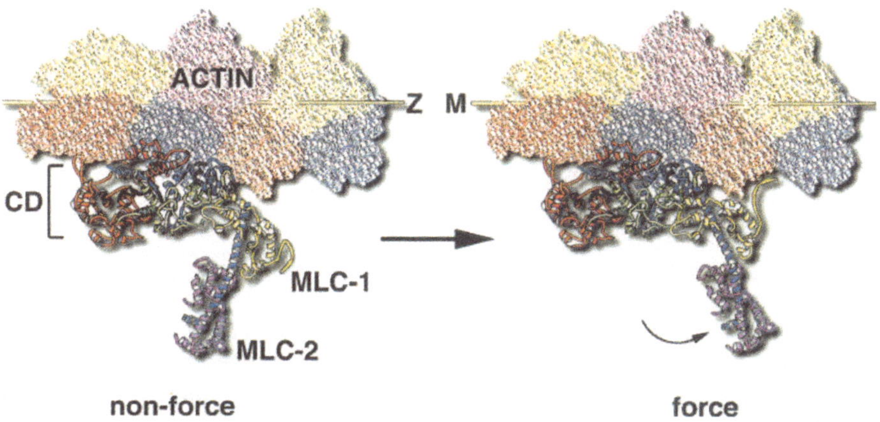

Fig. 1. Three-dimensional ribbon structure of myosin-S1 [46] associated with the actin filament (Z = towards Z-line, M = towards M-line). The myosin heavy chain consists of a 25 K N-terminal (green), 50 K (red), and a C-terminal joining 20 K (blue) domain. The pear-shaped head is called the catalytic domain (CD). Essential myosin light chain (MLC-1, yellow) and regulatory myosin light chain (MLC-2) are associated with the alpha-helical C-terminal part of the 20 K-domain (light chain-binding domain) (adapted from: Rayment I, Holden HM (1994) TIBS 19:129–134).
The catalytic domain (CD) of myosin-S1 binds to actin in a non-force generating state. Force generation is elicited by elastic bending of the light chain-binding domain, the lever arm rather than by rotation of the catalytic domain. In addition to the CD, the N-terminus of MLC-1 binds to a neighboring actin monomer in the force (high Ca^{2+}) but not in the non-force-generating (low Ca^{2+}) state.

crease in cross-bridge cycling rate and contractility [13]. The relative higher efficiency of essential MLC regulation in the human compared to the rodent ventricle could explain the evolutionary diverged types of cardiac adaptation mechanisms to increased work demand, namely MHC regulation in rodents and essential MLC regulation in man.

Mutations shed new light on essential MLC function

In patients with hypertrophic cardiomyopathy (HCM) with mid-left ventricular thickening, a Met149Val substitution in VLC-1 was observed [41]. Myosin with the mutated VLC-1 revealed an increased actin translocation velocity in the *in vitro* motility assay [41]. It is worth noting that Met149Val is at the binding interface with the myosin heavy chain [38]. As suggested above, tethering the myosin head to actin via MLC-1 seems to control force generation and cycling kinetics of the cross-bridge. Therefore, weakening the interaction between MHC and MLC-1 should produce the same enhancement of cross-bridge function as weakening the actin and MLC-1 interaction. It is not clear whether Met149Val mutation of VLC-1 really results in a weakening of MHC-MLC-1 interaction, but if so, it would explain the improved function of myosin with Met149Val mutation in VLC-1 in the *in vitro* motility assay [41]. Changing the MHC/MLC-1 interaction on the MHC site may be represented by a missense mutation close to the MHC/MLC-1 interface (Arg719Gln) [7]. Again, this mutation close to the MHC/actin tether increases actin translocation velocity. These results suggest that any deterioration of the MHC/actin tether at the MHC/MLC-1 interface (by mutation) or the MLC-1/actin interface (Ala substitution, peptide competition, MLC-1 isoform transition) increases myosin function.

Future prospects

A new therapeutic approach to improve cardiac contractility could be achieved by the development of drugs weakening the MHC/actin tether. Thus, molecules resembling the N-terminus of MLC-1 may inhibit the interaction between essential MLC and actin. Alternatively, gene constructs coding for N-terminal peptides of cardiac MLC-1 could be transferred into cardiomyocytes for ectopic expression, eventually increasing the inotropic state of the heart.

Both, pharmacological and the genetic approaches could improve power output of cardiac contraction and can represent future therapeutic approaches for treatment of cardiac failure.

Acknowledgments. This work was supported by DFG Mo 362/17-1/2.

References

1. Arndt H, Bletz C, Katus HA, Mall G, Rüegg JC (1989) Calcium sensitivity and unloaded shortening velocity of hypertrophied and non-hypertrophied skinned human atrial fibers. Pflügers Arch 415:209–213
2. Auckland LM, Lambert SJ, Cummins P (1986) Cardiac myosin light and heavy chain isotypes in Tetralogy of Fallot. Cardiovasc Res 20:828–863
3. Barton P, Buckingham ME (1985) The myosin alkali light chain proteins and their genes. Biochem J 231:249–261
4. Bouvagnet P, Leger J, Pons F, Dechesne C, Leger JJ (1984) Fiber types and myosin types in human atrial and ventricular myocardium. An anatomical description. Circ Res 55:794–804
5. Brenner B (1988) Effect of Ca^{2+} on cross-bridge turnover kinetics in skinned single rabbit psoas fibers: implications for regulation of muscle contraction. Proc Natl Acad Sci USA 85:3265–3269
6. Catala F, Wanner R, Barton P, Cohen A, Wright W, Buckingham M (1995) A skeletal muscle specific enhancer regulated by factors binding to E and CArG boxes is present in the promoter of the mouse myosin light chain 1A gene. Mol Cell Biol 15:4585–4596
7. Consevage MW, Salada GC, Baylen BG, Ladda RL, Rogan PK (1994) A new missense mutation, Arg719Gln in the β-cardiac myosin heavy chain gene of patients with familial hypertrophic cardiomyopathy. Hum Mol Genet 3:1025–1026
8. Cserjesi P, Brown D, Lyons GE, Olsdon EN (1995) Expression of the novel basic Helix-Loop-Helix gene eHAND in neural crest derivatives and extraembryonic membranes during mouse development. Dev Biol 170:664–678

9. Cummins P, Lambert SJ (1986) Myosin transitions in the bovine and human heart. A developmental and anatomical study of heavy and light subunits in the atrium and ventricle. Circ Res 58:846–858
10. Dantzig JA, Goldman YE, Millar NC, Lacktis J, Homsher E (1992) Reversal of the cross-bridge force-generating transition by photogeneration of phosphate in rabbit psoas muscle fibers. J Physiol (Lond) 451:247–278
11. Eisenberg E, Hill TL (1985) Muscle contraction and free energy transduction in biological systems. Science 227:999–1006
12. Epstein ND, Cohn GM, Cyran F, Fananapazir L (1992) Differences of clinical expression of hypertrophic cardiomyopathy associated with two distinct mutations in the β-myosin heavy chain gene: A908Leu-Val mutation and a 403Arg-Gln mutation. Circulation 86:345–352
13. Fewell JG, Hewett T, Sanbe A, Klevitsky R, Hayes E, Warshaw D, Maughan J, Robbins J (1998) Functional significance of cardiac essential light chain isoform switching in transgenic mice. J Clin Invest 101:2630–2639
14. Fodor WL, Darras B, Seharaseyon J, Falkenthal S, Francke U, Vanin EF (1989) Human ventricular/slow twitch myosin alkali light chain gene characterization, sequence, and chromosomal location. J Biol Chem 264:2143–2149
15. Gorza L, Mercadier JJ, Schwartz K, Thornell LE, Sartore S, Schiaffino S (1984) Myosin types in the human hearts. An immunofluorescence study of normal and hypertrophied atrial and ventricular myocardium. Circ Res 54:694–702
16. Hailstones D, Barton P, Chan-Thomas P, Sasse S, Sutherland C, Hardeman E, Gunning P (1992) Differential regulation of the atrial isoforms of the myosin light chains during striated muscle development. J Biol Chem 267:23295–23300
17. Hayashibara T, Miyanishi T (1994) Binding of the amino-terminal region of myosin alkali 1 light chain to actin and its effect on actin-myosin interaction. Biochem 33:12821–12827
18. Hirzel HO, Tuchschmid CR, Schneider J, Krayenbuehl, Schaub MC (1985) Relationship between myosin isoenzyme composition, hemodynamics and myocardial structure in various forms of human cardiac hypertrophy. Circ Res 57:729–740
19. Holmes KC (1997) The swinging lever-arm hypothesis of muscle contraction. Curr Biol 7:R112–R118
20. Hopkins SC, Sabido-David C, Corrie JET, Irving M, Goldman YE (1998) Fluorescence polarization transients from rhodamine isomers on the myosin regulatory light chain in skeletal muscle fibers. Biophys J 74:1039–3110
21. Howard J, Spudich JA (1996) Is the lever arm of myosin a molecular elastic element? Proc Natl Acad Sci USA 93:4462–4464
22. Huxley AF, Simmons R (1971) Proposed mechanism of force generation in striated muscle. Nature (Lond) 233:533–538
23. Irving M, Allen TS, Sabido-David C, Craik JS, Brandmeier B, Kendrick-Jones J, Corrie JET, Trentham DR, Goldman YE (1995) Tilting of the light chain region of myosin during step length changes and active force generation in skeletal muscle. Nature 375:688–691
24. Lankford EB, Epstein ND, Fananapazir L, Sweeney HL (1995) Abnormal contractile properties of muscle fibers expressing β-myosin heavy chain gene mutation in patients with hypertrophic cardiomyopathy. J Clin Invest 95:1409–1414
25. Lombardi V, Piazzesi G, Ferenci A, Thirlwell H, Dobbie I, Irving M (1995) Elastic distorsion of myosin heads and repriming of the working stroke in muscle. Nature 374:553–555
26. Lowes BD, Minobe W, Abraham WT, Rizeq MN, Bohlmeyer TJ, Quaife RA, Roden RL, Dutcher DL, Robertson AD, Voelkel NF, Badesch DB, Groves BM, Gilbert EM, Bristow MR (1997) Changes in gene expression in the intact human heart. Down-

regulation of α-myosin heavy chain in hypertrophied, failing ventricular myocardium. J Clin Invest 100:2315–2324
27. Macerea M, Szabo P, Wadgaonkar R, Siddiqui M, Verma R (1992) Localization of the gene encoding for ventricular regulatory light chain (Myl 2) to human chromosome 12q23q24.3. Genomics 13:765–772
28. Matsuda G, Maita T, Kato Y, Chen JI, Umegane T (1981) Amino acid sequence of the cardiac L-2A, L-2B and gizzard 10000Mr light chains of chicken muscle myosin. FEBS Lett 135:232–236
29. Mercadier JJ, Bouveret P, Gorza L, Schiaffino S, Clark WA, Zak R, Swynghedauw B, Schwartz K (1983) Myosin isoenzymes in normal and hypertrophied human ventricular myocardium. Circ Res 53:52–62
30. Molkentin JD, Lu JR, Markham B, Richardson J, Robins J, Olson EN (1998) A calcineurin-dependent transcriptional pathway for cardiac hypertrophy. Cell 93:215–228
31. Moncrief ND, Kretsinger RH, Goodman M (1990) Evolution of EF-hand calcium-modulated proteins: relationships based on amino acid sequences. J Mol Evol 30:522–562
32. Morano I (1999) Tuning the human heart molecular motors by myosin light chains. J Mol Med 77:544–555
33. Morano I, Bletz C, Wojciechowski R, Rüegg JC (1991) Modulation of cross-bridge kinetics by myosin isoenzymes in skinned human heart fibers. Circ Res 68:614–618
34. Morano I, Haase H (1997) Different actin affinities of human cardiac essential myosin light chain isoforms. FEBS Lett 408:71–74
35. Morano I, Hädicke K, Haase H, Böhm M, Erdmann E, Schaub MC (1997) Changes in essential myosin light chain isoform expression provide a molecular basis for isometric force regulation in the failing human heart. J Mol Cell Cardiol 29:1177–1187
36. Morano I, Ritter O, Bonz A, Timek T, Vahl CF, Michel G (1995) Myosin light-chain actin interaction regulates cardiac contractility. Circ Res 76:720–725
37. Morano M, Zacharzowski U, Maier M, Lange PE, Alexi-Meskishvili V, Haase H, Morano I (1996) Regulation of human heart contractility by essential myosin light chain isoforms. J Clin Invest 98:467–473
38. Mornet D, Pantel P, Audemard E, Kassab R (1979) The limited tryptic cleavage of chymotryptic S1: an approach to the characterization of the actin site in myosin heads. Biochem Biophys Res Comm 89:925–932
39. Nakao K, Minobe W, Roden R, Bristow MR, Leinwand LA (1997) Myosin heavy chain gene expression in human heart failure. J Clin Invest 100:2362–2370
40. Olson EN (1992) Interplay between proliferation and differentiation within the myogenic lineage. Dev Biol 154:261–272
41. Poetter K, Jiang H, Hassanzadeh S, Master SR, Chang A, Dalaka MC, Rayment I, Sellers JR, Fananapazir L, Epstein ND (1996) Mutation of either the essential or regulatory light chains of myosin are associated with a rare myopathy in human heart and skeletal muscle. Nat Genet 13:63–69
42. Price KN, Littler WA, Cummins P (1980) Human atrial and ventricular myosin light chain subunits in the adult and during development. Biochem J 191:571–580
43. Ritter O, Haase H, Schulte HD, Morano I (1999) Remodeling of the hypertrophic human myocardium by cardiac bHLH transcription factors. J Cell Biochem 74:551–561
44. Rayment I, Holden H, Sellers J, Fananapazir L, Epstein ND (1995) Structural interpretation of the mutations in the β-cardiac myosin that have been implicated in familial hypertrophic cardiomyopathy. Proc Natl Acad Sci 92:3864–3868
45. Rarick HM, Opgenorth TJ, Vongeldern TW, Wuwong JSR, Solaro RJ (1996) An essential myosin light chain peptide induces supramaximal stimulation of cardiac myofibrillar ATPase activity. J Biol Chem 271:27039–27043

46. Rayment I, Rypniewski WR, Schmidt-Bäse K, Smith R, Tomchick DR, Benning MM, Winkelmann DA, Wesenberg G, Holden HM (1993) Three-dimensional structure of myosin subfragment-1: a molecular motor. Science 261:50–58
47. Ritter O, Luther HP, Haase H, Baltas LG, Balzereit D, Baumann G, Schulte HD, Morano I (1999) Expression of atrial myosin light chains but not alpha-myosin heavy chains correlate with increased ventricular function in patients with HOCM in vivo. J Mol Med 77:677–685
48. Saez LJ, Gianola KM, McNally EM, Feghali R, Eddy R (1987) Human cardiac myosin heavy chain genes and their linkage in the genome. Nucleic Acids Res 15:5443–5459
49. Schaub MC, Tuchschmid CR, Srihari R, Hirzel HO (1984) Myosin isoenzymes in human hypertrophic hearts. Shift of atrial myosin heavy chains and ventricular light chains. Eur Heart J 5:85–93
50. Seharaseyon J, Bober E, Hsieh CL, Fodor WL, Francke U, Arnold HH, Vanin EF (1990) Human embryonic/atrial myosin alkali light chain gene: characterization, sequence, and chromosomal location. Genomics 7:289–293
51. Srivastava D, Cserjesi P, Olson EN (1995) A subclass of bHLH proteins required for cardiac morphogenesis. Science 270:1995–1999
52. Srivastava D, Thomas T, Lin Q, Kirby ML, Brown D, Olson EN (1997) Regulation of cardiac mesodermal and neural crest development by the bHLH transcription factor, dHAND. Nat Gen 16:154–160
53. Stepkowski D (1995) The role of the skeletal muscle myosin light chain N-terminal fragments. FEBS Lett 374:6–11
54. Sutoh K (1982) Identification of myosin binding sites on the actin sequence. Biochem 21:3654–3661
55. Sütsch G, Brunner UT, Von Schulthess C, Hirzel HO, Hess OM, Turina M, Krayenbuehl HP, Schaub MC (1992) Hemodynamic performance and myosin light chain 1 expression in the hypertrophied left ventricle in aortic valve disease before and after valve replacement. Circ Res 70:1035–1043
56. Sweeney HL (1995) Function of the N-terminus of the myosin essential light chain of vertebrate striated muscle. Biophys J 68:112–119
57. Timson DJ, Trayer HR, Trayer IP (1998) The N-terminus of A1-type myosin essential light chains binds actin and modulates myosin motor function. Eur J Biochem 255:654–662
58. Trayer IP, Trayer HP, Levine BA (1987) Evidence that the N-terminal region of the A1 light chain of myosin interacts directly with the C-terminal region of actin. Eur J Biochem 164:259–266
59. Uyeda T, Abramson PD, Spudich JA (1996) The neck region of the myosin motor domain acts as a lever arm to generate movement. Proc Natl Acad Sci USA 93:4459–4464
60. Vikstrom KL, Leinwand LA (1996) Contractile protein mutations and heart disease. Curr Op in Cell Biol 8:97–105
61. Westwood SA, Perry SV (1982) Two forms of the P-light chain of myosin in rabbit and bovine hearts. FEBS Lett 142:31–34

CHAPTER 19

Myocardial infarction, infarct repair, and strategies for muscle regeneration

C. E. MURRY, M. ZHANG, H. REINECKE
Department of Pathology,
University of Washington, Seattle WA, USA

Introduction

Despite impressive advances in the last decade at treating coronary atherosclerosis, myocardial infarction remains the number one cause of death and disability in industrialized countries. A great deal of effort has been expended over the last 25 years toward identifying strategies to limit the amount of myocardium lost to infarction [4, 5]. Although infarct size limitation remains a highly desirable goal, it has been extremely difficult to achieve clinically. Over the last 5 years, our group has become increasingly interested in working on strategies to enhance the repair phase of myocardial infarction [31–33, 42, 43]. Our long-term goals are to induce muscular regeneration of the infarcted region. An intermediate goal, however, is to understand the molecular biology of infarct healing and to find strategies to prevent complications of infarction such as ventricular dilation that contribute to heart failure. This chapter will review the pathobiology of myocardial infarction and infarct repair, and then summarize some of our recent work in cardiomyocyte transplantation for creation of new myocardium.

Pathobiology of myocardial infarction

Cell Injury during myocardial ischemia

In the great majority of cases, myocardial infarcts result from rupture of an atherosclerotic plaque in a coronary artery, resulting in an occlusive thrombus [8, 9]. A small percentage of infarcts result from vasospasm, thromboemboli, or vasculitis. Within seconds of the onset of severe ischemia contractile function rapidly diminishes, with the result that the ischemic tissue goes from actively contracting to passively bulging with each beat. Contractile failure serves an adaptive function by lowering the tissue's metabolic requirements. Nevertheless, ischemic myocardium still has a high metabolic rate, and the residual demand for high energy phosphates outstrips the ability of anaerobic glycolysis to synthesize ATP [15–18]. As a result, tissue high energy phosphate levels fall, concomitantly with accumulation of metabolic end-products such as lactic acid and inorganic phosphate. Depletion of

ATP and accumulation of metabolic products independently contribute to cell injury. Current evidence points to rupture of the sarcolemma as the event which causes cells to be irreversibly injured [19, 51].

In the dog, which probably mimics the collateralized, diseased human heart, irreversible ischemic injury begins within 15–20 min after the onset of severe ischemia [19, 40, 41]. Necrosis is first seen in the subendocardium (innermost layer), where collateral blood flow is lowest and metabolic demand highest. With increasing duration of ischemia there is a wavefront of cell death that sweeps from the subendocardium to the subepicardium (outermost layer). The lateral borders of the infarct are constant and extend to the interface of the ischemic and non-ischemic vascular beds. Irreversible injury is 80% complete within 3 hours of ischemia in the dog, and by 6 hours the infarct is 100% complete.

It should be clear, therefore, that once myocardium becomes ischemic, there are only a few hours during which one can intervene to salvage the muscle at risk. A fundamental problem is that most patients wait over 3 hours after coronary occlusion before seeking medical attention. To date, even the most potent anti-ischemic interventions (ischemic preconditioning and pretreatment with calcium channel blockers) cannot protect myocardium from a sustained ischemic insult of 3 hours [30, 39]. If human infarcts evolve like most animal studies suggest, there will be little myocardium left to salvage by reperfusion therapy by the time the patient is seen by a physician.

Infarct repair in the mammalian heart

Because infarct size limitation has proved to be such a difficult target to achieve clinically, our group has been interested in strategies to enhance myocardial infarct repair. Unlike many organs in the body, the heart cannot undergo regenerative healing after necrotizing injury. Two problems prevent regeneration. First, unlike smooth muscle, cardiomyocytes which survive the injury do not re-enter the cell cycle to any significant extent [1, 20, 34, 47, 48]. Although very low rates of cardiomyocyte proliferation have been reported in injured hearts by some investigators, this clearly does not occur to a physiologically meaningful extent. Second, unlike skeletal muscle, there are apparently no muscle stem cells in myocardium. Pluripotent somatic stem cells have recently been reported to exist in many tissues such as the brain [3, 54], bone marrow [37], and skeletal muscle [14], but to date none have been described in the heart. Similarly, circulating stem cells have not been shown to contribute to cardiac repair. The possibility remains that either resident or circulating stem cells could contribute to infarct repair, but, in any case, their contribution cannot be physiologically significant.

The events of myocardial infarct repair have been reviewed well by Reimer and Jennings [38] and will be covered only briefly here. The sequence of events is essentially the same in all mammalian species studied. The rates of repair differ considerably, however, with small species healing infarcts more quickly than large species. This may simply reflect the overall size of the necrotic region, since geometric factors (surface to volume ratio) require that large infarcts heal more slowly than small infarcts [29]. Myocardial necrosis elicits a vigorous inflammatory response, composed initially of neutrophils and later predominantly of macrophages. The macrophages persist throughout the repair process and likely serve as the major orchestrators of healing. Concomitant with phagocytosis of necrotic myocardium by macrophages, there is ingrowth of granulation tissue. Granulation tissue is the provisional tissue of wound repair, consisting of proliferating fibroblasts and angiogenic capillary sprouts, all contained within a hydrophilic matrix rich in proteoglycans.

Over the ensuing weeks, the infarct fibroblasts produce an increasingly fibrous matrix, containing predominantly collagen and a lesser amount of elastin, characteristic of mature scar tissue. Remodeling of granulation tissue into scar is accompanied by apoptosis of fibroblasts and endothelial cells [11, 52]. In small species such as mice and rats, necrotic myocardium is typically replaced by granulation tissue within a week, and scar formation is largely complete within 4 weeks. In larger species such as dogs and humans, all stages of infarct repair can be observed at once, with the outer regions containing young scar tissue, transitioning to granulation tissue and unresorbed necrotic myocardium in the center of the infarct. In humans, infarct repair is largely complete within 6 weeks [28].

Post-infarct ventricular remodeling

When infarct healing proceeds "well", the resulting product is a scar, which is smaller than the original myocardium it replaced and follows the normal contour of the left ventricular wall. Infarct repair can have significant complications, however. As healing progresses there is always some thinning of the infarct, and sometimes true aneurysms form. Current evidence indicates that ventricular dilation bodes poorly for the patient [36, 46]. Wall stress increases markedly with increasing radius; mechanical stress has been proposed to cause apoptosis of cardiomyocytes in the non-infarcted region, possibly exacerbating failure [6]. Furthermore, dilation is often progressive (probably due in part to increased wall stress). The constellation of scar thinning and left ventricular dilation, coupled with hypertrophy and interstitial fibrosis of the remaining non-ischemic myocardium, is referred to as "ventricular remodeling".

The mechanism of ventricular remodeling is under intensive investigation. Many of the events that take place in the infarct also occur to a lesser extent in the non-infarcted myocardium. For example, in the non-infarcted region fibroblasts also proliferate, synthesize new matrix, and eventually cause interstitial fibrosis [10]. In the infarct the collagen matrix is broken down by metalloproteinases, allowing "slippage" of necrotic myocyte bundles [35, 37]. Myocyte slippage causes ventricular dilation by reducing the number of myocytes across the wall and by increasing the apex-to-base chamber axis. Similarly, collagen breakdown and slippage of myocyte bundles also occur in the non-infarcted myocardium, exacerbating ventricular dilation. Finally, there is increasing evidence that the non-infarcted myocardium also undergoes apoptosis as it remodels to adapt to the infarct [6].

Strategies for Cardiac Regeneration

The ideal way to repair a myocardial infarct would be to induce the heart to regenerate new muscle instead of forming a scar. In theory there would be at least three ways that this could be accomplished. First, the surviving cardiomyocytes could be induced to divide and migrate into the wound. The mechanism of cardiac myocyte withdrawal from the cell cycle is being studied in other labs [21, 22, 26, 49] and will not be covered here. To our knowledge there have been no studies of cardiomyocyte chemotactic factors, or how cells at the periphery of infarcts might be induced to uncouple from the remaining cardiomyocytes and invade the infarct. Second, the fibroblasts of granulation tissue could be induced to differentiate into muscle cells. Our current understanding of cardiac differentiation does not permit transdifferentiation of wound fibroblasts to form cardiomyocytes. We have, however, recently induced cells in cardiac granulation tissue *in vivo* to form *skeletal myofibers* by adenoviral transfer of the myogenic determination gene, MyoD [31]. As molecular regulation of cardiac development becomes better understood, it may be possible to use a similar strategy to induce cardiomyocyte differentiation in healing infarcts. The final route toward muscle regeneration would be to graft cells into injured hearts to establish a new muscle tissue. In principle, these could be committed somatic cells such as cardiomyocytes or skeletal muscle cells, or they could be stem cells somehow programmed to differentiate *in vivo*. The remainder of this chapter will focus on creating new myocardium by grafting differentiated cardiomyocytes. Readers interested in skeletal muscle cell grafting for cardiac repair are referred to our accompanying chapter in this volume.

Cardiomyocyte engraftment

Initial studies of cell grafting into normal hearts were quite encouraging. Field's group showed that fetal cardiomyocytes can be grafted into normal mouse or dog hearts [23, 50], where they formed intercalated discs with host cardiomyocytes. The behavior of grafted cardiomyocytes in injured hearts, in contrast, is less well understood. Several groups have shown that cardiomyocytes can be grafted successfully into myocardial infarcts or cardiac cryoinjuries [7, 24, 25, 44]. In contrast, a recent publication by Claycomb and colleagues reported that fetal and neonatal pig cardiomyocytes, as well as the cardiac-derived cell line HL-1, did not survive after grafting into pig infarcts [55].

Among studies which showed graft survival, there is still discrepancy regarding the amount of differentiation that occurs in the grafts. For example, Leor et al. reported that embryonic human cardiomyocytes grafted into injured rat hearts did not differentiate into an adult phenotype, even when studied several months after grafting [24]. Similarly, in the study by Claycomb et al. the grafted fetal cardiomyocytes appeared to maintain their fetal phenotype in the normal host heart for the five weeks studied [55]. In contrast, Connold et al. reported that embryonic rat cardiomyocytes formed organized gap junctions with other graft cells when grafted into injured rat hearts, suggesting some differentiation could occur [7]. Importantly, there are no data demonstrating electromechanical coupling between graft and host myocardium after injury.

We proposed that much of the above discrepancy resulted from differences in the type of donor cells used or the status of the host myocardium at the time of grafting. We therefore systematically evaluated several key variables that may influence success of cardiomyocyte grafting, including

- developmental stage of the donor cell (fetal, neonatal, adult);
- the status of the host tissue (normal myocardium, acutely necrotic tissue, and granulation tissue);
- differentiation toward an adult phenotype.
- graft cell integration, i.e., formation of electrical and mechanical junctions with host cardiomyocytes.

Donor cell stage and time after injury

Initial studies were performed to address how the developmental stage of the grafted cardiomyocytes (adult, neonatal, E15 fetal rat) or the status of the host tissue (acute necrosis, granulation tissue, normal myocardium) influenced the success of engraftment. Adult Fischer 344 rats were subjected to cryoinjury as described [31, 33]. At the appropriate time, cardiomyocytes from syngeneic donors were injected directly into the normal or injured myocardium. Figure 1 summarizes the survival pattern of fetal, neonatal, and adult cardiomyocytes after grafting into normal myocardium, acutely injured myocardium, and granulation tissue (6 day-old injury). Adult cardiomyocyte grafts showed no survival at day 6 and hence were

Fig. 1. Survival of cardiomyocyte grafts. Fetal, neonatal or adult rat cardiomyocytes were grafted into normal myocardium, acutely cryoinjured myocardium, or granulation tissue (d 6 after injury). Fetal and neonatal grafts are shown at day 6, and the adult cardiomyocyte grafts at day 1 after transplantation. **A, B, C** Adult cardiomyocytes did not survive to a significant extent under any grafting condition. The inset in panel **C** shows a rarely observed X-GAL-positive adult cardiomyocyte at day 1 (bar = 25 μm). In contrast, fetal (**D, E, F**) and neonatal (**G, H, I**) cardiomyocytes formed viable grafts in all three kinds of host tissue. Close approximation to host cardiomyocytes was frequently observed in normal myocardium. In injured myocardium, however, graft and host were often separated by intervening wound tissue. All panels show hematoxylin and eosin (H&E) staining. Bar = 25 μm. *Abbreviations: Gr* graft cells; *Ho* host myocardium; *GT* granulation tissue. Reproduced from [43] with permission

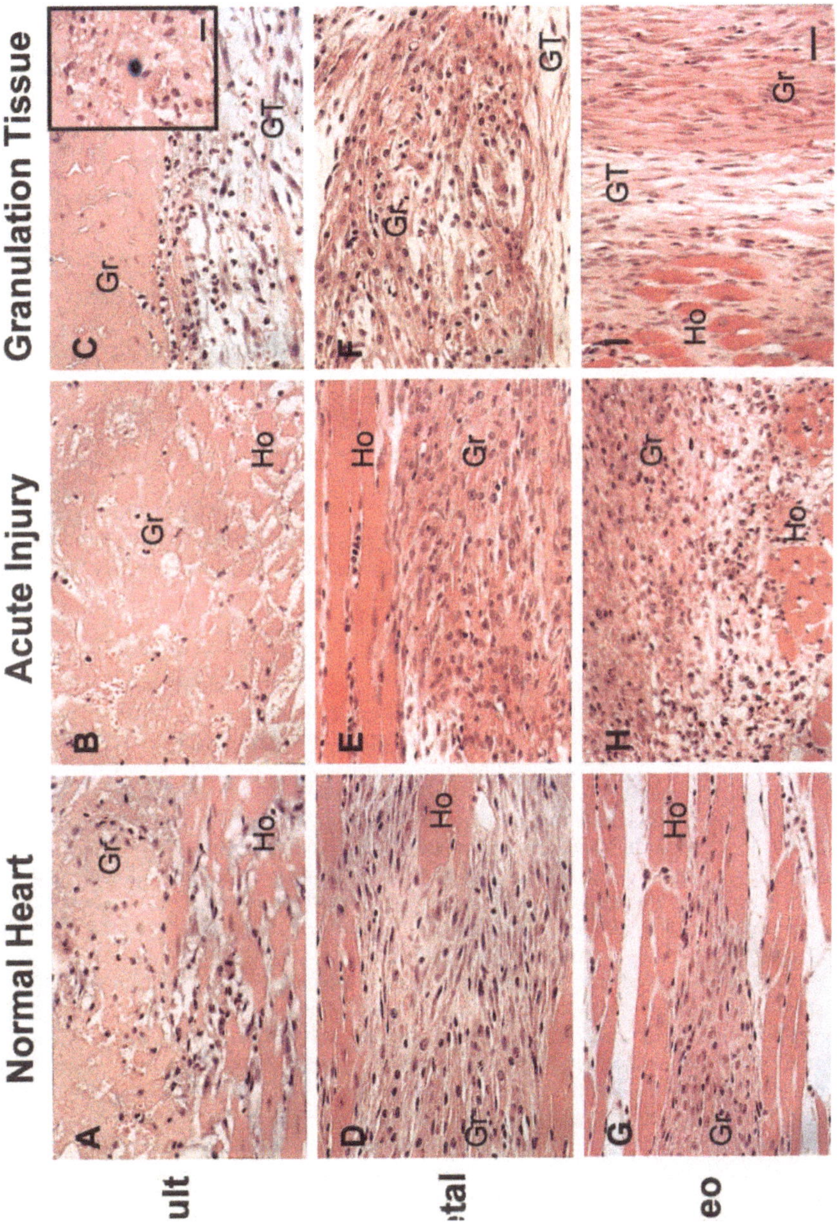
Normal Heart
Acute Injury
Granulation Tissue
A
B
C
D
E
F
G
H
I
Gr
Ho
GT
ult
tal
eo

studied at day 1 after grafting. Even at day 1 (Fig. 1 A–C) the vast majority of adult cardiomyocytes had features typical of coagulation necrosis, including loss of nuclei and more intensely eosinophilic cytoplasm. A few viable adult cardiomyocytes were found at day 1 after grafting into granulation tissue (Fig. 1 C, inset), but none were seen in any other group. Since adult cardiomyocytes remaining after injection survived *in vitro* and showed rod-shaped morphology after 24 hours in culture, it is clear that they were viable at the time of injection. In contrast, fetal and neonatal cardiomyocytes (Fig. 1 D–F, G–I) formed viable grafts after transplantation under all conditions. Since the cell yield from neonatal hearts was ~7 times higher than from embryonic hearts and no major differences in viability after grafting were observed, we chose neonatal cardiomyocytes for the time course study.

Differentiation of neonatal cardiomyocyte grafts

A time course study was done to define the biology of neonatal cardiomyocytes after grafting into acutely necrotic cryolesions. Four million donor cells were injected directly into the lesion immediately after myocardial

Fig. 2. Differentiation of neonatal cardiomyocyte grafts. Host myocardium is shown only in the day 3 panels (**B**, **F**, **J**, **N**). Each time point shows serial sections from the same heart. Bar = 35 μm.
H&E: **A** At day 1 the graft cardiomyocytes appeared small, round and undifferentiated. The graft area was mostly surrounded by necrotic host myocardium and interstitial hemorrhage. **B** At day 3 progressive wound healing was observed, and graft cardiomyocytes began to elongate. **C** At day 6 all of the necrotic host myocardium was removed. The graft cardiomyocytes began to enlarge and had early sarcomere formation (see also Fig. 3). **C inset** Potential proliferation of the graft neonatal cardiomyocytes was studied by double staining for proliferating cell nuclear antigen (PCNA, dark gray) and α-cardiac myosin heavy chain (light gray). PCNA-positive graft neonatal cardiomyocytes were observed from 3 days to 2 weeks, with a peak frequency of 2% double-positive cells occurring at 6 days (as shown). Bar = 10 μm. **D** By 8 weeks the graft cardiomyocytes had undergone progressive hypertrophy resulting in an adult-like rod-shaped phenotype with well-developed sarcomeres. **D inset** Anti-BrdU and eosin staining of a graft area at 8 weeks after grafting. BrdU-positive graft neonatal cardiomyocytes were identified by typical cross striations as demonstrated by eosin counterstaining. Bar = 10 μm. *Cadherin:* **E** At day 1 the graft cardiomyocytes were stained in a mostly circumferential or scattered fashion. **F** By day 3 graft cardiomyocytes appeared more elongated and cadherin was partially concentrated at the cell ends and sides. Note that in adult host cardiomyocytes (*arrowhead*) cadherin was exclusively concentrated in the intercalated disc. **G** At day 6 cadherin was progressively concentrated at the ends of the graft cells indicating the organization of newly formed intercalated discs. **H** By 8 weeks cadherin was almost exclusively concentrated in the newly formed intercalated disc.
Connexin43: At day 1 (**I**) and 3 (**J**) the graft cardiomyocytes were negative for connexin43. Note strong staining for connexin43 at the intercalated disc of adult host cardiomyocytes (*panel* **J**, *arrowhead*). **K** By day 6 the graft cardiomyocytes expressed connexin43 in a scattered, punctate fashion. **L** By 8 weeks connexin43 was mostly expressed in the newly formed intercalated discs.
BrdU: Graft cells were labeled with BrdU *in utero* prior to isolation, and BrdU staining later used to track them in the adult recipients. Graft cells were detected throughout the time course (**M** through **P**). The inset in panel **M** (Bar = 10 μm) shows nuclear fragmentation in some of the grafted neonatal cardiomyocytes (*arrowhead*) indicating cell death after transplantation. Reproduced from [43] with permission

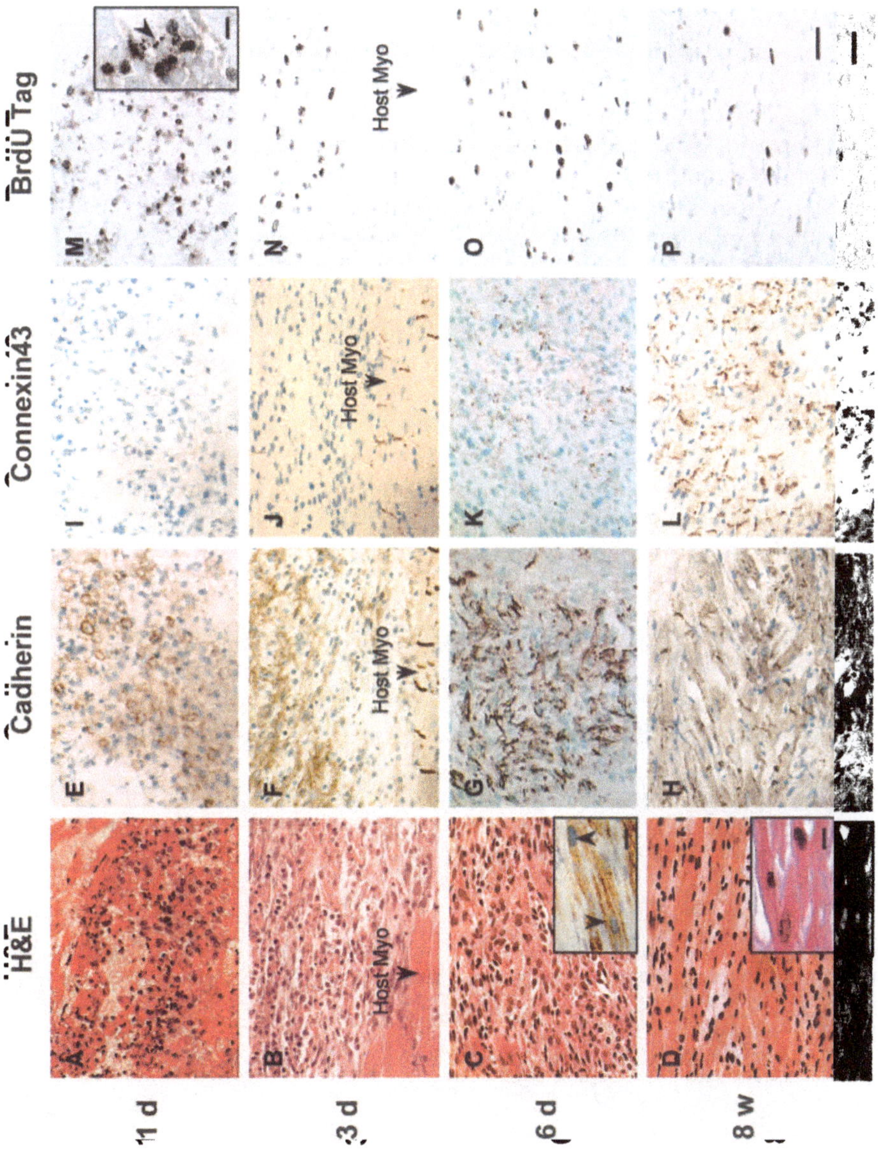
H&E
Cadherin
Connexin43
BrdU Tag
1 d
3 d
6 d
8 w
Host Myo
Host Myo
Host Myo
Host Myo
A
B
C
D
E
F
G
H
I
J
K
L
M
N
O
P

freeze-thaw. In all studies the cells to be grafted were identified by administering BrdU *in utero* to mark the nuclei prior to cell isolation. The graft cells later were identified in every case by BrdU immunostaining on serial sections. At day 1 after grafting the neonatal cardiomyocytes appeared small, round, and undifferentiated. The graft area was surrounded by necrotic host myocardium containing numerous inflammatory cells and interstitial hemorrhage (Fig. 2A). It should be noted that dead neonatal graft cells also were identified at day 1 by BrdU-positive cell fragments (Fig. 2M, inset). By day 3 wound healing was underway, characterized by phagocytosis of necrotic host cardiomyocytes, concomitant with ingrowth of fibroblasts and capillaries to form granulation tissue. The graft cardiomyocytes had elongated and frequently were in close approximation to intact host cardiomyocytes (Fig. 2B). By day 6 almost all of the necrotic host myocardium was removed. The graft cardiomyocytes appeared more differentiated in terms of cell elongation and the formation of sarcomeres (Figs. 2C and 3). At 2, 4 (data not shown), and 8 weeks there was progressive elongation into a rod-shaped morphology, and sarcomeres became increasingly well defined (Figs. 2D and 3).

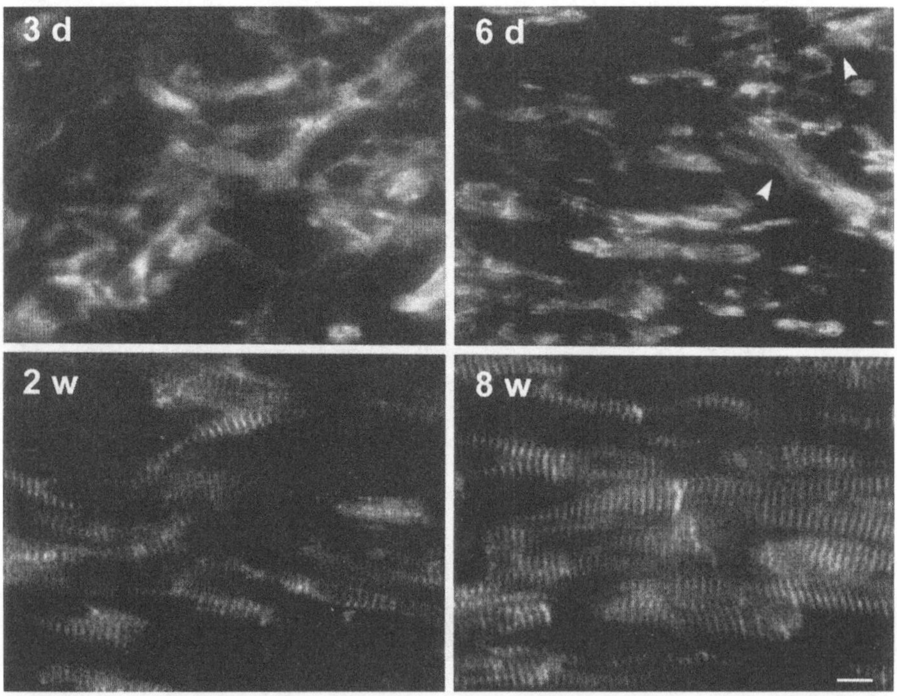

Fig. 3. Desmin immunostaining in cardiomyocyte grafts. Desmin was initially diffusely distributed in the cytoplasm (3 d). Rudimentary sarcomeres were detected at day 6 (*arrowheads*). By 2 weeks virtually all grafted cardiomyocytes had well-developed sarcomeres. Note the progressive hypertrophy between 2 and 8 weeks. Bar = 10 μm. Reproduced from [43] with permission

At all time points consecutive heart sections were stained for the BrdU tag in order to identify grafted cells reliably. Fig. 2 (M through P) shows that BrdU-positive cells were detected throughout the time course. Furthermore, BrdU-positive cardiomyocytes were readily demonstrated at 8 weeks and had typical rod-shaped morphology and well-defined sarcomeres (Fig. 2D *inset*). Development of sarcomeres in grafted cardiomyocytes was further studied by desmin immunofluorescence staining (Fig. 3). Rudimentary sarcomeres were detected as early as day 6 after grafting. By 2 and 8 weeks virtually all grafted cardiomyocytes had well-developed sarcomeres (Fig. 3) and had hypertrophied to ~65% of adult cell diameter.

Electromechanical coupling: N-cadherin and connexin43 expression patterns

To investigate electromechanical integration of grafted neonatal cardiomyocytes and host myocardium, immunostaining was performed for major components of the intercalated disc. At day 1, the graft cardiomyocytes expressed cadherin in a mostly circumferential or scattered fashion (Fig. 2E). In contrast, the connexin43 antibody did not stain the graft cardiomyocytes at day 1 (Fig. 2I). By 3 days, when the graft cardiomyocytes had elongated, cadherin was partially concentrated at the cell ends (Fig. 2F). At this time point, however, the vast majority of the graft cardiomyocytes still appeared negative for connexin43 (Fig. 2J). In contrast, in adult host cardiomyocytes cadherin and connexin43 were concentrated and co-localized in the intercalated disc (Fig. 2F, J). By day 6 there was progressive concentration of cadherin staining at the graft cell ends, indicating the organization of newly formed intercalated discs (Fig. 2G). Interestingly, by 6 days most of the graft cells expressed connexin43 in a scattered, punctate fashion (Fig. 2K). However, occasional graft cardiomyocytes showed partial concentration of connexin43 molecules in the forming intercalated disc (Fig. 2K).

Between 1 and 6 days neonatal graft cardiomyocytes were observed in close apposition to host myocardium. Adult host myocytes at the interface often extended cell processes toward the graft myocytes (Fig. 4A). Furthermore, using confocal microscopy we observed gap junctions between graft and host cardiomyocytes, suggesting electromechanical integration of the graft (Fig. 4B). In a minority of hearts at this time, however, graft cells were separated from host myocardium by intervening wound tissue. Over the ensuing weeks there was progressive concentration of cadherin and connexin43 in the intercalated disc while the graft cardiomyocytes developed a more rod-shaped (adult-like) appearance. By 8 weeks, cadherin and connexin43 were restricted to intercalated discs, virtually indistinguishable from the host myocardium (Fig. 2H, L). At the later time points we observed less frequent contact between graft and host (~40% of successful grafts). Furthermore, in the hearts with contact the interaction was restricted to the edges of the grafts, with most of the graft being separated from host by intervening scar tissue (Fig. 4C).

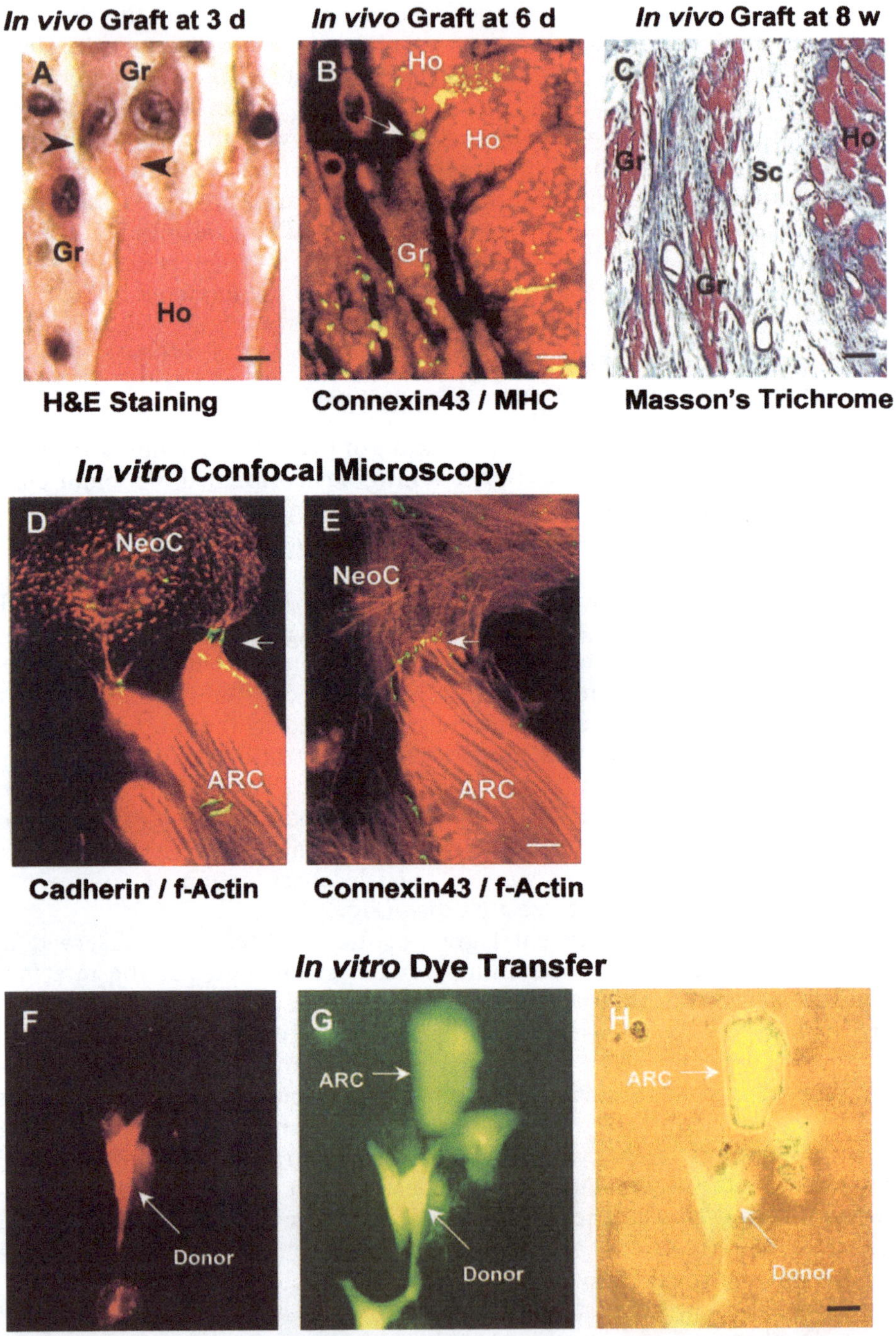

In vivo Graft at 3 d
In vivo Graft at 6 d
In vivo Graft at 8 w
A
Gr
Gr
Ho
B
Ho
Ho
Gr
C
Gr
Sc
Ho
Gr
H&E Staining
Connexin43 / MHC
Masson's Trichrome
In vitro Confocal Microscopy
D
NeoC
ARC
E
NeoC
ARC
Cadherin / f-Actin
Connexin43 / f-Actin
In vitro Dye Transfer
F
Donor
G
ARC
Donor
H
ARC
Donor

Gap junctions in neonatal and adult cardiomyocyte cocultures

Cocultures of adult and neonatal cardiomyocytes were studied to determine the capacity of the two cell populations to form electromechanical junctions. When the cells were placed in coculture they formed a synchronously beating network, indicating electrical coupling. Confocal microscopy showed that cadherin (Fig. 4D) and connexin43 (Fig. 4E) localized to contact sites between neonatal and adult cardiomyocytes. To test directly whether the two cell types were connected by gap junctions, we performed microinjection studies. Beating neonatal cardiomyocytes were microinjected with a combination of Lucifer yellow (~250 daltons), which readily passes through gap junctions [15], and rhodamine-dextran (~10000 daltons), which is not transferable through gap junctions. Figure 4 (F, G, H) shows dye transfer from a neonatal cardiomyocyte (donor) to adjacent neonatal cardiomyocytes and, most importantly, to an adult cardiomyocyte which was identified by its typical rod shape (Fig. 4H). These results clearly demonstrate that neonatal cardiomyocytes can form gap junctions with adult cardiomyocytes in coculture.

Cell death in cardiomyocyte grafts

The above studies showed that cardiomyocyte grafting could create new myocardium in injured hearts. The grafts, however, were relatively small and seemed unlikely to be capable of restoring regional contractile function. We therefore attempted to induce formation of larger amounts of new

Fig. 4. **A** H&E staining of graft cells at day 3. Cell processes of the host cardiomyocyte (Ho) appear to be in contact with graft cardiomyocytes (Gr) (*arrowheads*). Bar = 5 μm. **B** Confocal microscopy of a day 6 graft. Connexin43 staining in white, MHC staining (MF-20 antibody) in gray. Shown is the graft-host interface. A graft cardiomyocyte (Gr) appears to form a gap junction (*arrow*) with a host cardiomyocyte (Ho). Optical section = 100 nm thick; bar = 5 μm.
C Masson's trichrome staining of an 8 week graft. At time points >2 weeks host (Ho) and graft (Gr) often were separated by scar tissue (Sc). Bar = 40 μm.
D, E Confocal microscopy of cocultured neonatal and adult rat cardiomyocytes. **D** Cadherin (white) mediated adherens junctions (*arrow*) were readily observed after 24 h of coculture. **E** Connexin43 (white) mediated gap junctions (*arrow*) are shown at 48 h. The frequency of gap junction formation and the intensity of connexin43 immunofluorescence appeared to increase with coculture time. F-actin was used as a counterstain (gray). Note that sarcomeres in the adult cardiomyocytes have been obscured by the need to overexpose the image to detect f-actin in the neonatal cells. *NeoC*, neonatal cardiomyocyte; *ARC*, adult rat cardiomyocyte. Bar = 8 μm.
F, G, H Dye transfer between neonatal and adult cardiomyocytes *in vitro*. After 20 h of coculture a beating neonatal cardiomyocyte (donor) was microinjected with Lucifer yellow (transferable) and rhodamine-dextran (non-transferable). **F** (rhodamine filter) shows the microinjected donor cell. **G** (Lucifer yellow filter) identifies cells to which the Lucifer yellow has been transferred via gap junctions. Among these cells are adjacent neonatal cardiomyocytes and an adult rat cardiomyocyte (ARC) which is identified by its typical morphology in **H** by bright field exposure. Bar = 20 μm. Reproduced from [43] with permission

myocardium by grafting larger numbers of cells into acutely cryoinjured hearts. A dose-response curve was generated where the number of input cells ranged from 3 to 25 million, and graft size measured one week later. (For reference, morphometric studies indicate that there are ~20 million cardiomyocytes in the adult rat left ventricle [2].) Disappointingly, there was no significant increase in the size of cardiomyocyte grafts with increasing cell number. We reasoned that a substantial fraction of the injected cells must be dying. In fact, some cell death had been noted in the initial grafting experiments, but its magnitude could not be determined by the qualitative nature of the experiment. To quantify cell death, the cardiomyocytes were labeled with a red fluorescent dye prior to grafting. Cell death was determined by a TUNEL procedure, which added green-fluorescing nucleotides to the 3′ fragments of broken DNA strands. Representative data from this experiment are shown in Fig. 5. This analysis showed that

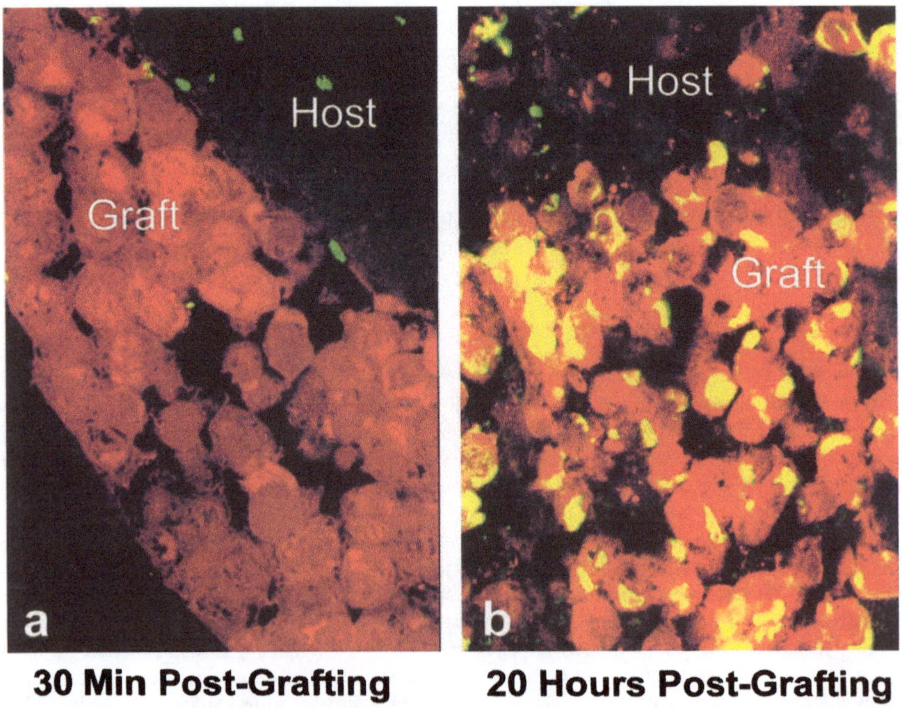

Fig. 5. Cell death in cardiomyocyte grafts. Neonatal cardiomyocytes were labeled in culture dishes with Orange Cell Tracker (Molecular Probes), which form covalent adducts with intracellular proteins. The labeled cardiomyocytes were grafted into acutely cryoinjured hearts, and the rats were killed either 30 min (**a**) or 20 h (**b**) after grafting. Cells with fragmented DNA were identified by a fluorescent TUNEL method in paraffin sections and examined with a confocal microscope. The Cell Tracker signal in graft cells appears gray in this figure, while the TUNEL signal appears white.
a At 30 min after grafting a cluster of graft cardiomyocytes is identified, but none of the cells is TUNEL-positive. Note the TUNEL-positive cells in the injured host myocardium. **b** At 20 h after grafting numerous graft cardiomyocytes have TUNEL-positive nuclei, indicating cell death has occurred

graft cells had intact DNA 30 min after grafting, indicating that cells were initially viable. At 1 day after grafting, however, there was extensive DNA fragmentation in the graft cells. An average of 32% of the graft cells were TUNEL-positive, indicating that a large fraction of the grafted cells died within the first day.

Summary and future directions

Myocardium has a high metabolic rate and dies quickly after the onset of severe ischemia. By the time most patients present for medical attention they probably have lost most of the cardiomyocytes at risk. This presents a fundamental problem for strategies to limit myocardial infarct size. On the other hand, once an infarct has occurred there are weeks during which one can intervene and influence the way in which it heals. We view the healing infarct as a "plastic" tissue which can be manipulated therapeutically. The best example to date is the fact that angiotensin converting enzyme inhibitors prevent left ventricular remodeling after infarcts, improve cardiac performance, and save lives. While highly significant, this may be only the first step in enhancing cardiac repair.

The ultimate form of infarct repair would be the induction of muscle regeneration and restoration of contractile function. This repair could be achieved through activating cardiomyocyte cell division, inducing cardiac transdifferentiation of cells in the infarct, or by grafting muscle cells or their precursors. Cardiomyocyte grafting is one strategy that shows potential for regenerative healing. It is clear that cardiomyocyte grafting can create new myocardium in injured hearts and that the new muscle can electromechanically couple with host myocardium. If the amount of new myocardium can be increased, it should be possible to restore contractile function in the injured region.

There are several significant challenges to this strategy, however, which must be overcome before it could be clinically useful. To begin with, the source of cells for human therapy has not been identified. Obtaining cardiomyocytes from adult hearts is unlikely to yield sufficient cells, unless one can solve the cell cycle problem and induce them to proliferate. Furthermore, we have shown that adult cardiomyocytes do not survive after grafting. Human fetal cardiomyocytes are also unlikely to be available in sufficient numbers, due to both ethical and practical considerations. Recent advances in stem cell biology show significant promise toward addressing the cell sourcing question. The development of human embryonic stem cells [12, 45, 53] opens one new route for *in vitro* derivation of cardiomyocytes. Also, somatic stem cells in the bone marrow and other tissues are capable of differentiating into multiple lineages, including skeletal [56] and smooth muscle [13]. Preliminary experiments also suggest that bone marrow-derived cells may also differentiate into cardiac myocytes [27]. Stem cell approaches certainly bear further investigation for cardiac repair.

A second major challenge to cardiomyocyte grafting is enhancing cell survival. We observed that ~35% of cardiomyocytes had fragmented DNA on the first day after grafting. Given the kinetics of TUNEL labeling, it is likely that substantially more cells than this die after placement into the injured heart. Given the low proliferative capacity of cardiomyocytes, it is imperative that as many of them survive as possible after grafting. The cause of their death is not known at present. Possible causes include ischemia, injury by inflammatory cells, and activation of apoptotic pathways, e.g., through loss of matrix attachments or activation of death receptors.

A third challenge to address will be scar formation. In the studies detailed here, we observed good apposition between graft and host cardiomyocytes during the first week after grafting. As healing proceeded, however, the grafts became splayed apart by fibrous tissue, and scar tissue typically separated the grafts from the host myocardium. This scar tissue could prevent electromechanical coupling between graft and host. Additionally, entrapment by scar tissue could interfere with the mechanics of graft contraction and relaxation cycles. Most worrisome would be the possibility of scarring creating anatomical substrates that lead to arrhythmias. We know surprisingly little about the factors that lead to fibrosis after myocardial infarction. An anti-fibrogenic regimen could be a significant asset to forming new myocardium, however.

Finally, the ultimate test of a regenerative therapy is not morphological repair, but rather whether it restores contractile function. Future studies will need to address whether creating new myocardium through cardiomyocyte grafting improves regional wall motion or the global performance of the injured heart.

Acknowledgment. This work was supported in part by grants from the National Heart, Lung, and Blood Institutes, the American Heart Association, and Collateral Therapeutics, Inc. Most of the experiments reported here were done while Dr. Murry was the recipient of a Burroughs Wellcome Career Award in the Biomedical Sciences.

References

1. Anversa P, Kajstura J (1998) Ventricular myocytes are not terminally differentiated in the adult mammalian heart. Circ Res 83(1):1–14
2. Anversa P, Olivetti G, Loud AV (1980) Morphometric study of early postnatal development in the left and right ventricular myocardium of the rat. I. Hypertrophy, hyperplasia, and binucleation of myocytes. Circ Res 46(4):495–502
3. Bjornson CR, Rietze RL, Reynolds BA, Magli MC, Vescovi AL (1999) Turning brain into blood: a hematopoietic fate adopted by adult neural stem cells in vivo [see comments]. Science 283(5401):534–537
4. Braunwald E (1974) Editorial: Reduction of myocardial-infarct size. N Engl J Med 291(10):525–526
5. Braunwald E, Maroko PR (1974) The reduction of infarct size – an idea whose time (for testing) has come. Circulation 50(2):206–209

6. Cheng W, Li B, Kajstura J, Li P, Wolin MS, Sonnenblick EH, Hintze TH, Olivetti G, Anversa P (1995) Stretch-induced programmed myocyte cell death. J Clin Invest 96:2247–2259
7. Connold AL, Frischknecht R, Dimitrakos M, Vrbov'a G (1997) The survival of embryonic cardiomyocytes transplanted into damaged host rat myocardium. J Muscle Res Cell Motil 18(1):63–70
8. Davies MJ (1995) Acute coronary thrombosis – the role of plaque disruption and its initiation and prevention. Eur Heart J 16 (Suppl L):3–7
9. Davies MJ, Thomas AC (1985) Plaque fissuring – the cause of acute myocardial infarction, sudden ischemic death, and crescendo angina. Br Heart J 53:363–373
10. De Carvalho Frimm C, Sun Y, Weber KT (1997) Angiotensin II receptor blockade and myocardial fibrosis of the infarcted rat heart. J Lab Clin Med 129(4):439–446
11. Desmouliere A, Redard M, Darby I, Gabbiani G (1995) Apoptosis mediates the decrease in cellularity during the transition between granulation tissue and scar. Am J Pathol 146:56–66
12. Doetschman TC, Eistetter H, Katz M, Schmidt W, Kemler R (1985) The *in vitro* development of blastocyst-derived embryonic stem cell lines: Formation of visceral yolk sac, blood islands and myocardium. J Embryol Exp Morphol 87:27–45
13. Galmiche MC, Koteliansky VE, Briere J, Herve P, Charbord P (1993) Stromal cells from human long-term marrow cultures are mesenchymal cells that differentiate following a vascular smooth muscle differentiation pathway. Blood 82(1):66–76
14. Gussoni E, Soneoka Y, Strickland CD, Buzney EA, Khan MK, Flint AF, Kunkel LM, Mulligan RC (1999) Dystrophin expression in the mdx mouse restored by stem cell transplantation. Nature 401(6751):390–394
15. Hoffmeister HM, Mauser M, Schaper W (1985) Effect of adenosine and AICAR on ATP content and regional contractile function in reperfused canine myocardium. Basic Res Cardiol 80(4):445–458
16. Jennings RB, Murry CE, Reimer KA (1991) Energy metabolism in preconditioned and control myocardium: effect of total ischemia. J Mol Cell Cardiol 23:1449–1458
17. Jennings RB, Murry CE, Steenbergen C Jr, Reimer KA (1990) Development of cell injury in sustained acute ischemia. Circulation 82 (3 Suppl):II2–12
18. Jennings RB, Reimer KA (1981) Lethal myocardial ischemic injury. Am J Pathol 102:241–255
19. Jennings RB, Reimer KA, Steenbergen C (1986) Myocardial ischemia revisited. The osmolar load, membrane damage, and reperfusion. J Mol Cell Cardiol 18(8): 769–780
20. Kajstura J, Leri A, Finato N, Di Loreto C, Beltrami CA, Anversa P (1998) Myocyte proliferation in end-stage cardiac failure in humans. Proc Natl Acad Sci USA 95(15):8801–8805
21. Kim KK, Soonpaa MH, Daud AI, Koh GY, Kim JS, Field LJ (1994) Tumor suppressor gene expression during normal and pathologic myocardial growth. J Biol Chem 269(36):22607–22613
22. Kirshenbaum LA, Schneider MD (1995) Adenovirus E1A represses cardiac gene transcription and reactivates DNA synthesis in ventricular myocytes, via alternative pocket protein- and p300-binding domains. J Biol Chem 270(14):7791–7794
23. Koh GY, Soonpaa MH, Klug MG, Pride HP, Cooper BJ, Zipes DP, Field LJ (1995) Stable fetal cardiomyocyte grafts in the hearts of dystrophic mice and dogs. J Clin Invest 96:2034–2042
24. Leor J, Patterson M, Quinones MJ, Kedes LH, Kloner RA (1996) Transplantation of fetal myocardial tissue into the infarcted myocardium of rat. A potential method for repair of infarcted myocardium? Circulation 94 (9 Suppl):II332–336

25. Li RK, Jia ZQ, Weisel RD, Mickle DA, Zhang J, Mohabeer MK, Rao V, Ivanov J (1996) Cardiomyocyte transplantation improves heart function. Ann Thorac Surg 62(3):654–600
26. Liu Y, Kitsis RN (1996) Induction of DNA synthesis and apoptosis in cardiac myocytes by E1A oncoprotein. J Cell Biol 133(2):325–334
27. Makino S, Fukuda K, Miyoshi S, Konishi F, Kodama H, Pan J, Sano M, Takahashi T, Hori S, Abe H, Hata J, Umezawa A, Ogawa S (1999) Cardiomyocytes can be generated from marrow stromal cells in vitro. J Clin Invest 103(5):697–705
28. Mallory GK, White PD, Salcedo-Salgar J (1939) The speed of healing of myocardial infarction: a study of the pathologic anatomy in 72 cases. Am Heart J 18:647–671
29. Miura T, Shizukuda Y, Ogawa S, Ishimoto R, Iimura O (1991) Effects of early and later reperfusion on healing speed of experimental myocardial infarct. Can J Cardiol 7(3):146–154
30. Murry CE, Jennings RB, Reimer KA (1986) Preconditioning with ischemia: a delay of lethal cell injury in ischemic myocardium. Circulation 74:1124–1136
31. Murry CE, Kay MA, Bartosek T, Hauschka SD, Schwartz SM (1996) Muscle differentiation during repair of myocardial necrosis in rats via gene transfer with MyoD. J Clin Invest 98(10):2209–2217
32. Murry CE, Kay MA, Covin CW, Bartosek T, Schwartz SM (1994) MyoD-based gene therapy for myocardial infarction. Circulation 90 (Suppl):1–518 (abstr)
33. Murry CE, Wiseman RW, Schwartz SM, Hauschka SD (1996) Skeletal myoblast transplantation for repair of myocardial necrosis. J Clin Invest 98(11):2512–2523
34. Olivetti G, Anversa P, Melissari M, Loud A (1980) Morphometry of medial hypertrophy in the rat thoracic aorta. Lab Invest 2:559–565
35. Olivetti G, Capasso JM, Sonnenblick EH, Anversa P (1990) Side-to-side slippage of myocytes participates in ventricular wall remodeling acutely after myocardial infarction in rats. Circ Res 67(1):23–34
36. Pfeffer JM, Fischer TA, Pfeffer MA (1995) Angiotensin-converting enzyme inhibition and ventricular remodeling after myocardial infarction. Annu Rev Physiol 57P805-26:805–826
37. Pittenger MF, Mackay AM, Beck SC, Jaiswal RK, Douglas R, Mosca JD, Moorman MA, Simonetti DW, Craig S, Marshak DR (1999) Multilineage potential of adult human mesenchymal stem cells. Science 284(5411):143–147
38. Reimer KA, Jennings RB (1992) Myocardial ischemia, hypoxia, and infarction. In: Fozzard HA, Haber E, Jennings RB, Katz AM, Morgan HE (eds) The Heart and Cardiovascular System. Raven Press, New York, pp 1875–1973
39. Reimer KA, Jennings RB (1984) Verapamil in two reperfusion models of myocardial infarction. Temporary protection of severely ischemic myocardium without limitation of ultimate infarct size. Lab Invest 51(6):655–666
40. Reimer KA, Lowe JE, Rasmussen MM, Jennings RB (1977) The wavefront phenomenon of ischemic cell death. 1. Myocardial infarct size vs duration of coronary occlusion in dogs. Circulation 56(5):786–794
41. Reimer KA, Jennings RB (1979) The "wavefront phenomenon" of myocardial ischemic cell death. II. Transmural progression of necrosis within the framework of ischemic bed size (myocardium at risk) and collateral blood flow. Lab Invest 40:633–644
42. Reinecke H, Murry CE (1998) Electromechanical coupling between cardiac and skeletal muscle cells. Implications for infarct repair. Circulation 98(17):I-757–I-758
43. Reinecke H, Zhang M, Bartosek T, Murry CE (1999) Survival, integration, and differentiation of cardiomyocyte grafts: a study in normal and injured rat hearts. Circulation 100(2):193–202

44. Scorsin M, Marotte F, Sabri A, Le Dref O, Demirag M, Samuel JL, Rappaport L, Menasch'e P (1996) Can grafted cardiomyocytes colonize peri-infarct myocardial areas? Circulation 94 (9 Suppl):II337–340
45. Shamblott MJ, Axelman J, Wang S, Bugg EM, Littlefield JW, Donovan PJ, Blumenthal PD, Huggins GR, Gearhart JD (1998) Derivation of pluripotent stem cells from cultured human primordial germ cells [published erratum appears in Proc Natl Acad Sci USA (1999) 96(3):1162]. Proc Natl Acad Sci USA 95(23):13726–13731
46. The SOLVD Investigators (1991) Effect of enalapril on survival in patients with reduced left ventricular ejection fractions and congestive heart failure [see comments]. N Engl J Med 325(5):293–302
47. Soonpaa MH, Field LJ (1998) Survey of studies examining mammalian cardiomyocyte DNA synthesis. Circ Res 83(1):15–26
48. Soonpaa MH, Field LJ (1997) Assessment of cardiomyocyte DNA synthesis in normal and injured adult mouse hearts. Am J Physiol 272 (Ipt 2):H220–H226
49. Soonpaa MH, Field LJ (1994) Assessment of cardiomyocyte DNA synthesis during hypertrophy in adult mice. Am J Physiol 266(4):t 2H1439–1445
50. Soonpaa MH, Koh GY, Klug MG, Field LJ (1994) Formation of nascent intercalated disks between grafted fetal cardiomyocytes and host myocardium. Science 264:98
51. Steenbergen C, Hill ML, Jennings RB (1987) Cytoskeletal damage during myocardial ischemia: changes in vinculin immunofluorescence staining during total in vitro ischemia in canine heart. Circ Res 60(4):478–486
52. Takemura G, Ohno M, Hayakawa Y, Misao J, Kanoh M, Ohno A, Uno Y, Minatoguchi S, Fujiwara T, Fujiwara H (1998) Role of apoptosis in the disappearance of infiltrated and proliferated interstitial cells after myocardial infarction [see comments]. Circ Res 82(11):1130–1138
53. Thomson JA, Itskovitz-Eldor J, Shapiro SS, Waknitz MA, Swiergiel JJ, Marshall VS, Jones JM (1998) Embryonic stem cell lines derived from human blastocysts [see comments] [published erratum appears in Science (1998) 282(5395):1827]. Science 282(5391):1145–1147
54. Vescovi AL, Snyder EY (1999) Establishment and properties of neural stem cell clones: plasticity in vitro and in vivo. Brain Pathol 9(3):569–598
55. Watanabe E, Smith DM Jr, Delcaprio JB, Sun J, Smart FW, Van MC Jr, Claycomb WC (1998) Cardiomyocyte transplantation in a porcine myocardial infarction model. Cell Transplant 7(3):239–246
56. Wakitani S, Saito T, Caplan AI (1995) Myogenic cells derived from rat bone marrow mesenchymal stem cells exposed to 5-azacytidine. Muscle Nerve 18(12): 1417–1426
57. Weisman HF, Bush DE, Mannisi JA, Weisfeldt ML, Healy B (1988) Cellular mechanisms of myocardial infarct expansion. Circulation 78(1):186–201

Chapter 20

Cardiomyocytes can induce rhythmic contraction of skeletal muscle cells. Potential use for infarct repair

H. Reinecke, G.H. MacDonald[1], S.D. Hauschka[2], C.E. Murry

Department of Pathology, [1]Department of Otolaryngology, [2]Department of Biochemistry, University of Washington, Seattle, Washington

Summary

Skeletal myoblasts form viable grafts of mature muscle in injured hearts, and these grafts contract when exogenously stimulated. It is not known, however, whether cardiac muscle can form electromechanical junctions with skeletal muscle and induce its synchronous contraction. Here we report that undifferentiated skeletal myoblasts expressed N-cadherin and connexin43, major adhesion and gap junction proteins of the intercalated disk. Both proteins were markedly down-regulated after the cells differentiated into myotubes. Similarly, differentiated skeletal muscle grafts in injured hearts had no detectable N-cadherin or connexin43; hence, electromechanical coupling did not occur after *in vivo* grafting. Surprisingly, however, skeletal myotubes contracted in synchrony with cardiomyocytes in coculture. Isoproterenol increased myotube contraction rates by 25% in coculture without affecting myotubes in monoculture, indicating that cardiomyocytes were the pacemakers. The gap junction inhibitor heptanol aborted myotube contractions but left spontaneous contractions of individual cardiomyocytes intact, suggesting gap junction-dependent myotube activation. Confocal microscopy revealed the expression of cadherin and connexin43 at junctions between myotubes and cardiomyocytes *in vitro*. Microinjection studies showed that myotubes were capable of dye transfer via gap junctions. Calcium imaging revealed that the contraction of cardiomyocytes induced synchronous, calcium-dependent contractions in myotubes. Thus, cardiomyocytes form electromechanical junctions with skeletal myotubes in coculture, and induce their synchronous contraction via gap junctions. The induction of similar junctions *in vivo* may be sufficient to make skeletal muscle grafts beat synchronously with the host myocardium.

Introduction

Mature cardiomyocytes are terminally differentiated and do not reenter the cell cycle to a significant extent after injury [1, 27]. Hence, the loss of myocardium, e.g., due to myocardial infarction, is irreversible. Since the heart lacks functional repair mechanisms, we have begun to explore skeletal muscle as a possible replacement tissue. In fact, several aspects favor skeletal muscle rather than cardiac muscle as a source of graft cells for cardiac repair. First, skeletal muscle is much more resistant to ischemia than cardiac muscle [9, 32]. Second, skeletal myoblasts might establish satellite cells, thereby providing resident muscle stem cells for future self-repair [20]. Third, autologous skeletal muscle satellite cells could be isolated from muscle biopsies and reimplanted into the infarct, thereby circumventing graft rejection. We and others have shown that skeletal myoblasts will form viable grafts of differentiated skeletal muscle in normal and injured hearts [5, 15, 20, 26, 30, 33].

In the heart the cardiomyocytes are electromechanically coupled by specialized cell-cell junctions, the intercalated disks, which contain adherens and gap junctions for mechanical and electrical coupling, respectively. The major adherens junction protein in the heart is N-cadherin [31], whereas connexin43 is the major gap junction protein in the mature mammalian heart [4]. Electromechanical coupling between cardiomyocytes is a basic requirement for coordinated mechanical activity in the myocardium (functional syncitium). There is, however, a main theoretical drawback to skeletal muscle for cardiac repair, that is the different electrical properties of skeletal muscle cells. In contrast to heart muscle cells, skeletal muscle fibers represent a true syncitium: mononucleated myoblasts fuse under withdrawal of growth factors (e.g., basic FGF) to form multinucleated muscle fibers which mature, become innervated and electrically isolated from one other during skeletal muscle development. Electrical isolation of skeletal muscle fibers is a prerequisite for fine motor control. This is achieved by the down-regulation of N-cadherin and connexin43 as skeletal muscle matures [2, 16], and probably also by the basement lamina and thin endomysial connective tissue layer surrounding adjacent muscle fibers. However, functional gap junctions have been detected during the early stages of skeletal muscle development. Furthermore, gap junctional intercellular communication was shown to play an important role in myoblast fusion [18, 21], and an equally important role in myoblast fusion was described for N-cadherin [7, 10, 12, 17, 21, 22].

In summary, skeletal myoblast grafting into the injured heart has potential for cardiac repair. Little is known, however, about the capability of graft cells to form electromechanical junctions with each other and with host cardiomyocytes. Therefore, the goals of the current study were 1) to investigate the formation of electromechanical junctions between cardiac and skeletal muscle, and 2) to test whether cardiac muscle can provide excitation to skeletal muscle and induce its synchronous contraction.

Methods

Cell isolations and rat cardiac injury model

These studies were approved by the University of Washington Animal Care Committee and were conducted in accordance with federal guidelines. Neonatal skeletal myoblasts and neonatal cardiomyocytes were isolated by enzymatic dispersion from 1–2 day old Fischer 344 rats (Simonsen Labs, Gilroy, CA) and cultured as previously described [20, 25]. Under these conditions about 50% and 90% of the cells in skeletal and cardiac muscle-derived cultures are myogenic. Fischer 344 is an inbred strain and was used to avoid graft rejection. Myoblasts were grown in F10 medium (GIBCO BRL, Grand Island, NY) in the presence of 15% horse serum and 6 ng/ml bFGF. Myogenic differentiation was induced by switching the cells to a medium containing 1.5% horse serum, 6 μg/ml insulin and no bFGF.

Neonatal cardiomyocytes were grown in DMEM/M199 (4:1) supplemented with 10% horse serum, 5% fetal bovine serum (HyClone, Logan, UT), penicillin G (100 U/ml), streptomycin (100 μg/ml), and amphotericin B (0.25 μg/ml). Both cell types were cultured in gelatin-coated dishes [20].

Hearts of adult male Fischer 344 rats were cryoinjured by placing a 6 mm aluminum rod, precooled with liquid nitrogen, in contact with the surface of the anterior left ventricular wall as previously described [20, 25]. Normal control and acutely cryoinjured hearts were injected with 3×10^6 skeletal myoblasts. Rats were sacrificed at timed intervals (1 and 3 days; 1, 2, and 4 weeks; 3 months; n=4/group). Hearts were perfusion fixed with methyl Carnoy's solution (60% methanol, 30% chloroform, 10% glacial acetic acid), transversely sectioned, and embedded in paraffin.

Immunocytochemistry and Western blot analysis

Immunostaining was performed using immunoperoxidase and immunofluorescent methods as described [20, 25]. Expression of cadherin and connexin43 in undifferentiated myoblasts and differentiated myotubes was determined by Western blot analysis. Skeletal myotubes were maintained in differentiation medium for 10 days before lysis. On day 5 cytosine arabinofuranoside (5 μM) (Sigma, St. Louis, MO) was added to kill proliferating cells (e.g., fibroblasts). Cells were lysed in standard sample buffer containing protease inhibitors (1 mM Pefabloc® SC, 10 μg/ml leupeptin, 10 μg/ml aprotinin) (Boehringer Mannheim, Indianapolis, IN). Twenty micrograms of total soluble protein was separated via SDS-polyacrylamide gel electrophoresis (Bio-Rad, Hercules, CA) using a 7.5% resolving gel for cadherin and a 12% resolving gel for connexin43 detection. Proteins were electroblotted to Hybond-ECL nitrocellulose membrane (Amersham Corp., Arlington Heights, IL) and immunoreactions were carried out as described using the ECL detection kit [23, 24]. N-cadherin was detected using an anti-pancadherin mouse monoclonal antibody [29] (Sigma), diluted 1:2000 for light microscopy, 1:200 for immunofluorescence, and 1:1000 for Western blotting). Connexin43 was detected using a mouse monoclonal antibody [13] (Chemicon, Temecula, CA), diluted 1:200 for light and fluorescence microscopy and 1:1000 for Western blotting.

Coculture of neonatal cardiomyocytes and skeletal muscle cells

Neonatal cardiomyocytes and skeletal myoblasts were mixed in ratios of 1:3 and 1:1 in DMEM/M199 with 10% horse serum and 5% fetal bovine serum and plated at a total cell density between 6×10^3 and 1×10^4 per cm^2. It appeared that the best results were obtained when 1×10^4 total cells per cm^2 were plated at a ratio of 1:1, allowing formation of smaller, unbranched myotubes and enough surrounding cardiomyocytes to provide excitation (note that the fusion of myoblasts into multinucleated myotubes leads to a substantially lower number of myotubes compared to the original number of myoblasts). Sixty-mm gelatin-coated tissue culture plates (Falcon, Franklin Lakes, NJ) were used for video analysis and microinjection studies; Lab-Tek II glass chamber slides (Nunc, Naperville, IL) for confocal microscopy; and Lab-Tek II chambered coverglass (Nunc) for calcium imaging. All surfaces were coated with gelatin (Difco, Detroit, MI). Neonatal cardiomyocytes and skeletal myoblasts were mixed and cocultured in 60 mm plates for 2 days, by which time the myoblasts had fused to form multinucleated myotubes. Cocultures then were evaluated under an inverted microscope equipped with a heated chamber (37 °C) and a video camera. Isoproterenol (25 nM) (Sigma) was used as a β-adrenergic agonist and 1-heptanol (0.5 mM) (Sigma) as a gap junction inhibitor [6]. Plates were incubated with the respective drug for 20 min before the analysis. For statistical quantification, 3 different plates were evaluated and the contraction frequencies of 8 different fields on each plate were counted. The field areas were encircled with a marker pen, and specific morphological characteristics were noted in order to find the same fields before and after treatments. Monocultures of cardiomyocytes and skeletal myotubes, respectively, served as controls.

Confocal microscopy

For confocal microscopy neonatal cardiomyocytes and skeletal myoblasts were cocultured for 2–3 days. Cells were fixed for 2 min in 3% paraformaldehyde in PBS, 0.2% Triton X-100, 5 mmol/L EGTA (pH 7.2) followed by fixation with 3% paraformaldehyde in PBS for 20 min. Slides were incubated with pan-cadherin or connexin43 antibodies for 60 min. Primary antibodies were detected with a rabbit anti-mouse FITC-conjugated secondary antibody (DAKO, Carpinteria, CA). Counterstaining for f-actin was performed using rhodamine-phalloidin (Molecular Probes, Eugene, OR). Vectashield (Vector, Burlingame, CA) was used as mounting medium. Optical sections of 0.1 µm thickness were obtained using a BioRad MRC 600 confocal microscope (Hercules, CA) equiped with a krypton-argon laser.

Microinjection studies

Gap junctions were evaluated functionally by microinjecting cells with gap junction-permeable dye, Lucifer yellow (Molecular Probes). Pilot studies showed that injecting cardiac myocytes resulted in excessive dilution of the dye after transfer into the much larger myotubes, so we chose to inject myotubes instead. It was necessary to inject quiescent instead of actively contracting myotubes, since injecting beating myotubes often caused hypercontracture and cell death. Therefore, beating cocultures were rendered quiescent by pretreatment with the calcium chelator BAPTA-AM (40 μM, 30 min) (Sigma), and subsequent addition of the cross-bridge cycle inhibitor 2,3-butanedione monoxime (BDM; 5 mM) (Sigma) to the medium. Microinjections were performed as described [25]. The dye solution was composed of Lucifer yellow (gap junction permeable) and tetramethyl-rhodamine-dextran (gap junction impermeable) (Molecular Probes). Skeletal myotubes in close approximation to cardiomyocytes were pressure-injected (time setting 0.4 s, pressure setting 180 kPa). In order to visualize cell nuclei, cocultures were vitally counter-stained with Hoechst 33342 (4 μg/ml). Dye transfer was evaluated under a Olympus BH-2 fluorescence microscope.

Calcium imaging of cocultures

For calcium imaging [34, 35] neonatal cardiomyocytes and skeletal myoblasts were cocultured for 5 days. Beating cocultures were loaded with the membrane-permeant acetoxymethyl ester derivative of the fluorescent calcium indicator, calcium green. Cells were loaded with 5 μM calcium green-AM (Molecular Probes), 0.02% Pluronic® F-127 (Molecular Probes) and 0.15% dimethylsulfoxide (Sigma) in DMEM/M199 with 10% horse serum and 5% fetal bovine serum for 45 min at 37 °C/5% CO_2. The cultures were gently given two changes of fresh medium at the end of dye loading to remove extracellular dye. Cells were imaged on a Diaphot TMD (Nikon) inverted microscope equipped with a 40X, NA 1.3 Fluor objective, Nikon B-2E fluorescent filter set and a 75 W Xenon lamp. The dye was excited at 450 to 490 nm while an emission band from 520 to 560 nm was directed to a Hamamatsu II Intensifier coupled to a Hamamatsu CCD-77 camera. The intensified images were recorded directly onto an optical memory disk recorder (OMDR, Panasonic TQ-3038F) at 30 frames per second. Black level and gain were set at each imaging session and blank images were collected for flat field correction prior to analysis. The analog OMDR images were converted to TIFF files with Image/1 (version 4.17, Universal Imaging Corp.), then transferred to a Macintosh PPC9600/200MP computer for analysis and movie conversion. To address the question whether myotube contractions were induced by stretch, cocultures were mechanically arrested with BDM. BDM was present during loading with calcium green and throughout the evaluation. Pretreatment with BAPTA-AM was omitted in the latter experiments since the calcium chelator seemed to interfere with calcium green activation.

Results

Differentiation and electromechanical integration of skeletal muscle grafts

The histology and differentiation pattern of skeletal myoblast grafts were described in a previous study from our group [20]. Briefly, at day 1 after grafting the myoblasts were undifferentiated. By day 3, the grafted cells fused into multinucleated myotubes and expressed structural proteins such as myosin heavy chain. At 1 week the myotubes had developed recognizable cross striations, while at 2 weeks many had peripheral nuclei and clearly identifiable sarcomeres, signs of maturation. Progressive hypertrophy was observed over the entire time course, and by 3 months the grafts appeared very similar to normal adult skeletal muscle. Interestingly, the skeletal muscle grafts began to express the slow fiber marker, β-myosin heavy chain, between 2 and 4 weeks after grafting. This suggests the grafts were converting to a more fatigue-resistant phenotype in the cardiac environment [20].

To investigate electromechanical integration of grafted skeletal muscle and normal or injured host myocardium, immunostaining was performed for components of the intercalated disk. Figure 1 shows a representative graft

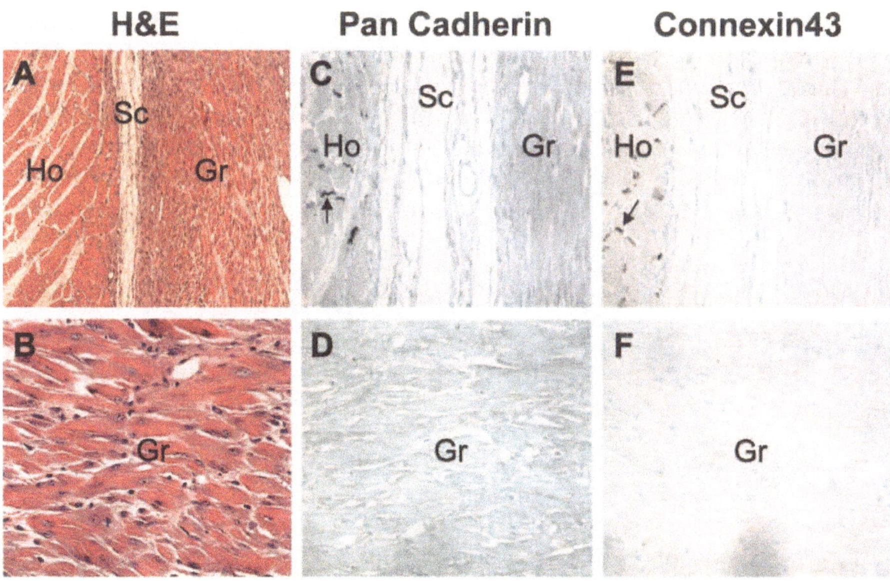

Fig. 1. Skeletal muscle cell grafting into the injured heart at 2 weeks. **A, B** Hematoxylin & eosin staining. Skeletal muscle cells formed a viable graft (Gr) that was often separated from the host myocardium (Ho) by scar tissue (Sc). No immunostaining for cadherin (**C, D**) or connexin43 (**E, F**) was found in the skeletal muscle graft. In contrast, the host myocardium showed a typical staining pattern for both molecules as they co-localize in the intercalated disc (arrows). Panels **B, D, F** show high power micrographs of the graft area [25a].

at 2 weeks, when the grafted myoblasts had already fused and differentiated (Fig. 1, panel A, B). An antibody to the C-terminus of N-cadherin ("anti pan-cadherin"), the principle component of the cardiac adherens junction, did not stain graft cells (Fig. 1, panel C, D). Similarly, antibodies to connexin43, the principal gap junction protein of ventricular myocytes, did not stain grafted skeletal muscle cells (Fig. 1, panel E, F). Both antibodies, however, gave intense staining at the intercalated disks of host cardiomyocytes where N-cadherin and connexin43 typically colocalize. The skeletal muscle grafts did not contain detectable amounts of N-cadherin or connexin43 at any time up to 3 months after grafting into normal or injured myocardium. Hence, the grafts did not form electromechanical junctions *in vivo*.

Electromechanical coupling *in vitro*

Western blot analysis of skeletal muscle cells *in vitro* showed that undifferentiated primary rat myoblasts expressed N-cadherin and connexin43 at high levels (Fig. 2). In contrast, cultures containing differentiated myotubes showed markedly decreased (but still detectable) levels of both N-cadherin and connexin43 at day 10 of differentiation (Fig. 2). It should be mentioned that our primary myoblast cultures contained contaminating non-myocytes, which may partially contribute to the signal of both proteins. For the differentiated myotubes, proliferating non-myocytes were killed with cytosine arabinofuranoside and are unlikely to confound the experiment. To verify that cadherin and connexin43 were expressed by myoblasts, the Western blot analysis was also repeated with the mouse myoblast line C2C12. As expected both cadherin and connexin43 were abundantly expressed in C2C12 myoblasts. In C2C12 myotubes, however, only connexin43 expression was down-regulated to levels similar to those observed in primary myotubes, whereas cadherin continued to be expressed

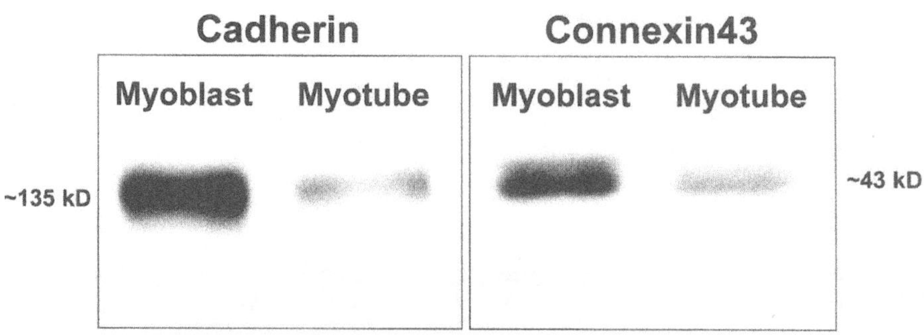

Fig. 2. Western blot analysis of N-cadherin and connexin43 in undifferentiated myoblasts and differentiated myotubes. N-cadherin and connexin43 were expressed at high levels in myoblasts; however, the differentiated myotubes showed a marked down-regulation of both molecules at day 10 after induction of differentiation. Cytosine arabinofuranoside (5 μM) was added to myotube cultures on day 5 to prevent fibroblast overgrowth [25a].

at high levels (data not shown), displaying a phenotypic divergence of an established cell line from primary muscle cells.

Given the lower N-cadherin and connexin43 levels with ongoing differentiation, it seemed unlikely that skeletal myotubes would form electromechanical junctions with cardiomyocytes. To our surprise, however, when skeletal myoblasts and neonatal cardiomyocytes were cocultured, some of the resulting skeletal myotubes contracted in synchrony with the cardiomyocyte network. Clearly identifiable synchronous contractions were observed in $\sim 10\%$ of myotubes, although there was some variation among cultures, with differing cell densities etc.

Myotube formation occurred over the first 2 days of coculture, and synchronous contractions were noted shortly thereafter. Synchronously contracting networks were observed for as long as 15 days of coculture, the longest time tested.

Monocultures of primary skeletal myotubes can contract or twitch erratically when plated at high density. In striking contrast to skeletal myotube monocultures, however, the contractions of myotubes in coculture with cardiomyocytes were very regular ("heart beat"-like) and the frequency of contractions appeared highly synchronized. For example, myotubes and cardiomyocytes would skip the same beat and then resume contracting again in synchrony.
(Note to the reader: A video tape of these cells in coculture was shown at the conference.)

We hypothesized that some of the cardiomyocytes had electrically captured closely adjacent myotubes and were pacing them via gap junctions. Pharmacological experiments to test this hypothesis are summarized in Fig. 3. Isoproterenol, a well-known β-adrenergic agonist, caused approximately a 25% increase in the contraction frequency of beating myotubes in cocultures. A similar effect of isoproterenol was observed in cardiomyocyte monocultures, whereas no effect was seen in typically non-contracting skeletal myotube monocultures (data not shown). These data implicate cardiomyocytes as the pacemakers. In contrast, the gap junction inhibitor 1-heptanol completely aborted myotube contractions but left spontaneous contractions of individual cardiomyocytes intact, suggesting that excitation of the myotubes required gap junctions. Wash-out of the drugs returned the contraction frequencies to baseline levels (Fig. 3). Interestingly, heptanol also inhibited the spontaneous irregular contractions in high density skeletal myotube monocultures. This suggests that low levels of connexin43 in differentiated myotubes may be sufficient for the formation of functional gap junctions between myotubes as well (data not shown).

If electromechanical coupling had indeed occurred between cardiomyocytes and skeletal myotubes, the responsible molecules should be detectable at myotube-cardiomyocyte interfaces. Therefore, immunofluorescent staining for N-cadherin and connexin43 in conjunction with confocal microscopy was performed. Figure 4 (panel A) shows abundant expression of N-cadherin at contact sites between a cardiomyocyte and a myotube at day

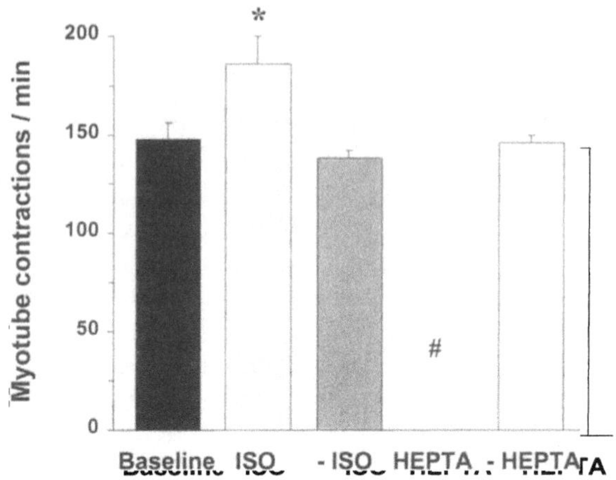

Fig. 3. Contraction frequencies of myotubes cocultured with neonatal cardiomyocytes for 6 days. Isoproterenol (ISO; 25 nM) caused a significant increase of the contraction frequency of putative cardiomyocyte-paced myotubes (+25% versus baseline). In contrast, heptanol (HEPTA; 0.5 mM) completely inhibited myotube contractions. Myotube contractions returned to baseline levels after wash-out (-ISO and -HEPTA). Values represent means ±SD from 8 fields of 3 different cocultures (24 fields total) for each treatment; statistical analysis by ANOVA followed by Bonferroni t-test; *$p<0.05$ vs baseline and -ISO, #$p<0.05$ vs baseline and -HEPTA. (Mean contraction rates varied from experiment to experiment and were often lower than the rates observed in this experiment; e.g., note in Fig. 5 that the rate is about 120/min) [25a].

2. The adherens junction was often seen as N-cadherin positive, finger-like cell processes extending from the actin cytoskeleton. Similarly, connexin43 was detected at contact sites between cardiomyocytes and myotubes shown at day 3 (Fig. 4, panel B). The formation of gap junctions between cardiomyocytes and skeletal myotubes appeared to lag somewhat behind the formation of adherens junctions and appeared to increase with coculture time. No cadherin or connexin43 proteins were detected in myotubes in areas remote from contacts with cardiomyocytes.

To test directly whether skeletal myotubes can form functional gap junctions, we performed microinjection studies. Skeletal myotubes were microinjected with a combination of Lucifer yellow (~250 Daltons), which readily passes through gap junctions [3], and rhodamine-dextran (~10000 Daltons), which is not transferable through gap junctions. Dye transfer from a myotube to a different cell type after 4 days of coculture is shown in Fig. 4 (panels C, D, E). Even though the "beating" criterion was not available to identify the recipient cell unambiguously (microinjections were carried out in mechanically quiescent cultures), the binucleation and second order dye transfer (recipient to adjacent cell) strongly suggest a cardiomyocyte as the recipient cell. It is also notable that first order dye transfer (myotube to recipient) was only observed to this cell and not to any other of the many adjacent cells (see Fig. 4 E, Hoechst nuclei staining), likely fibroblasts. The experiment proves that even differentiated skeletal muscle cells are capable of forming

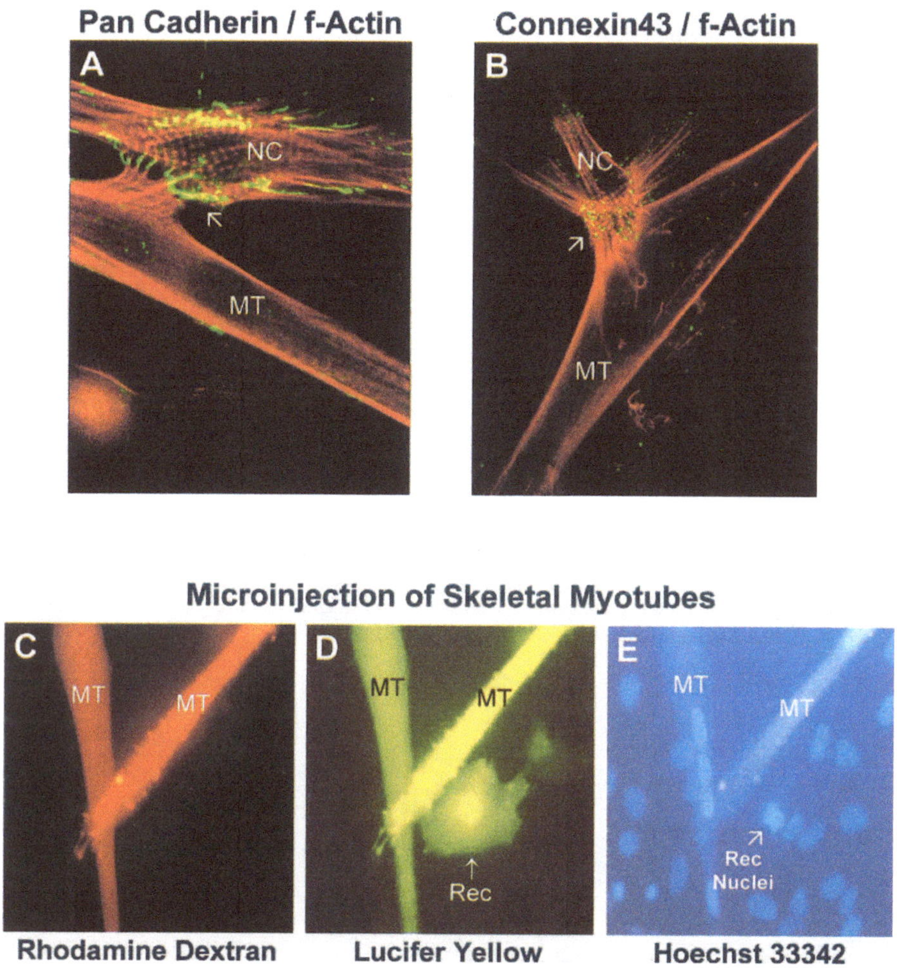

Fig. 4. Confocal microscopy of cardiomyocyte-skeletal myotube cocultures stained for N-cadherin (**A**) and connexin43 (**B**). N-cadherin and connexin43 are shown in light gray, f-actin counterstained with rhodamine phalloidin (dark gray). Expression of N-cadherin and connexin43 was detected at the interfaces between cardiomyocytes and myotubes (*arrows*). N-cadherin is shown at day 2, connexin43 at day 3 of coculture. Note that myotubes express N-cadherin and connexin43 only at the point of cardiomyocyte contact. **C**, **D**, **E** Dye transfer studies in cocultures of skeletal and cardiac muscle cells. Shown are cocultures at day 4. Two skeletal myotubes (MT) were microinjected with Lucifer yellow (gap junction permeable) and rhodamine-dextran (gap junction impermeable). (**C**) Rhodamine filter: microinjected donor myotubes (MT). (**D**) Lucifer yellow filter: recipient cell (Rec) to which the Lucifer yellow has been transferred via gap junctions. Note the more faintly fluorescent cell which has been the recipient of second order dye transfer from the first recipient. (**E**) Nuclear staining by Hoechst 33342. Even though the "beating" criterion was not available to identify the recipient cell unambiguously, binucleation (*arrow*) and second order dye transfer to an adjacent cell strongly suggest a cardiomyocyte as the recipient cell. It is also notable that the dye was not transferred to any of the other adjacent cells (see Fig. 4E, Hoechst staining), likely fibroblasts [25a].

functional gap junctions with other cell types *in vitro*. Dye transfer between myotubes and adjacent, presumptive cardiomyocytes was less frequent than the observation of synchronous beating. This likely reflects a greater difficulty for the passage of the 250 Dalton lucifer molecule versus ions involved in action potential propagation. Technical artifacts induced by microinjection also could have inhibited gap junction transfer in some cells.

We employed calcium imaging to ensure that the motions observed in the skeletal myotubes were calcium-dependent contractions and not due to passive tethering by beating cardiomyocytes. Figure 5 shows that cardio-

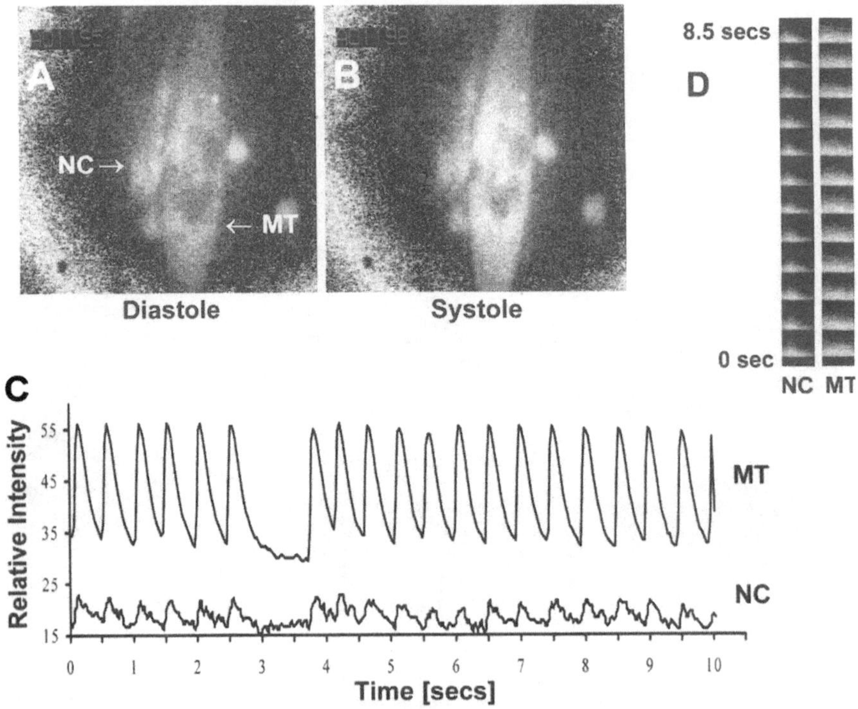

Fig. 5. Calcium imaging in cardiomyocyte-skeletal myotube cocultures at day 4. (**A**, **B**) Cells were loaded with calcium green, and intracellular calcium release-induced fluorescence was evaluated. Panel (**A**) shows the cardiomyocyte (NC) and the adjacent skeletal myotube (MT) in "diastole" (low $[Ca^{2+}]_i$), and panel (**B**) in "systole" (high $[Ca^{2+}]_i$). (**C**) The graphs represent the relative fluorescent intensity of a single myotube (*upper graph*, MT) and an adjacent cardiomyocyte (*lower graph*, NC) over a time period of 10.2 s. The frequencies of the cardiomyocyte and the myotube were significantly synchronized (correlation coefficient $r=0.85$). Note that even in a period of skipped beats around the 3 s time point the synchrony persisted. The lower overall intensity of the cardiomyocyte is due to its smaller size versus the skeletal myotube. Panel **D** shows image analysis of calcium fluxes from an adjacent neonatal cardiomyocyte (NC) and myotube (MT) pair. A 24×24 pixel region was sampled, and the average light signal along one of the 24 pixel line segments is shown for each cell. Each contraction was initiated by rapid calcium release that decayed slowly, giving a sharp lower border and a fuzzy upper border to the light signal. The calcium releases are precisely synchronized in the two cell types, indicating tight coupling [25a].

myocyte calcium transients induced highly synchronized calcium transients in an adjacent skeletal myotube. As noted previously with analysis of contractile activity, occasional pauses in calcium cycling occurred synchronously in the two cell types, indicating tight coupling. These data show that the myotube contractions are an active process requiring action potential-induced calcium transients. An alternate analysis of the synchrony of calcium transients is shown in Fig. 5D. A square was drawn over the region of maximal fluorescence in an adjacent neonatal cardiomyocyte (NC) and myotube (MT). The average light signal along one side of the square is shown for each cell over an 8.5-second interval. The rapid upstroke of the calcium transient is followed by a slow decay of the signal, giving a ladder-like appearance with sharp lower borders and fuzzy upper borders. The rapid upstrokes of the two calcium transients are precisely aligned. Minor variation in the beat-to-beat interval is also identical in the two cells. Taken together these data show that the calcium transients are highly synchronized in the cardiomyocytes and skeletal myotubes.

To address the possibility that myotube contractions occurred in response to stretch rather than action potential propagation through gap junctions, cocultures were mechanically arrested by the presence of 2,3-butanedione monoxime throughout the experiment. 2,3-Butanedione monoxime acts as an inhibitor of actin-myosin cross-bridge cycling [11, 28]. We found that synchronous calcium cycles persisted after mechanical arrest, indicating that myotube contractions were not induced by passive stretch. Taken together, these experiments demonstrate that skeletal myotubes and cardiomyocytes can indeed achieve electromechanical coupling via N-cadherin mediated adherens junctions and connexin43-mediated gap junctions.

Discussion

The major findings of the current study are

- skeletal myoblasts express significant amounts of N-cadherin and connexin43 but down-regulate these proteins as they differentiate into myotubes;
- mature skeletal muscle grafts in the injured heart do not express significant amounts of N-cadherin and connexin43 and, therefore, do not form electromechanical junctions with host myocardium;
- skeletal and cardiac muscle cells form N-cadherin and connexin43-mediated electromechanical junctions *in vitro*;
- cardiomyocytes can pace skeletal muscle cells via these gap junctions, resulting in synchronized "heart beat-like" contractions.

Comparison with previous studies

The finding that skeletal muscle grafts did not express N-cadherin and connexin43 agrees with our previous physiological studies [20]. We found that the grafts exhibited recruitment of contractile units with increasing voltage, indicating that the muscle fibers were not coupled through gap junctions [20]. Our results differ somewhat from a recent study in mice by Robinson et al. [26]. These authors injected LacZ-tagged C2C12 myoblasts into the systemic circulation, and a subset engrafted into the myocardium, mostly as isolated cells rather than as a multicellular tissue. Electron microscopy showed apparent junctions, with some characteristics of adherens junctions and gap junctions between LacZ-labeled cells and cardiomyocytes. Connexin43 was detected by immunostaining at interfaces between implanted cells (identified by SERCA-1 staining) and cardiomyocytes. Unfortunately, these connexin43-positive cells were not definitively identified as graft by double staining for LacZ. Despite some ambiguities, these data appeared clearly different from our results. We do not think the difference lies in the cells used for grafting, because our cell culture experiments showed identical down-regulation of connexin43 in C2C12 myoblasts and primary rat myoblasts after differentiation *in vitro*. Similar data showing down-regulation of N-cadherin and connexin43 expression in skeletal muscle cells during development have been reported by other groups as well [2, 8, 14, 16]. Additionally, we have grafted C2C12 myoblasts into injured rat hearts (albeit with cyclosporine immunosuppression) and could not detect either N-cadherin or connexin43 in differentiated myotubes *in vivo* (H. Reinecke and C.E. Murry, unpublished results). One possibility is that isolated skeletal muscle cells without fusion partners, as observed in Robinson's study, might retain high levels of connexin43 expression similar to myoblasts, while multinucleated myotubes down-regulate this protein.

A recent study from Taylor et al. reported improved systolic and diastolic function after autologous satellite cell implantation in cryoinjured rabbit hearts [30]. In this study the grafts formed multicellular tissues which were insulated from the surrounding myocardium by scar tissue. The authors reported that the graft cells appeared mononucleated by electron microscopy and were joined to one another by intercalated disk-like structures. They concluded that the skeletal muscle cells had trans-differentiated into a cardiac muscle phenotype. Other groups have suggested cardiac differentiation of skeletal muscle grafts [5, 33] based on morphological criteria. Our studies have found no such evidence for transdifferentiation. Our skeletal muscle grafts formed multinucleated myofibers with no intercalated disks, expressed myosin isoforms specific to skeletal muscle, failed to express cardiac α-myosin, did not express cardiac junctional proteins, and showed contractile properties specific to skeletal muscle (fiber recruitment by voltage, ability to induce tetanus) [20]. Possible explanations for the discrepancies include species differences, their use of adult satellite cells versus our use of neonatal myoblasts, and the lack of definitive markers to delineate grafted skeletal muscle from host myocardial cells.

Electromechanical coupling between cardiac and skeletal muscle

Before performing these studies it was unknown whether cardiac muscle could excite skeletal muscle, even if the cells were electrically coupled via gap junctions. Cardiac muscle cells usually have a very high input resistance and use quite small currents for excitation, whereas skeletal muscle cells have low input resistance and require large currents for excitation. Thus, it seemed possible that cardiac muscle currents might be insufficient to depolarize skeletal muscle cells to threshold. The current experiments, however, clearly indicate that cardiac muscle cells can trigger depolarization in skeletal muscle. Furthermore, our evidence suggests that the cardiac muscle cells pass depolarizing current directly to the skeletal myotubes via gap junctions.

The question remains why we see such a discrepancy between our *in vivo* and *in vitro* results. Electromechanical coupling requires the proper junctional molecules to be expressed at the correct anatomical location. It seems that *in vivo* there are problems both with gene expression and with anatomy. We believe the critical difference in gene expression lies in the extent to which skeletal muscle cells differentiate. In grafts, the skeletal muscle cells become almost indistinguishable from normal adult skeletal muscle, whereas in culture the myotubes remain relatively immature. We propose that the low levels of connexin43 and N-cadherin which persist in the cultured myotubes are physiologically significant and permit them to make homotypic molecular junctions with cardiomyocytes. When grafted, however, these junctional molecules are down-regulated as the cells mature, leaving the graft muscle fibers electrically insulated. Another possibility, which we consider less likely, is that *neonatal* cardiomyocytes can form junctions with skeletal myotubes, but that *adult* cardiomyocytes (which of course are present *in vivo*) are somehow unable to form these junctions. A previous study from our laboratory has shown, however, that adult cardiomyocytes can extend cell processes and establish junctions with neonatal cardiomyocytes *in vitro* and *in vivo*, indicating that both developmental stages of cardiomyocytes preserve the capabilities to form new intercellular junctions [25]. The anatomical problem stems from formation of a scar tissue barrier which can separate graft from host. It is possible that even with proper expression of junctional molecules, the skeletal muscle grafts could be insulated from host myocardium by scar tissue. Future studies will be required to address both of these issues.

Summary

The current study has presented structural and functional evidence for the formation of electromechanical junctions between skeletal and cardiac muscle cells *in vitro*. Furthermore, we have shown that these junctions permit the cardiac muscle cells to trigger synchronous, calcium-dependent contraction of the skeletal muscle cells. We hypothesize that these junctions do not occur after grafting *in vivo* due to down-regulation of N-cadherin and connexin43 in skeletal myofibers. If this hypothesis is correct, it is possible that inducing persistent expression of these two junctional proteins in skeletal muscle cells and by devising strategies for limiting scar tissue barriers may cause electromechanical coupling between skeletal and cardiac muscle cells *in vivo*.

Acknowledgments. The authors are indebted to Dr. John Angello for assistance with the microinjection system. We thank Ms. Veronica Poppa for expert assistance with confocal microscopy. This work was supported by NIH grants K08-HL03094, P01-HL03174, R01-HL61553, and a fellowship grant from Collateral Therapeutics, Inc. C.E. Murry is the recipient of a Burroughs Wellcome Career Award in the Biomedical Sciences.

References

1. Anversa P, Olivetti G, Loud AV (1980) Morphometric study of early postnatal development in the left and right ventricular myocardium of the rat. I. Hypertrophy, hyperplasia, and binucleation of myocytes. Circ Res 46(4):495–502
2. Balogh S, Naus CC, Merrifield P (1993) Expression of gap junctions in cultured rat L6 cells during myogenesis. Dev Biol 155(2):351–360
3. Becker DL, Evans WH, Green CR, Warner A (1995) Functional analysis of amino acid sequences in connexin43 involved in intercellular communication through gap junctions. J Cell Sci 108 (Pt4):1455–1467
4. Beyer EC, Paul DL, Goodenough DA (1987) Connexin43: a protein from rat heart homologous to a gap junction protein from liver. J Cell Biol 105 (6 Pt I): 2621–2629
5. Chiu RC, Zibaitis A, Kao RL (1995) Cellular cardiomyoplasty: myocardial regeneration with satellite cell implantation [see comments]. Ann Thorac Surg 60(1):12–18
6. Christ GJ, Spektor M, Brink PR, Barr L (1999) Further evidence for the selective disruption of intercellular communication by heptanol. Am J Physiol 276 (6Pt2):H1911–H1917
7. Cifuentes-Diaz C, Nicolet M, Goudou D, Rieger F, Mege RM (1993) N-cadherin and N-CAM-mediated adhesion in development and regeneration of skeletal muscle. Neuromuscul Disord 3(5–6):361–365
8. Dahl E, Winterhager E, Traub O, Willecke K (1995) Expression of gap junction genes, connexin40 and connexin43, during fetal mouse development. Anat Embryol (Berl) 191(3):267–278
9. Eckert P, Schnackerz K (1991) Ischemic tolerance of human skeletal muscle. Ann Plast Surg 26(1):77–84
10. George-Weinstein M, Gerhart J, Blitz J, Simak E, Knudsen KA (1997) N-cadherin promotes the commitment and differentiation of skeletal muscle precursor cells. Dev Biol 185(1):14–24
11. Hajjar RJ, Ingwall JS, Gwathmey JK (1994) Mechanism of action of 2,3-butanedione monoxime on contracture during metabolic inhibition. Am J Physiol 267 (IPt2):H100–H108

12. Holt CE, Lemaire P, Gurdon JB (1994) Cadherin-mediated cell interactions are necessary for the activation of MyoD in Xenopus mesoderm. Proc Natl Acad Sci USA 91(23):10844–10848
13. Kanter HL, Laing JG, Beau SL, Beyer EC, Saffitz JE (1993) Distinct patterns of connexin expression in canine Purkinje fibers and ventricular muscle. Circ Res 72(5):1124–1131
14. Knudsen KA, Myers L, McElwee SA (1990) A role for the Ca^{2+}-dependent adhesion molecule, N-cadherin, in myoblast interaction during myogenesis. Exp Cell Res 188(2):175–184
15. Koh GY, Klug MG, Soonpaa MH, Field LJ (1993) Differentiation and long-term survival of C2C12 myoblast grafts in heart [see comments]. J Clin Invest 92(3): 1548–1554
16. MacCalman CD, Bardeesy N, Holland PC, Blaschuk OW (1992) Noncoordinate developmental regulation of N-cadherin, N-CAM, integrin, and fibronectin mRNA levels during myoblast terminal differentiation. Dev Dyn 195(2):127–132
17. Mege RM, Goudou D, Diaz C, Nicolet M, Garcia L, Geraud G, Rieger F (1992) N-cadherin and N-CAM in myoblast fusion: compared localisation and effect of blockade by peptides and antibodies. J Cell Sci 103 (Pt 4):897–906
18. Mege RM, Goudou D, Giaume C, Nicolet M, Rieger F (1994) Is intercellular communication via gap junctions required for myoblast fusion? Cell Adhes Commun 2(4):329–343
19. Murry CE, Kay MA, Bartosek T, Hauschka SD, Schwartz SM (1996) Muscle differentiation during repair of myocardial necrosis in rats via gene transfer with MyoD. J Clin Invest 98(10):2209–2217
20. Murry CE, Wiseman RW, Schwartz SM, Hauschka SD (1996) Skeletal myoblast transplantation for repair of myocardial necrosis. J Clin Invest 98(11):2512–2523
21. Proulx A, Merrifield PA, Naus CC (1997) Blocking gap junctional intercellular communication in myoblasts inhibits myogenin and MRF4 expression. Dev Genet 20(2):133–144
22. Redfield A, Nieman MT, Knudsen KA (1997) Cadherins promote skeletal muscle differentiation in three-dimensional cultures. J Cell Biol 138(6):1323–1331
23. Reinecke H, Studer R, Vetter R, Holtz J, Drexler H (1996) Cardiac Na^+/Ca^{2+} exchange activity in patients with end-stage heart failure. Cardiovasc Res 31(1):48–54
24. Reinecke H, Vetter R, Drexler H (1997) Effects of alpha-adrenergic stimulation on the sarcolemmal Na^+/Ca^{2+}-exchanger in adult rat ventricular cardiocytes. Cardiovasc Res 36(2):216–222
25. Reinecke H, Zhang M, Bartosek T, Murry CE (1999) Survival, integration, and differentiation of cardiomyocyte grafts: a study in normal and injured rat hearts. Circulation 100(2):193–202
25a. Reinecke H, MacDonald GH, Hamchka SD, Murry CE (2000) Electromechanical coupling between skeletal and cardiac muscle. Implications for infarct repair. J Cell Biol 149:731–740
26. Robinson SW, Cho PW, Levitsky HI, Olson JL, Hruban RH, Acker MA, Kessler PD (1996) Arterial delivery of genetically labelled skeletal myoblasts to the murine heart: long-term survival and phenotypic modification of implanted myoblasts. Cell Transplant 5(1):77–91
27. Rumyantsev PP (1991) Differentiation of cardiomyocytes. In: Carlson BM (ed) Growth and Hyperplasia of Cardiac Muscle Cells. Harwood, New York, pp 3–68
28. Seow CY, Shroff SG, Ford LE (1997) Detachment of low-force bridges contributes to the rapid tension transients of skinned rabbit skeletal muscle fibres. J Physiol (Lond) 501(Pt 1):149–164

29. Takeichi M (1988) The cadherins: cell-cell adhesion molecules controlling animal morphogenesis. Development 102 (4):639–655
30. Taylor DA, Atkins BZ, Hungspreugs P, Jones TR, Reedy MC, Hutcheson KA, Glower DD, Kraus WE (1998) Regenerating functional myocardium: improved performance after skeletal myoblast transplantation [published erratum appears in Nat Med (1998) 4 (10):1200]. Nat Med 4 (8):929–933
31. Volk T, Geiger B (1984) A 135-kd membrane protein of intercellular adherens junctions. EMBO J 3 (10):2249–2260
32. Wolff KD, Stiller D (1993) Ischemia tolerance of free-muscle flaps: an NMR-spectroscopic study in the rat. Plast Reconstr Surg 91 (3) 485–491
33. Yoon PD, Kao RL, Magovern GJ (1995) Myocardial regeneration. Transplanting satellite cells into damaged myocardium. Tex Heart Inst J 22 (2):119–125
34. Zirpel L, Rubel EW (1996) Eighth nerve activity regulates intracellular calcium concentration of avian cochlear nucleus neurons via a metabotropic glutamate receptor. J Neurophysiol 76 (6):4127–4139
35. Zirpel L, Lippe WR, Rubel EW (1998) Activity-dependent regulation of $[Ca^{2+}]_i$ in avian cochlear nucleus neurons: roles of protein kinases A and C and relation to cell death. J Neurophysiol 79 (5):2288–2302

CHAPTER 21

Strategies to identify cardiomyocyte cell cycle regulatory genes

K. B. S. PASUMARTHI, L. J. FIELD
The Wells Center for Pediatric Research
and the Krannert Institute of Cardiology,
Indiana University School of Medicine,
Indianapolis, IN, USA

Introduction

Cardiomyocyte death is a common event in many forms of heart disease. The ability to increase the number of functional cardiomyocytes in a diseased heart should a priori lead to improved cardiac function. This hypothesis has prompted a number of investigators to attempt to identify genes which regulate cardiomyocyte proliferation, with the hope that modulating the activity of such genes might engender regenerative growth in diseased hearts. Several basic strategies have been employed for the identification and subsequent testing of putative cardiomyocyte cell cycle regulatory genes. Here we provide a review of these strategies and, where appropriate, provide experimental results from our laboratory which support the feasibility of the general approach.

Strategy 1: candidate gene approaches

The candidate gene approach has been the most common strategy used to identify genes capable of inducing cardiomyocyte proliferation, and many variations of this theme have been reported. In its simplest form, the approach is based on the premise that genes known to be associated with proliferation in other cell types are likely to have a similar role in the myocardium. The advent of various cardiomyocyte gene transfer techniques, as for example DNA transfection, viral transduction [26, 42, 52], direct DNA microinjection [3, 36], and the generation of transgenic animals [11, 12], has made it feasible to directly test the ability of specific candidate gene products to induce myocardial proliferation either *in vitro* or *in vivo.*

As more and more fundamental cell cycle regulatory proteins have been identified, it has become imperative to develop strategies with which to stratify the likely importance of a given candidate. One approach entails the careful assessment of the cardiac expression profile for the candidate gene during developmental stages characterized by markedly different rates of cardiomyocyte proliferation [4, 35, 47]. Concordance between candidate gene expression and the rate of cardiomyocyte DNA synthesis and/or cytokinesis provides a good first approximation for a potential role of that gene in cardiomyocyte cell cycle regulation [20, 47].

Characterization of genes expressed during pathophysiologic cardiac growth has also been used in an effort to identify cardiomyocyte cell cycle regulators. In most instances, this has entailed the analysis of gene expression during pharmacologic- or work-induced cardiac hypertrophy. A priori, this would appear to be counter intuitive as cardiac hypertrophy is not accompanied by overt cardiomyocyte proliferation. Nonetheless many of the genes activated during hypertrophic myocardial growth have proven to be cell cycle regulators (as for example proto-oncogenes). These observations have led to the notion that hypertrophic myocardial growth may reflect an abortive attempt of terminally differentiated cardiomyocytes to re-enter the cell cycle. However, mixed results have been observed in experiments where proto-oncogene expression was targeted to the heart in transgenic animals. For example, overexpression of c-myc produced mild cardiomyocyte developmental hyperplasia which resulted in hypercellular adult hearts comprised of smaller cardiomyocytes [18, 19]. Although ras overexpression in transgenic animals can induce cardiac hypertrophy, the low penetrance and segregating pattern of the phenotype suggests that additional, cooperating genes are required [13].

Advances in elucidating fundamental cell cycle regulatory pathways has afforded an alternative candidate gene strategy. For example, it is now established that transition through the various cell cycle check points is regulated in part by the activity of a family of protein kinases (the cyclin-dependent kinases or CDKs) and their activating partners (the cyclins). Initiation of DNA synthesis in cultured cells requires transit through the so-called restriction point, which is near the G1 → S boundary of the cell cycle. Transit through the restriction point is largely regulated by CDK4 and the D-type cyclins (reviewed in [14, 17]). CDK4/cyclin D-mediated phosphorylation of members of the retinoblastoma (RB) gene family disrupts RB-E2F binding, thereby permitting E2F-mediated transcription of multiple genes involved in regulating DNA synthesis [7, 9].

Since it is generally believed that terminally differentiated cardiomyocytes are arrested in G_0/G_1 [4], forced expression of proteins which regulate G1 → S transit might provide a means to reactivate proliferation in the myocardium. Towards that end Schneider and colleagues have used adenoviral delivery of E2F-1 to attempt to reactivate cardiomyocyte DNA synthesis *in vitro* and *in vivo.* Forced expression of E2F-1-induced DNA synthesis in cultures of neonatal rat cardiomyocytes, with many of the transfected cells apparently reaching G2/M prior to undergoing apoptosis [27]. The cytotoxic effect of E2F-1 was partially abated by co-expression of E1B (which, among other functions, abrogates p53 activity) or Bcl-2. Analogous results were observed following viral delivery of E2F-1 to cultured adult ventricular myocytes, and following direct viral injection into the adult myocardium [1].

Using a somewhat different approach, our laboratory has generated transgenic mice which express cyclin D1 under the regulation of the α-cardiac myosin heavy chain (MHC) promoter [49]. Our initial microinjections yielded twenty-four MHC-CYCD1 transgenic founders; no obvious morbidity was apparent in these animals. Eight mice were randomly selected and placed in breeding cages. These animals gave rise to six independent transgenic lineages, and three were selected for detailed analysis. Transgene expression was initially established by Western blot analyses (Fig. 1). High levels of cyclin D1 expression was observed in adult mice from MHC-CYCD1 lines 7, 12 and 21. Elevated expression of CDK4, the cognate D-type cyclin-dependent kinase, was also apparent in the transgenic hearts (Fig. 1). Other studies have documented increased kinase activity in cyclin D1 immune complex prepared from adult MHC-CYCD1 transgenic hearts as compared to the nontransgenic controls [49]. Thus, the kinase activity required for G1/S transit is present in the adult transgenic myocardium.

To determine if the presence of sustained cyclin D1/CDK4 kinase activity was sufficient to drive cardiomyocyte DNA synthesis in adult hearts, the MHC-CYCD1 mice were crossed with MHC-nLAC mice (which express a nuclear localized β-galactosidase reporter gene under the regulation of the cardiac MHC promoter, see [45, 48]). Cardiomyocyte nuclei in mice expressing the MHC-nLAC reporter gene are readily identified by simple X-GAL staining of histologic sections. Mice produced by these crosses carrying either the MHC-nLAC transgene alone or both the MHC-nLAC and the MHC-CYCD1 transgenes were identified and sequestered. At 11 weeks of age, the mice received a bolus injection of tritiated thymidine, were sacrificed and the hearts were processed and sectioned. The sections were stained with X-GAL to visualize the cardiomyocyte nuclei and processed for autoradiography. A marked increase in the number of ventricular cardiomyocyte nuclei was apparent in low power views of sections of hearts

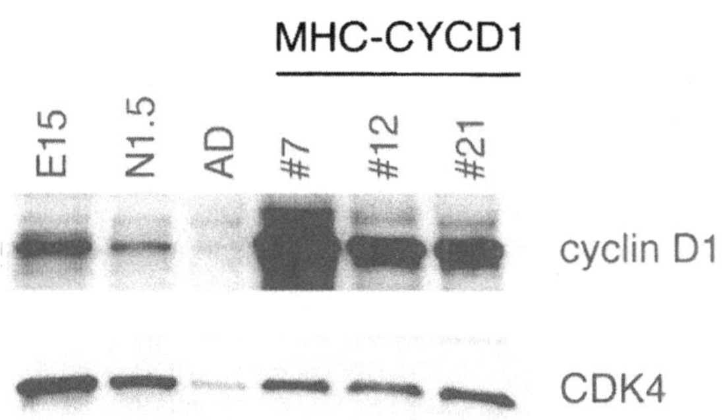

Fig. 1. Up-regulation of cyclin D1 and CDK4 in MHC-CYCD1 transgenic hearts. Protein was prepared from the hearts of adult mice from MHC-CYCD1 lines 7, 12 and 21. Control samples were prepared from nontransgenic embryonic, neonatal and adult hearts. Note the increased expression of cyclin D1 and CDK4 in the samples from the transgenic mice (adapted from [49])

expressing the MHC-CYCD1 transgene as compared to control hearts (Fig. 2A vs. B, respectively). Examination of the sections under higher magnification revealed a relatively high incidence of ventricular cardiomyocyte DNA synthesis in the mice expressing the MHC-CYCD1 transgene, as evidenced by the presence of silver grains over blue nuclei (Fig. 2C and D). The MHC-CYCD1 mice exhibited a ventricular cardiomyo-

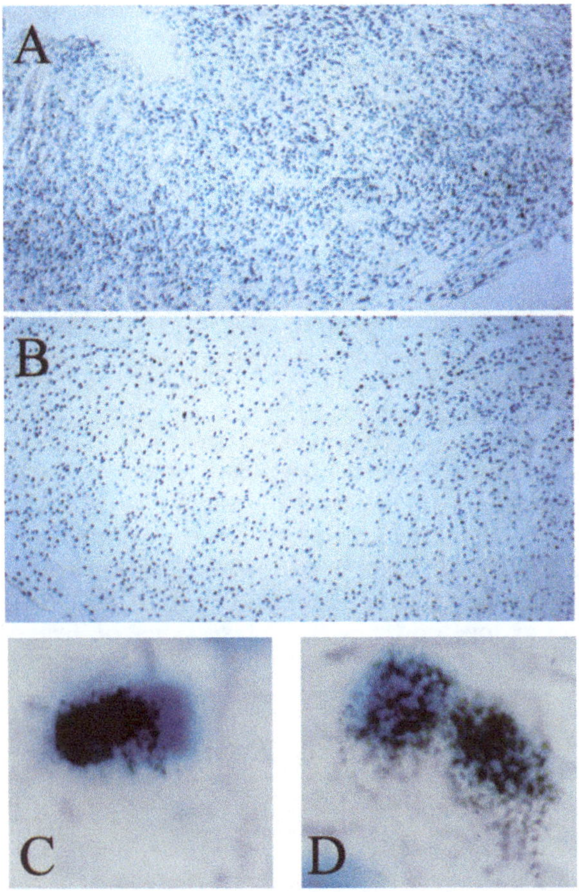

Fig. 2. Panel **A** shows a survey micrograph of the left ventricular wall of an adult mouse carrying both the MHC-nLAC and the MHC-CYCD1 transgenes, stained with X-GAL. Note relative density of the cardiomyocyte nuclei (blue staining). Panel **B** shows a survey photomicrograph of the left ventricular wall of a control adult MHC-nLAC transgenic mouse stained with X-GAL. Note the marked decrease in nuclear density as compared to the MHC-CYCD1 litter mate shown in panel **A**. Panels **C** and **D** show autoradiographs of sections prepared from transgenic mice carrying both the MHC-nLAC and the MHC-CYCD1 transgenes. The mice received an injection of tritiated thymidine, and the hearts were harvested, sectioned, stained with X-GAL and processed for autoradiography. Note the presence of silver grains over the blue nuclei, which is indicative of cardiomyocyte DNA synthesis. Panel **D** shows two putative daughter cardiomyocyte nuclei (adapted from [49])

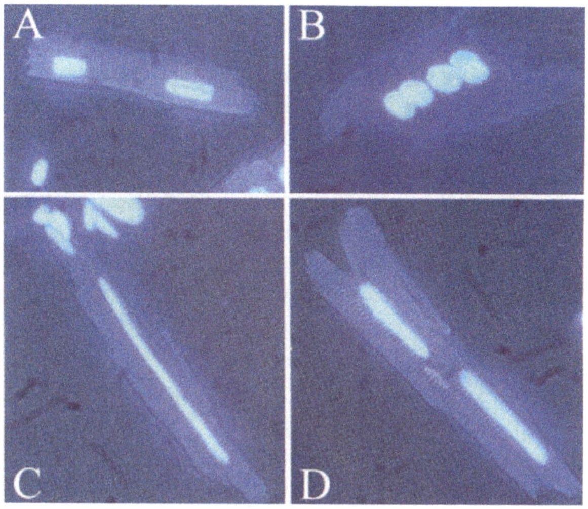

Fig. 3. Cardiomyocyte morphology in MHC-CYCD1 transgenic mice. Dispersed cell preparations were generated by collagenase digestion. Cells were affixed to glass slides, stained with Hoechst 33342 and photographed under fluorescent illumination. Panel **A** shows a typical bi-nucleated adult cardiomyocyte. Panel **B** shows a typical tetra-nucleated adult transgenic cardiomyocyte from a MHC-CYCD1 mouse. Panel **C** shows a transgenic cardiomyocyte with abnormally elongated nucleus, suggestive of genomic duplication without karyokinesis. Panel **D** shows a transgenic cardiomyocyte with two normal and one abnormal nucleus (adapted from [49])

cyte ^{3}H-thymidine labeling index of 0.12±0.011% (SEM, n=20000 nuclei), as compared to 0.0005% for non-transgenic animals (1 synthetic nucleus in 180000, see [43, 45]).

Dispersed cell suspensions were prepared from the MHC-CYCD1 transgenic hearts to determine if transgene expression had an overt effect on cardiomyocyte nuclear ploidy, or alternatively if there was an increase in the number of nuclei present in the cardiomyocytes. The preponderance of cells prepared from nontransgenic hearts were bi-nucleated. Bi-nucleated cardiomyocytes were also present in the MHC-CYCD1 transgenic hearts (Fig. 3A). In addition, a high percentage of the transgenic cardiomyocytes (approaching 50%) were tetra-nucleated (Fig. 3B). Cardiomyocytes with abnormal nuclear content were also apparent: for example, cells with abnormally long nuclei suggestive of nuclear replication in the absence of karyokinesis were seen (Fig. 3C). Cardiomyocytes with apparently partially replicated nuclei (Fig. 3D) were also observed. There was no evidence of ongoing apoptosis in the transgenic hearts. Current studies with this model are aimed at attempting to drive the tetra-nucleated ventricular cardiomyocytes through the M phase.

Strategy 2: clinical approaches

Several clinical disorders are associated with hyperplastic myocardial growth. For example, Tuberous Sclerosis Complex (TSC) is characterized by the formation of benign growths in a variety of tissues, including the heart. Fifty percent of all primary myocardial tumors occur in TSC patients, and fifty percent of all TSC patients exhibit primary cardiac tumors (56). Given the prominent cardiac phenotype in TSC, identification and cloning of genes associated with this disorder should provide insight into cardiomyocyte cell cycle regulation.

TSC can occur spontaneously as a result of de novo mutation. There is also a familial form of the disease wherein a mutant gene is inherited from one parent. The familial form of TSC exhibits an autosomal dominant pattern of inheritance, and genetic studies have identified two disease-causing loci (designated TSC1 and TSC2). The etiology of tumors in patients with mutation in TSC1 or TSC2 are indistinguishable, suggesting that these two genes are involved in the same biochemical pathway. The TSC1 gene, located at chromosome 9q34, encodes a 130 kD protein called hamartin [54], while the TSC2 gene, located at chromosome 16p13.3, encodes a 198 kD protein called tuberin [8]. Molecular analyses of tumor material from TSC patients indicated that disease progression is associated with loss of heterozygosity at either locus [15, 16], confirming earlier predictions based on genetic analyses that the TSC genes function as tumor suppressors.

Given the apparent role of tuberin in cardiomyocyte cell cycle regulation, we have cloned the complete cDNA and gene encoding the murine TSC2 gene ([23], Tsai, Pajak and Field, in preparation). This study revealed a high degree of homology between the deduced amino acid sequence of the murine and human proteins. Northern blot surveys demonstrated widespread TSC2 expression, and cardiac expression of the gene was developmentally regulated with relatively low levels of mRNA in fetal hearts and high levels in adult hearts [46].

It has recently been shown that Eker rats, a genetic model for renal carcinoma, carry a germ-line TSC2 mutation [30, 59]. The mutation comprises the fortuitous insertion of a repetitive DNA element (an IAP element) into intron 30 of the Eker rats. This insertion causes an aberrant splicing event which results in premature chain termination of the tuberin protein. Rats heterozygous for the mutation ($TSC2^{EK/+}$) are predisposed to renal carcinoma. Tumor progression in the heterozygous Eker rats is accompanied by loss of heterozygosity at the TSC2 locus, and expression of a transgene encoding a wild-type TSC2 cDNA blocks renal carcinoma in this model [32]. Rats homozygous for the mutation ($TSC2^{EK/EK}$) die in utero during mid-gestation.

The availability of this model allowed us to experimentally determine if tuberin activity is required for normal cardiomyocyte terminal differentiation [40]. Towards that end, we crossed heterozygous Eker rats and harvested the resulting embryos at day 12.5 of development. Whole embryo cultures were then prepared individually from each fetus. Spontaneously contractile cardiomyocytes were observed after multiple passages of the whole embryo cultures prepared from fetuses homozygous for the mutant TSC2 allele, but not from cultures prepared from heterozygous or wild-type fetuses (Fig. 4A).

To confirm that the contractile cells were cardiomyocytes, immune cytologic analyses were performed with an anti-sarcomeric myosin heavy chain (MHC) antibody and an anti-nebulin antibody. Previous studies have shown that the presence of MHC immune reactivity in the absence of nebulin immune reactivity can be used to distinguish cardiomyocytes from other striated muscle cells [29]. Examination of passage 4 $TSC2^{EK/EK}$ whole embryo cultures revealed the presence of cells with abundant sarcomeric MHC immune reactivity (Fig. 4B, green signal), but lacking nebulin immune reactivity (Fig. 4C, secondary antibody would yield red signal). Thus, the beating cells present in the whole embryo cultures were cardiomyocytes.

Thymidine incorporation, in conjunction with anti-MHC and anti-nebulin immune cytology, was used to monitor cardiomyocyte DNA synthesis in whole embryo cultures prepared from the $TSC2^{EK/EK}$ fetuses. Silver grains were readily detected over the nuclei of sarcomeric MHC-positive, nebulin-negative cells (Fig. 4D and E, respectively). Thus loss of tuberin activity resulted in sustained cardiomyocyte DNA synthesis in whole embryo Eker rat cultures. The overall cardiomyocyte labeling index was 3.4% in passage 4 cultures and 4.2% in passage 8 cultures. Recently this observation has been partially corroborated in mice. Although disruption of the TSC2 gene resulted in embryonic lethality, histologic analyses suggested the presence of enhanced ventricular myocardial proliferation in the homozygous mutant fetuses [31].

Given the impact of loss of tuberin activity on cardiomyocyte terminal differentiation, further characterization of the molecular activity of TSC2 might suggest a strategy to promote regenerative growth in adult hearts. Molecular analyses have identified several structural motifs which may be important for tuberin activity. An alternatively spliced region encoding a leucine zipper is located at amino acid residues 81–102 [8]. Inter-digitation of leucine zipper motifs, which consist of a periodic array of leucine residues on an α-helix, has been shown to facilitate protein-protein binding [33]. Given the importance of this structural motif in protein multimerization, TSC2 splice variants lacking the leucine zipper motif would likely have altered binding activities. Amino acid residues 346–371 were recently shown to mediate binding to hamartin, the product of the TSC1 gene [55]. The demonstration that the TSC1 and TSC2 gene products directly interact with one another provides compelling circumstantial evidence that these two proteins are involved in a common biochemical pathway.

Amino acid residues 1617–1655 of tuberin exhibit homology to the GTPase-activating protein rap1GAP [8, 38]; rap1GAP is a negative regulator of rap1, a ras superfamily member which appears to diminish the transforming activity of the Ki-ras mutant in co-transfected cells [28]. Tuberin and rap1a are both localized in the Golgi apparatus [57], and tuberin can stimulate the rap1A GTPase activity in co-transfected cells [57]. These observa-

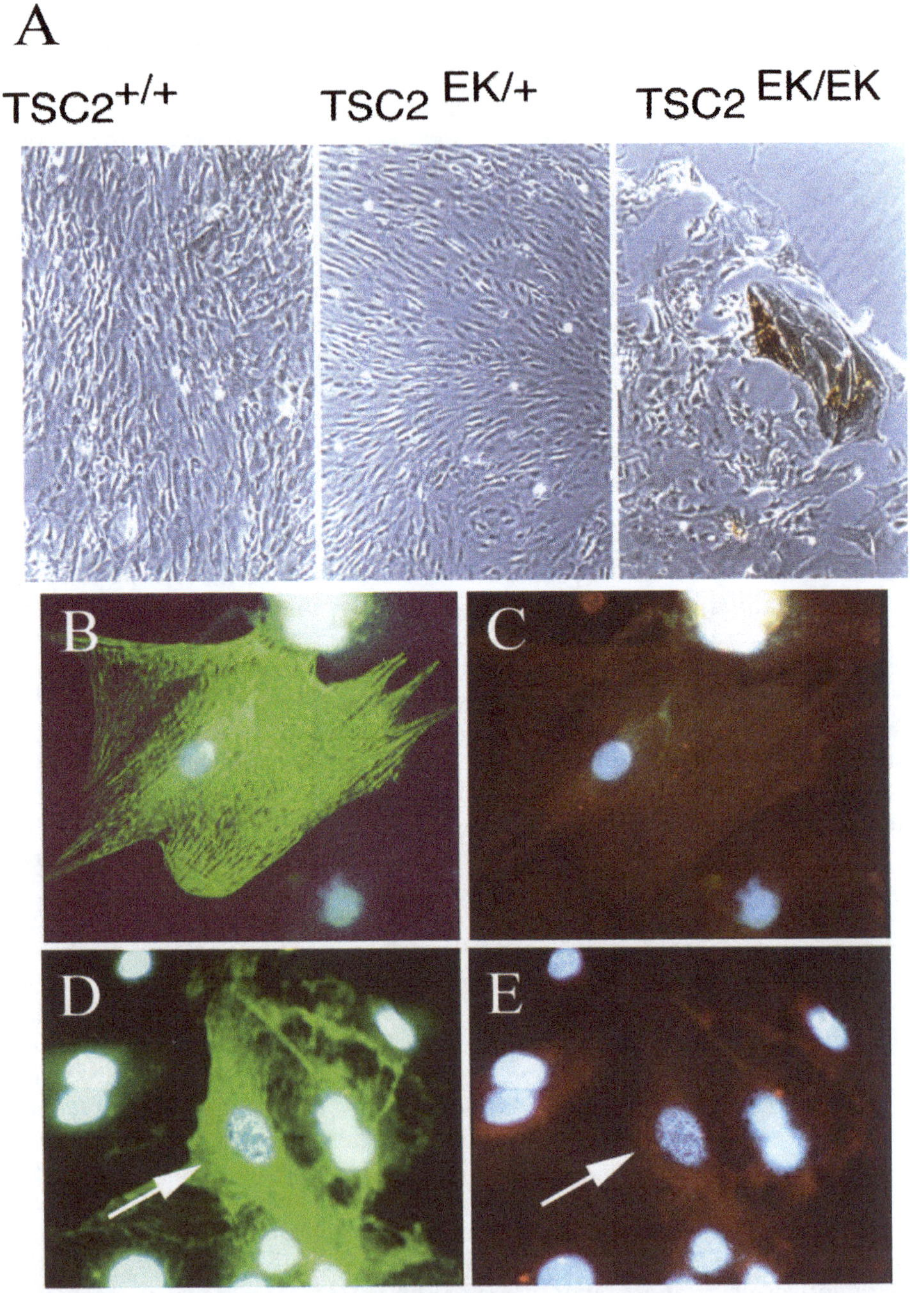
A
TSC2+/+
TSC2 EK/+
TSC2 EK/EK
B
C
D
E

tions strongly suggest that this motif is important for normal tuberin activity. Finally, two-hybrid screens identified a rabaptin-5-binding domain at amino acid residues 1668–1726 [58]. Rabaptin-5 regulates the activity of rab5, a small GTPase which is the rate-limiting component of the endocytotic membrane-docking apparatus [51]. Biochemical studies revealed that tuberin possesses potent rab5 GAP activity, and abnormally high levels of endocytosis were present in tuberin-deficient cells (presumably as a consequence of aberrant endocytotic membrane function, see [58]).

Current efforts have focused on attempting to generate modified TSC2 cDNAs which exhibit dominant negative activity. Towards that end, we have produced a series of tuberin cDNAs in which one or more of the structural motifs described above were deleted. These constructs were then tested for their ability to enhance growth rate, increase endocytosis and promote aberrant protein trafficking (all characteristics of tuberin-deficient cells). Indeed, several of these cDNAs mimicked tuberin-deficiency when expressed in NIH-3T3 cells [41]. The cDNA with the greatest growth-promoting activity in cell culture was tested for its ability to alter cardiomyocyte cell cycle regulation *in vivo*. Transgenic mice were produced wherein the MHC promoter was used to target expression of a tuberin cDNA in which the leucine zipper and Rabaptin 5 domains were deleted. Although cardiac development was normal in these animals, ventricular cardiomyocyte DNA synthesis following isoproterenol-induced hypertrophy was ca. 35-fold greater than that observed in non-transgenic siblings. These results suggest that modulation of tuberin activity in adult hearts, in concert with β-adrenergic stimulation, might be exploited to induce regenerative growth. It is, however, important to stress that the overall rates of cardiomyocyte DNA synthesis in these animals was still quite low.

Strategy 3: functional approaches

The approaches outlined above rely on the use of known gene products that were selected based on their activity in other cell types, their patterns of expression during normal and/or pathologic myocardial growth, or their

Fig. 4. Panel **A** shows sarcomeric myosin heavy chain (MHC) immune reactivity (horse radish peroxidase-conjugated secondary antibody, brown signal) in passage 4 whole embryo cultures prepared from $TSC2^{+/+}$, $TSC2^{EK/+}$, or $TSC2^{EK/EK}$ fetuses. Muscle cells are present only in the $TSC2^{EK/EK}$ cultures. Panels **B** and **C** show simultaneous immune fluorescence analysis of sarcomeric MHC expression (panel **B**, green signal) and nebulin (panel **C**, red signal) in passage 4 $TSC2^{EK/EK}$ cultures. The sample was counter-stained with Hoechst 33342 to visualize nuclei. Note that the $TSC2^{EK/EK}$ cell expresses MHC but not nebulin, indicating that it is a cardiac myocyte. Panels **D** and **E** show analyses of a similar culture processed simultaneously for MHC (panel **D**, green signal) and nebulin (panel **E**, red signal) immune reactivity, and then processed for autoradiography. The sample was counter-stained with Hoechst 33342 to visualize nuclei. The presence of silver grains over the nuclei (arrows) indicates that the cardiomyocytes continue to synthesize DNA (adapted from [40]) genetic association with clinical cardioproliferative disorders. An alternative strategy entails producing model systems in which cardiomyocyte proliferation is experimentally induced, with the hope that the proliferating cells could then be used as a reagent for gene discovery.

Towards that end, a number of groups have monitored cardiomyocyte proliferation in normal, diseased, and/or experimentally injured adult hearts. Cardiomyocyte proliferation is typically approximated by monitoring for the presence of cytologic landmarks associated with cell division (i.e., mitotic figures, cytokinesis), the expression of gene products required for cell cycle progression (i.e., PCNA, which is induced during DNA synthesis), or by monitoring DNA synthesis (by directly determining nuclear DNA content or by monitoring de novo DNA synthesis by tritiated thymidine or BrdU incorporation). The advantages and limitations of each of these approaches have recently been reviewed [44].

We had originally developed the MHC-nLAC model described above to provide an unequivocal means with which to monitor cardiomyocyte DNA synthesis in adult mouse hearts. Using this approach we observed a ventricular cardiomyocyte-tritiated thymidine labeling index of 0.0004% in the adult mouse heart. Induction of cardiac hypertrophy or myocardial damage resulting from cautery injury did not result in a significant increase in the cardiomyocyte-labeling index in this model [45]. Thus it would appear that the rates of cardiomyocyte DNA synthesis (and, by inference, proliferation) is exceedingly low in the normal and injured adult mouse heart: such low rates preclude biochemical and molecular analyses thereby making novel gene discovery very difficult in this species. There are however persistent reports of higher rates of DNA synthesis and cytokinesis in other species (reviewed in [2]), raising the possibility that gene discovery could be performed if enriched populations of the proliferating cardiomyocytes could be obtained.

Given the inherently low rates of active cardiomyocyte DNA synthesis in the adult mouse heart, we have strived to generate genetically modified model systems with aberrantly high rates of cardiomyocyte proliferation with the hope that they could be used to functionally identify cell cycle regulatory proteins. Our initial approach entailed generating transgenic mice expressing the SV40 Large T Antigen (T-Ag) oncoprotein under the regulation of the atrial natriuretic factor (ANF) promoter [10]. Based on paradigms established in other cell types [37, 39], we hypothesized that if the transgenic mice (designated ANF-TAG) developed cardiac tumors, the cardiomyocyte T-Ag-binding proteins were likely to be important cell cycle regulators. The ANF promoter was selected because ANF expression in normal adult hearts is limited to the atria; we reasoned that mice would more likely be able to tolerate atrial tumorigenesis than ventricular tumorigenesis.

Figure 5A shows a typical heart from an adult ANF-TAG transgenic mouse. The ANF-TAG transgenic mice exhibited pervasive right atrial hyperplasia, and in older animals the mass of the resulting tumors could easily exceed that of the ventricles. The hyperplastic response in the left atria was markedly diminished or absent in these animals. Interestingly, the level of left atrial T-Ag expression was similar to that observed in the tumorigenic right atria, as evidenced by both immune histology and Western blotting [10]. Subsequent developmental studies have indicated that right atrial T-Ag expression precedes left atrial expression, and that the onset of right atrial expression is temporally coincident with atrial cardiomyocyte cell cycle withdrawal (Field, unpublished and [46]). These observations are consistent with the notion that the cardiomyocytes must still be actively proliferating for T-Ag to induce sustained hyperplasia. We have recently confirmed this notion using a temperature-sensitive T-Ag mutant: thymidine incorporation in the fetal transgenic cardiomyocytes cultured at the permissive temperature was markedly greater than that observed for neonatal transgenic cardiomyocytes (Pajak and Field in preparation).

In other experiments, T-Ag expression was targeted to the ventricles with either the rat or mouse α-cardiac MHC promoters ([21], Field, unpublished results). As anticipated, viability of mice expressing T-Ag in the ventricles was quite low. Of a total of 15 founder animals generated with these constructs, only one survived long enough to transmit the transgene. That particular animal exhibited a highly mosaic pattern of ventricular expression due to transgene imprinting (Fig. 5B, see also [21]). Surface ECGs from mice in this lineage revealed the presence of ectopic ventricular pacemakers apparently originating from the tumor mass, suggesting that decreased viability may have resulted from lethal tumor-induced arrhythmias.

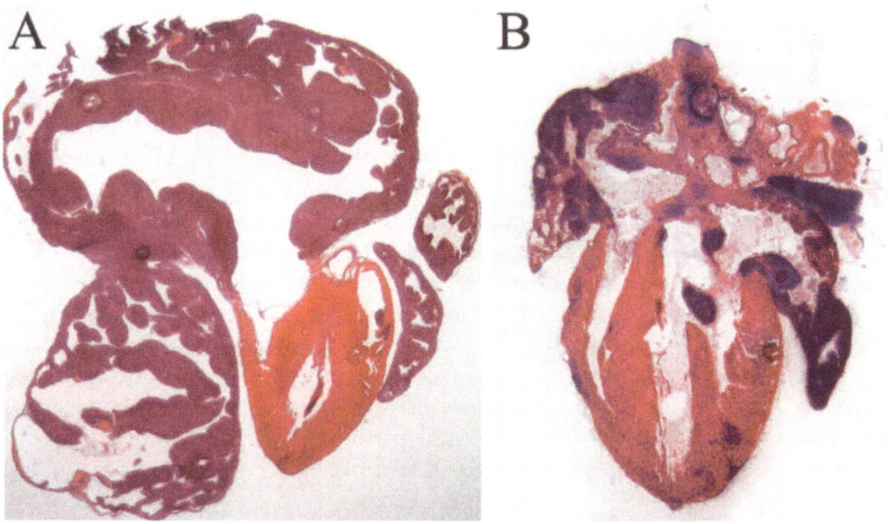

Fig. 5. Panel **A** shows a survey photomicrograph of an adult ANF-TAG transgenic mouse heart with a large right atrial tumor. The section was stained with H and E. Note that the right atrium is several-fold larger than the ventricles in this heart. Left atrial involvement is minimal. Panel **B** shows a survey photomicrograph of an adult MHC-TAG transgenic mouse heart stained with H and E. Note the bilateral atrial tumorigenesis, and the mosaic ventricular involvement (adapted from [10, 21])

Primary cultures of the transgenic tumor cardiomyocytes were viable and exhibited sustained spontaneous contractile activity. However the yield of cells per tumor was both low and highly variable. Two experiments were undertaken to remedy this. First, minced preparations of primary ANF-TAG atrial tumors were injected subcutaneously into syngeneic mice. About 10% of the recipient animals developed ectopic tumors which were comprised of differentiated cardiomyocytes. After several rounds of passage in syngeneic animals, a tumor cell line designated AT-1 was obtained [6, 34, 50]. Ultrastructural analyses of typical cultured AT-1 cells are shown in Fig. 6. Panel C shows a low power electron micrograph of an AT-1 cell; well-formed myofibrils are present throughout the cytoplasm. In culture the AT-1 cardiomyocytes form synchronously beating sheets, and gap junction and intercalated discs (Panels A and B, respectively) are readily seen between adjacent cells. Abundant secretory granules and a well-formed transverse tubule system are also apparent (Panels D and E, respectively). Although these cells still retained only limited capacity for passage in culture, they proved to be extremely useful in that large amounts of highly differentiated tumor cardiomyocytes were routinely and reproducibly obtainable (ca. 10–15 grams of tissue per animal as opposed to 200–500 mg of tissue from the primary atrial tumors). In a second experiment, primary cultures prepared from an MHC-TAG atrial tumor were subjected to continual passage. After approximately 30 passages, a relatively dedifferentiated T-Ag-positive cell line (designated AT-2) was established.

We have used the AT-2 cardiomyocyte cell cultures as a reagent to identify T-Ag-binding proteins [5]. Towards that end, cultures metabolically labeled with ^{35}S-methionine were lysed with non-ionic detergents which did not disrupt protein-protein interactions. The lysates were pre-cleared by absorption to protein A sepharose beads, and then reacted with either anti-T-Ag, anti-p53 or non-specific control antibodies. Immune complex was then collected by absorption to protein A sepharose beads, displayed on standard Laemmli SDS polyacrylamide gels and visualized by autoradiography (Fig. 7 A). Proteins of ca. 193, 120 and 53 kD were present in anti-T-Ag immune complexes but not in negative control (i.e., non-specific) immune complex. These proteins were designated as binding proteins.

The 53 kD protein present in anti-T-Ag immune complex was the p53 tumor suppressor. Since p53 binds avidly to T-Ag, it was anticipated that all of the binding proteins present in anti-T-Ag immune complexes would also present in an anti-p53 immune complex. Indeed, this was the case, as is shown for an immune complex generated with two different anti-p53 antibodies (Fig. 7 A). Note that an additional protein with a molecular weight of ca. 180 kD was also present in the 421 immune complex, but not in other anti-T-Ag or anti-p53 immune complexes.

The absence of RB in the anti-T-Ag and anti-p53 immune complexes was rather puzzling, particularly as non-phosphorylated RB protein can be detected in total protein from AT-2 cardiomyocytes (see [24]). To further address this issue, the RB signal was compared between total AT-2 lysate and lysate immune precipitated with an anti-T-Ag monoclonal antibody

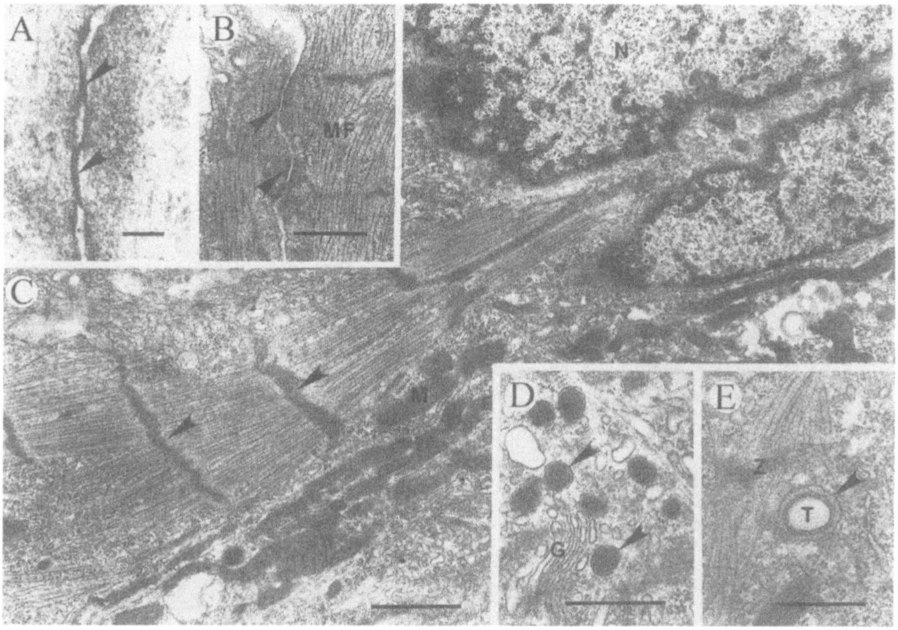

Fig. 6. Ultrastructural analysis of cultured AT-1 cardiomyocytes. Panel **A** shows numerous gap junctions between adjacent AT-1 cells; bar = 0.1 μm. Panel **B** shows fascia adherens between two adjacent AT-1 cardiomyocytes; bar = 0.5 μm. Panel **C** shows the well-developed myofibrils and active euchromatic nuclei typical of cultured AT-1 cells; bar = 1 μm. Panel **D** shows the presence of abundant ANF secretory granules; bar = 0.1 μm. Panel **E** shows the presence of a well developed transverse tubule system in the cultured cells; bar = 0.1 μm (adapted from [50])

(Fig. 7 B). No RB was detected in the anti-T-Ag immune precipitation by Western blot analysis. Reprobing the blot with an anti-T-Ag antibody indicated that T-Ag was quantitatively immune precipitated in this experiment. These results corroborate the studies above which failed to detect significant levels of T-Ag/RB immune complex in lysate from AT-2 cardiomyocytes. Other Western studies have demonstrated that there are no obvious shifts in the status of RB phosphorylation correlating with cardiomyocyte cell cycle withdrawal in the mouse when whole heart extracts are examined [46]. While these results collectively do not rule out a role for RB in cardiac development and/or terminal differentiation, they do strongly suggest that T-Ag/RB binding is not a prerequisite for T-Ag-induced cardiomyocyte proliferation in our cardiomyocyte cell lines.

Although RB was not a prominent T-Ag-binding protein in AT-2 cardiomyocytes, p107 (an RB family member) was readily detected (Fig. 7 A). We have cloned the murine p107 cDNA, determined the chromosomal location of the gene, and established its pattern of expression during mouse development. The p107 mRNA levels paralleled closely cardiomyocyte cell cycle withdrawal, with high levels in fetal hearts and low levels in adult hearts [25]. Our initial cDNA cloning study identified two p107 transcripts of 4.9 and 2.4 kb.

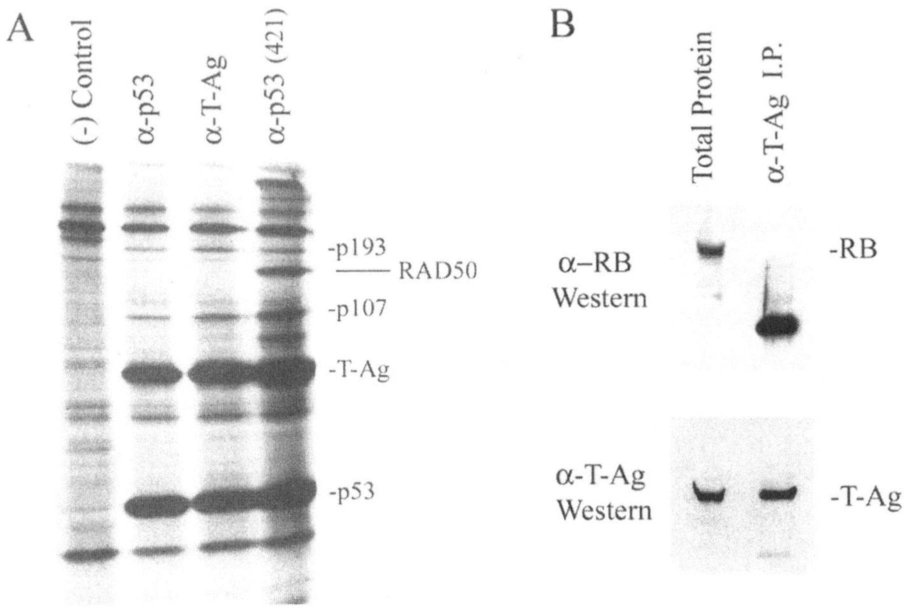

Fig. 7. Panel **A** shows a typical immune precipitation experiment from AT-2 cardiomyocytes. Cells grown in the presence of ^{35}S-methionine were homogenized and the resulting protein extract was immunoprecipitated with various antibodies. Immune complex was collected on protein A sepharose beads, resolved on 10% denaturing polyacrylamide gels and visualized by autoradiography. Immune complex generated with non-specific negative control antibody, anti-p53 and anti-T-Ag antibodies are shown. The position and identity of the cardiomyocyte T-Ag-binding proteins is shown on the right. Panel **B** shows immune precipitation (I.P.)/Western blot analysis of AT-2 protein. Total protein (50 μg) or anti-T-Ag immune complex (from 50 μg total protein) were run on a 10% polyacrylamide gel and transferred to Genescreen. The blots were then probed with anti-RB antibody and anti-T-Ag antibody. A strong RB signal is seen in total AT-2 lysate, but none in the anti-T-Ag-immunoprecipitated material, indicating that the preponderance of RB in AT-2 cells is not bound to T-Ag. Equivalent signals were seen in the anti-T-Ag Western, indicating that the T-Ag immune precipitation was quantitative (adapted from [5, 24])

The 4.9 kb transcript encodes the full length p107 molecule. The 2.4 kb transcript arises by alternative splicing and encodes a 68 kD (p68) protein which is co-linear with the N-terminus of p107 from amino acid residue 1 through 598. Beyond this point the deduced amino acid sequences were divergent, with the 68 kD protein terminating after only 3 additional amino acids. It is of interest to note that this breakdown in homology occurred immediately downstream of the A motif of the pocket domain. We have generated transgenic mice which constitutively overexpress p107 in the myocardium, and preliminary results indicated that these animals are resistant to isoproterenol-induced hypertrophy (Tsai and Field, in preparation).

We have also sequenced, cloned and characterized the 180 kD protein identified in AT-2 cardiomyocyte immune complexes generated with anti-p53 monoclonal antibody 421 (Fig. 7 A). This protein does not bind to T-

Ag or to p53; rather it cross reacts with the p53 antibody. Our interest in this protein was piqued by the observation that its steady-state levels were dramatically influenced by the confluence of the cell cultures and that it shared epitopic homology to p53 [5]. Accordingly, we isolated and sequenced the 180 kD protein. cDNA clones were then isolated using an oligonucleotide probe based on the least degenerate proteolytic peptide sequence data available. Sequence analysis of these cDNA clones indicated that this protein had significant regional homology to the yeast RAD50 gene [22]. RAD50 is a member of the RAD52 epistasis group and is required for the repair of double-stranded DNA breaks as well as for synaptinemal complex formation in sporulating cultures. Importantly, expression of the mouse cDNA rescued the MMS-sensitive phenotype in rad50 mutant yeast, indicating that the cardiomyocyte phosphoprotein is the mammalian homologue of the yeast RAD50 gene product. High levels of RAD50 expression were evident in the adult myocardium, a somewhat surprising observation given the absence of DNA synthesis in adult cardiomyocytes.

Summary

The approaches described above provide a generalized strategy to identify cardiomyocyte cell cycle regulatory proteins. Although it is clear from the candidate gene studies that gene transfer can be used to reactivate cardiomyocyte DNA synthesis *in vitro* and *in vivo*, several obstacles remain before this approach can be exploited for regenerative myocardial growth. In the case of E2F-1, anti-apoptotic strategies must be employed concomitantly. Moreover, deregulation of an apparently strong G2/M block will be required for either the E2F-1 or cyclin D1 approaches to be successful. It is also clear that genes identified from cardioproliferative clinical disorders can be exploited to deregulate the cardiomyocyte cell cycle. Although loss of TSC2 activity or expression of modified TSC2 activity result in sustained fetal cardiomyocyte proliferation or activation of adult cardiomyocyte cell cycle, respectively, these manipulations do not result in overt deregulation of the cardiomyocyte cell cycle. This result was largely predictable as the cardiac tumors in TSC patients are benign. Identification of additional genes which act in concert with the tuberin pathway will be required for successful regenerative growth.

Because the functional model approach requires a model system which exhibits deregulated cardiomyocyte proliferation, it will by default identify important cell cycle regulatory proteins. Our efforts with this approach have focused on identifying the cardiomyocyte T-Ag-binding proteins in cardiomyocyte cell lines derived from transgenic mouse tumors. Although the studies described above centered on p53 and p107 (both previously identified and well characterized T-Ag-binding proteins), this approach has the potential to identify novel regulatory proteins. This point is perhaps best illustrated by a recent study in which the 193 kD T-Ag-binding protein was cloned and characterized [53]. Surprisingly, molecular and functional analyses indicated that this protein, designated p193, is a new member of the BH3 only pro-apoptosis gene family. Current work is centered on determining if abrogation of the p193 signal transduction pathway can ameliorate the apoptotic activities induced by inappropriate cell cycle activation.

Despite the limitations encountered to date with cell cycle reactivation in adult cardiomyocytes, there is a reasonable level of optimism that the current hurdles (inappropriate induction of apoptosis, G2/M blockade) will ultimately be overcome. Progress towards this end will undoubtedly be fueled by the rapid advances in our knowledge of fundamental cell cycle regulators which act in other cell types, as well as by results emanating from the type of experimental approaches outlined in this review. Once regenerative growth is possible, research efforts will be refocused to determine the extent to which experimentally increased myocardial mass impacts on cardiac function in diseased hearts. Although restoration of systolic function in an injured heart constitutes the ultimate goal for these experimental interventions, other less rigorous endpoints might be of considerable value. Successful experimental validation of these models will determine the potential clinical value of regenerative myocardial growth. It is hoped that the initial models to test these hypotheses will be forthcoming.

Acknowledgments. We thank the NHLBI (LJF) and American Heart Association, Indiana Affiliate (KBSP) for support.

References

1. Agah R, Kirshenbaum LA, Abdellatif M, Truong LD, Chakraborty S, Michael LH, Schneider MD (1997) Adenoviral delivery of E2F-1 directs cell cycle reentry and p53 independent apoptosis in postmitotic adult myocardium in vivo. J Clin Invest 100:2722–2728
2. Anversa P, Kajstura J (1998) Ventricular myocytes are not terminally differentiated in the adult mammalian heart. Circ Res 83(1):1–14
3. Buttrick PM, Kass A, Kitsis RN, Kaplan ML, Leinwand LA (1992) Behavior of genes directly injected into the rat heart in vivo. Circ Res 70:193–198
4. Clubb FJ Jr, Bishop SP (1984) Formation of binucleated myocardial cells in the neonatal rat. An index for growth hypertrophy. Lab Invest 50:571–577
5. Daud AI, Lanson Jr NA, Claycomb WC, Field LJ (1993) Identification of SV40 large T-antigen-associated proteins in cardiomyocytes from transgenic mice. Am J Physiol 264:H1693–1700
6. Delcarpio JB, Lanson NA Jr, Field LJ, Claycomb WC (1991) Morphological characterization of cardiomyocytes isolated from a transplantable cardiac tumor derived from transgenic mouse atria (AT-1 cells). Circ Res 69:1591–1600
7. Dowdy SF, Hinds PW, Louie K, Reed SI, Arnold A, Weinberg RA (1993) Physical interaction of the retinoblastoma protein with human D cyclins. Cell 73:499–511
8. The European Chromosome 16 Tuberous Sclerosis Consortium (1993) Identification and characterization of the tuberous sclerosis gene on chromosome 16. Cell 75:1305–1315

9. Ewen ME, Sluss HK, Sherr CJ, Matsushime H, Kato J, Livingston DM (1993) Functional interactions of the retinoblastoma protein with mammalian D-type cyclins. Cell 73:487–497
10. Field LJ (1988) Atrial natriuretic factor-SV40 T antigen transgenes produce tumors and cardiac arrhythmias in mice. Science 239:1029–1033
11. Field LJ (1993) Transgenic mice in cardiovascular research. Ann Rev Physiol 55:97–114
12. Field LJ (1991) Cardiovascular research in transgenic animals. Trends in Cardiovascular Medicine 1:141–146
13. Gottshall KR, Becker KD, Hunter JJ, Chien KR (1996) A genetic based model of cardiac hypertrophy in MLC-ras mice. J Cardiac Failure 2:S28–34
14. Grana X, Reddy EP (1995) Cell cycle control in mammalian cells: role of cyclins, cyclin dependent kinases (CDKs), growth suppressor genes and cyclin-dependent kinase inhibitors (CKIs). Oncogene 11:211–219
15. Green AJ, Johnson PH, Yates JR (1994) The tuberous sclerosis gene on chromosome 9q34 acts as a growth suppressor. Hum Mol Gen 3:1833–1834
16. Green AJ, Smith M, Yates JR (1994) Loss of heterozygosity on chromosome 16p13.3 in hamartomas from tuberous sclerosis patients. Nat Genetics 6:193–196
17. Hunter T, Pines J (1994) Cyclins and cancer. II: Cyclin D and CDK inhibitors come of age. Cell 79:573–582
18. Jackson T, Allard MF, Sreenan CM, Doss LK, Bishop SP, Swain JL (1991) Transgenic animals as a tool for studying the effect of the c-myc proto-oncogene on cardiac development. Mol Cell Biochem 104:15–19
19. Jackson T, Allard MF, Sreenan CM, Doss LK, Bishop SP, Swain JL (1990) The c-myc proto-oncogene regulates cardiac development in transgenic mice. Mol Cell Biol 10:3709–3716
20. Kang MJ, Koh GY (1997) Differential and dramatic changes of cyclin-dependent kinase activities in cardiomyocytes during the neonatal period. J Mol Cell Cardiol 29:1767–1777
21. Katz E, Steinhelper ME, Daud A, Delcarpio JB, Claycomb WC, Field LJ (1992) Ventricular cardiomyocyte proliferation in transgenic mice expressing α-Cardiac Myosin Heavy Chain-SV40 T antigen fusion genes. Am J Physiol 262 (Heart and Circulatory Physiology 31):H1867–1876
22. Kim KK, Daud AI, Wong SC, Pajak L, Tsai S-C, Wang H, Henzel WJ, Field LJ (1996) Mouse RAD50 has limited epitopic homology to p53 and is expressed in the adult myocardium. J Biol Chem 271:29255–29264
23. Kim KK, Pajak L, Wang H, Field LJ (1995) Cloning, developmental expression, and evidence for alternative splicing of the murine tuberous sclerosis (TSC2) gene product. Cell & Mol Biol Res 41:515–526
24.] Kim KK, Soonpaa MH, Daud AI, Koh GY, Kim JS, Field LJ (1994) Tumor suppressor gene expression during normal and pathologic myocardial growth. J Biol Chem 269:22607–22613
25. Kim KK, Soonpaa MH, Wang H, Field LJ (1995) Developmental expression of p107 mRNA and evidence for alternative splicing of the p107 (RBL1) gene product. Genomics 28:520–529
26. Kirshenbaum LA (1997) Adenovirus mediated-gene transfer into cardiomyocytes. Molecular Cellular Biochemistry 172:13–21
27. Kirshenbaum LA, Abdellatif M, Chakraborty S, Schneider MD (1996) Human E2F-1 reactivates cell cycle progression in ventricular myocytes and represses cardiac gene transcription. Dev Biol 179:402–411
28. Kitayama H, Sugimoto Y, Matsuzaki T, Ikawa Y, Noda M (1989) A ras-related gene with transformation suppressor activity. Cell 56:77–84

29. Klug MG, Soonpaa MH, Field LJ (1995) DNA synthesis and multinucleation in embryonic stem cell-derived cardiomyocytes. Am J Physiol 269:H1913–1921
30. Kobayashi T, Hirayama Y, Kobayashi E, Kubo Y, Hino O (1995) A germline insertion in the tuberous sclerosis (Tsc2) gene gives rise to the Eker rat model of dominantly inherited cancer. Nat Genetics 9:70–74
31. Kobayashi T, Minowa O, Kuno J, Mitani H, Hino O, Noda T (1999) Renal carcinogenesis, hepatic hemangiomatosis, and embryonic lethality caused by a germ-line Tsc2 mutation in mice. Cancer Res 59:1206–1211
32. Kobayashi T, Mitani H, Takahashi R, Hirabayashi M, Ueda M, Tamura H, Hino O (1997) Transgenic rescue from embryonic lethality and renal carcinogenesis in the Eker rat model by introduction of a wild-type Tsc2 gene. Proc Natl Acad Sci USA 94:3990–3993
33. Landschulz WH, Johnson PF, McKnight SL (1989) The DNA binding domain of the rat liver nuclear protein C/EBP is bipartite. Science 243:1681–1688
34. Lanson NA Jr, Glembotski CC, Steinhelper ME, Field LJ, Claycomb WC (1992) Gene expression and atrial natriuretic factor processing and secretion in cultured AT-1 cardiac myocytes. Circulation 85:1835–1841
35. Li F, McNelis MR, Lustig K, Gerdes AM (1997) Hyperplasia and hypertrophy of chicken cardiac myocytes during posthatching development. Am J Physiol 273:R518–526
36. Lin H, Parmacek MS, Morle G, Bolling S, Leiden JM (1990) Expression of recombinant genes in myocardium in vivo after direct injection of DNA. Circulation 82:2217–2221
37. Ludlow JW, Skuse GR (1995) Viral oncoprotein binding to pRB, p107, p130 and p300. Virus Res 35:113–121
38. Maheshwar MM, Cheadle JP, Jones AC, Myring J, Fryer AE, Harris PC, Sampson JR (1997) The GAP-related domain of tuberin, the product of the TSC2 gene, is a target for missense mutations in tuberous sclerosis. Human Mol Genet 6:1991–1996
39. Moran E (1993) Interaction of adenoviral proteins with pRB and p53. FASEB J 7:880–885
40. Pajak L, Jin F, Xiao GH, Soonpaa MH, Field LJ, Yeung RS (1997) Sustained cardiomyocyte DNA synthesis in whole embryo cultures lacking the TSC2 gene product. Am J Physiol 273:H1619–1627
41. Kishore B, Pasumarthi S, Nakajima H, Nakajima HO, Jing S, Field LJ (2000) Enhanced cardiomyocyte DNA synthesis during myocardial hypertrophy in mice expressing a modified TSC2 transgene. Circ Res 86:1069–1077
42. Snyder RO, Spratt SK, Lagarde C, Bohl D, Kaspar B, Sloan B, Cohen LK, Danos O (1997) Efficient and stable adeno-associated virus-mediated transduction in the skeletal muscle of adult immunocompetent mice. Human Gene Therapy 8:1891–1900
43. Soonpaa MH, Field LJ (1994) Assessment of cardiomyocyte DNA synthesis during hypertrophy in adult mice. Am J Physiol 266:H1439–1445
44. Soonpaa MH, Field LJ (1998) Survey of studies examining mammalian cardiomyocyte DNA synthesis. Circ Res 83:15–26
45. Soonpaa MH, Field LJ (1997) Assessment of cardiomyocyte DNA synthesis in normal and injured adult mouse hearts. Am J Physiol 272:H220–226
46. Soonpaa MH, Kim KK, Franklin M, Pajak L, Field LJ (1996) Cardiomyocyte DNA synthesis and multinucleation during murine development. Am J Physiol 271:H2183–2189
47. Soonpaa MH, Kim KK, Pajak L, Franklin M, Field LJ (1996) Cardiomyocyte DNA synthesis and binucleation during murine development. Am J Physiol 271:H2183–2189

48. Soonpaa MH, Koh GY, Klug MG, Field LJ (1994) Formation of nascent intercalated disks between grafted fetal cardiomyocytes and host myocardium. Science 264:98–101
49. Soonpaa MH, Koh GY, Pajak L, Jing S, Wang H, Franklin M, Kim KK, Field LJ (1997) Cyclin D1 over-expression promotes cardiomyocyte DNA synthesis and multinucleation in transgenic mice. J Clin Invest 99:2644–2654
50. Steinhelper ME, Lanson N, Dresdner K, Delcarpio JB, Wit A, Claycomb WC, Field LJ (1990) Proliferation in vivo and in culture of differentiated adult atrial cardiomyocytes from transgenic mice. Am J Physiol 259 (Heart and Circulatory Physiology 28):H1826–H1834
51. Stenmark H, Vitale G, Ullrich O, Zerial M (1995) Rabaptin-5 is a direct effector of the small GTPase Rab5 in endocytic membrane fusion. Cell 83:423–432
52. Tripathy SK, Black HB, Goldwasser E, Leiden JM (1996) Immune responses to transgene-encoded protein limit the stability of gene expression after injection of replication-defective adenovirus vectors. Nature Med 2:545–550
53. Tsai S-C, Pasumarthi KBS, Pajak L, Franklin M, Patton B, Wang H, Henzel WJ, Stults JT, Field LJ (2000) SV40 Large T Antigen binds a novel BH3 containing pro-apoptosis protein in the cytoplasm. J Biol Chem 275:3239–3246
54. van Slegtenhorst M, de Hoogt R, Hermans C, Nellist M, Janssen B, Verhoef S, Lindhout D, van den Ouweland A, Halley D, Young J, Burley M, Jeremiah S, Woodward K, Nahmias J, Fox M, Ekong R, Osborne J, Wolfe J, Povey S, Snell RG, Cheadle JP, Jones AC, Tachataki M, Ravine D, Kwiatkowski DJ, et al (1997) Identification of the tuberous sclerosis gene TSC1 on chromosome 9q34. Science 277:805–808
55. van Slegtenhorst M, Nellist M, Nagelkerken B, Cheadle J, Snell R, van den Ouweland A, Reuser A, Sampson J, Halley D, van der Sluijs P (1998) Interaction between hamartin and tuberin, the TSC1 and TSC2 gene products. Human Mol Genet 7:1053–1057
56. Watson GH (1991) Cardiac rhabdomyomas in tuberous sclerosis. Ann NY Acad Sci 615:50–57
57. Wienecke R, Maize JC Jr, Shoarinejad F, Vass WC, Reed J, Bonifacino JS, Resau JH, de Gunzburg J, Yeung RS, DeClue JE (1996) Co-localization of the TSC2 product tuberin with its target Rap1 in the Golgi apparatus. Oncogene 13:913–923
58. Xiao GH, Shoarinejad F, Jin F, Golemis EA, Yeung RS (1997) The tuberous sclerosis 2 gene product, tuberin, functions as a Rab5 GTPase activating protein (GAP) in modulating endocytosis. J Biol Chem 272:6097–6100
59. Yeung RS, Xiao GH, Jin F, Lee WC, Testa JR, Knudson AG (1994) Predisposition to renal carcinoma in the Eker rat is determined by germ-line mutation of the tuberous sclerosis 2 (TSC2) gene. Proc Natl Acad Sci USA 91:11413–11416

Subject Index

FSC
www.fsc.org
MIX
Papier | Fördert gute Waldnutzung
FSC® C083411

Kolibri 360 GmbH
Ferdinand-Jühlke-Straße 7
99095 Erfurt, Deutschland
produktsicherheit@kolibri360.de